Clinical Pathology for Athletic Trainers

RECOGNIZING SYSTEMIC DISEASE

Second Edition

Clinical Pathology for Athletic Trainers

RECOGNIZING SYSTEMIC DISEASE

Second Edition

Daniel P. O'Connor, PhD, ATC
Laboratory of Integrated Physiology
University of Houston
Houston, Texas

A. Louise Fincher, EdD, ATC, LAT
Department of Kinesiology
University of Texas at Arlington
Arlington, Texas

SLACK
INCORPORATED
Delivering the best in health care information and education worldwide

www.slackbooks.com

ISBN: 978-1-55642-770-1

Instructors: *Clinical Pathology for Athletic Trainers: Recognizing Systemic Disease, Second Edition, Instructor's Manual,* is also available from SLACK Incorporated. Don't miss this important companion to *Clinical Pathology for Athletic Trainers: Recognizing Systemic Disease, Second Edition*. To obtain the *Instructor's Manual*, please visit http://www.efacultylounge.com.

The procedures and practices described in this book should be implemented in a manner consistent with the professional standards set for the circumstances that apply in each specific situation. Every effort has been made to confirm the accuracy of the information presented and to correctly relate generally accepted practices. The authors, editor, and publisher cannot accept responsibility for errors or exclusions or for the outcome of the material presented herein. There is no expressed or implied warranty of this book or information imparted by it. Care has been taken to ensure that drug selection and dosages are in accordance with currently accepted/recommended practice. Due to continuing research, changes in government policy and regulations, and various effects of drug reactions and interactions, it is recommended that the reader carefully review all materials and literature provided for each drug, especially those that are new or not frequently used. Any review or mention of specific companies or products is not intended as an endorsement by the author or publisher.

SLACK Incorporated uses a review process to evaluate submitted material. Prior to publication, educators or clinicians provide important feedback on the content that we publish. We welcome feedback on this work.

Published by: SLACK Incorporated
6900 Grove Road
Thorofare, NJ 08086 USA
Telephone: 856-848-1000
Fax: 856-853-5991
www.slackbooks.com

Contact SLACK Incorporated for more information about other books in this field or about the availability of our books from distributors outside the United States.

Library of Congress Cataloging-in-Publication Data

O'Connor, Daniel P.
Clinical pathology for athletic trainers : recognizing systemic disease / Daniel P. O'Connor, A. Louise Fincher. -- 2nd ed.
p. ; cm.
Includes bibliographical references and index.
ISBN 978-1-55642-770-1 (alk. paper)
1. Internal medicine--Handbooks, manuals, etc. 2. Athletic trainers--Handbooks, manuals, etc. 3. Sports medicine--Handbooks, manuals, etc. I. Fincher, A. Louise, 1961- II. Title.
[DNLM: 1. Signs and Symptoms. 2. Pathology, Clinical--methods. 3. Sports Medicine. WB 143 O18c 2007]

RC55.O36 2007
616.0024'796--dc22

2007043149

Printed in the United States of America.

Last digit is print number: 10 9 8 7 6 5 4 3 2 1

Dedication

For Mitzi, always.
—DPO

To my students, past, present, and future.
—ALF

Contents

Acknowledgments

A special thanks to Mitzi Laughlin, who has more patience than I deserve. I thank my parents, Dan and Mary, for who I am and what I have. Also, to Michael E. Cooley, ASMI, our medical illustrator, a very special thanks for the figures. To Bill Wissen, Dale Spence, and Allen Eggert, my personal and professional mentors and good friends, thanks for your time. Finally, I want to acknowledge my colleagues in the Greater Houston Athletic Trainers' Society, the Texas State Athletic Trainers' Association, and the Southwest Athletic Trainers' Association (NATA District 6): the best athletic trainers anywhere.

—DPO

To René, thank you for your endless patience and support throughout what I am sure seemed like a never-ending project. Without your support through the cancer battle, my part in this book would never have been a possibility. To my family, friends, and colleagues, thank you for your continuous support and encouragement through the cancer fight and beyond. Although they both left this earth too soon, my parents continue to influence my life today. I thank them for teaching me the importance of always doing my best, the value in giving to others, and the need for life-long learning. Lastly, I sincerely thank Dan O'Connor and SLACK Incorporated for giving me the opportunity to contribute to this Second Edition. Although it has been a long journey, I have enjoyed the ride.

—ALF

About the Authors

Daniel P. O'Connor, PhD, ATC, has published numerous journal articles and book chapters in addition to the First Edition of *Clinical Pathology for Athletic Trainers: Recognizing Systemic Disease.* He has served as an adjunct faculty member at Rice University and Texas Woman's University and was the Director of the Joe W. King Orthopedic Institute in Houston, Texas for 7 years. Dan is currently an Assistant Professor in the Laboratory of Integrated Physiology and the Department of Health and Human Performance at the University of Houston.

A. Louise Fincher, EdD, ATC, LAT, is an Associate Professor in the Department of Kinesiology and the Director of the Athletic Training Education Program at The University of Texas at Arlington. She also serves as the Associate Chair for the Department of Kinesiology. Lou has more than 23 years of experience as an athletic trainer and an educator. She has spent countless hours developing didactic and clinical education materials for both students and athletic training educators. Lou's research publications are focused in the areas of orthopedic outcomes and the effectiveness of therapeutic modalities. Her other publications include a book chapter, a column series on the management of athletic injuries, and an article on the use of the otoscope in evaluating ear injuries and illnesses. She has served on several National Athletic Trainers' Association (NATA) and Southwest Athletic Trainers' Association (SWATA) committees and currently serves on the NATA Education Council's Entry-Level Education Committee.

Introduction

The goal of this Second Edition of *Clinical Pathology for Athletic Trainers: Recognizing Systemic Disease* is the same as the first: to enable the athletic trainer and athletic training student to recognize, evaluate, and differentiate common systemic diseases. Our book has been thoroughly updated to address the Fourth Edition of the National Athletic Trainers' Association's (NATA) *Athletic Training Educational Competencies* related to the domains of pharmacology, pathology, and general medical illnesses and disorders.

Three new chapters have been added to this edition: Pharmacology (Chapter Three); Eye, Ear, Nose, Throat, and Mouth Disorders (Chapter Eleven); and Dermatological Conditions (Chapter Twelve). A significant number of new graphics have been added throughout the text along with photos to better illustrate the pathology and examination procedures. A color atlas has also been added to enhance the recognition of dermatological conditions. The content in several of the existing chapters has been substantially expanded: Pathophysiology (Chapter Two), Oncology (Chapter Five), Cardiovascular and Hematological Systems (Chapter Six), and Endocrine and Metabolic Systems (Chapter Ten). The chapter order has also been restructured to present a more logical and organized sequencing of information. The physical examination sections within each chapter have been expanded along with the addition of new lab exercises.

We have also added several new features to the Second Edition that we believe will further enhance student learning. Each chapter begins with a topical outline that incorporates the chapter's learning objectives. This feature will enable the student to better understand the scope and structure of each chapter and to help organize his or her thought processes relative to the material. The beginning of each chapter also contains a list of the specific cognitive and psychomotor competencies that will be addressed (based on the new Fourth Edition of the *Athletic Training Educational Competencies*). To assist the student in recognizing the conditions that warrant medical referral, physician (caduceus) and emergency referral (911) icons have been included in the margins of the text. The caduceus icon means that the patient should see his or her physician at his or her earliest convenience, whereas the 911 icon means that the patient should see a physician immediately. The 911 icon does not necessarily mean that the patient must be transported via ambulance; however, in some instances this would be best. And finally, Chapters Three through Fourteen contain case studies with critical thinking questions. These case studies are designed to provide students with an opportunity to apply the new content to real world situations and to develop their critical thinking skills.

Ancillary instructional materials for the Second Edition have been updated and revised to include an *Instructor's Manual*, a test bank, and PowerPoints. The *Instructor's Manual* provides chapter outlines with reference to the corresponding PowerPoints, as well as instructional tips for organizing the lab activities and teaching the psychomotor skills. The test bank contains more than 480 questions broken down by chapter and categorized by item type: multiple choice, short answer/essay, and application/critical thinking items. PowerPoints are provided for Chapters One through Fourteen and include many of the graphics and photos from the Second Edition.

Clinical Pathology for Athletic Trainers: Recognizing Systemic Disease, Second Edition, was written by athletic trainers specifically for athletic trainers, acknowledging their unique role in health care. It is intended to be a textbook for athletic training students in accredited athletic training educational programs and a reference book for certified athletic trainers. It emphasizes the clinical recognition and management of non-orthopedic pathology, which allows athletic trainers to recognize systemic illnesses and injuries.

The information in this text was drawn not only from standard medical reference books, but also from research and reviews published over the past 25 years in the sports medicine literature. In addition, the comments of many athletic training educators regarding the First Edition have been incorporated into this Second Edition. Those suggestions were invaluable in revising the book, and we are grateful for that input.

Chapter One

Principles of Clinical Pathology and Decision Making

Chapter Outline and Objectives

Introduction

- ❖ Define terminology used to discuss pathology.
  - Pathology in Sports Medicine and Athletic Training
  - Signs and Symptoms
  - Diagnosis
- ❖ Review the theoretical and scientific bases of clinical pathology.
  - Theories of Disease and Pathogenesis
- ❖ Discuss the role of the athletic trainer with respect to identifying general medical pathology.
  - Role of Athletic Trainers in Disease Prevention

Diagnostic Reasoning and Clinical Decision Making

Medical History

- ❖ Introduce questions included in a medical history relevant to general medical pathology.

Symptoms

- ❖ Review the behavior and characteristics of symptoms relevant to general medical pathology.

Physical Examination Techniques: Differentiating Normal and Abnormal Responses

- ❖ Introduce methods of physical examination relevant to general medical pathology.

This chapter addresses the following competencies from the *Athletic Training Educational Competencies, Fourth Edition*[1]:

Domain	Cognitive	Psychomotor
Acute Care of Injuries and Illnesses	4	
Medical Conditions and Disabilities	1–3	
Pathology of Injuries and Illnesses	4–6	

Introduction

The patient population with which athletic trainers work has changed significantly over the past 10 to 15 years. In addition to the traditional settings of secondary schools, universities, and professional sports, athletic trainers now also work within hospitals, sports medicine clinics, physicians' offices, the military, and corporate and industrial settings. Because of the diverse patient population within these varied practice settings, athletic trainers must be familiar with the common general medical conditions that may occur in these individuals.

Athletic trainers should be aware of the possible origins of an injury or illness, particularly symptoms that cannot be associated with specific trauma. Knowledge of pathology and mechanisms of disease will improve athletic trainers' clinical decision-making skills. Certain clinical skills, including taking a medical history, performing a physical examination, analyzing clinical information, and making a medical referral, also depend on this knowledge. Most of the general medical disorders or diseases encountered by the athletic trainer will involve one or more of the anatomical systems (cardiovascular, pulmonary, etc). In most cases, the signs and symptoms will point toward the involvement of a particular organ or system.

This textbook uses a systems approach for discussing pathology. Each chapter will address an individual system and the common injuries or illnesses associated with that system.

Pathology in Sports Medicine and Athletic Training

Pathology, a special field of medical science, focuses on the study of the biological causes, effects, and processes of disease.[2] *Pathogenesis* refers either to the underlying cause of a disease or the development of a disease. *Etiology* describes and studies pathogenesis to explain the mechanisms of disease.[2]

Signs and Symptoms

A *sign* is an observable indication of pathology, usually discovered during physical examination. A *symptom* is any abnormal function, appearance, or sensation that is experienced by the patient.[2] Thus, signs are objective and can be measured by the clinician, whereas symptoms are subjective and reported by the patient. Medical conditions often produce characteristic patterns of signs and symptoms.

Each patient's *clinical presentation* is the overall "picture" of signs, symptoms, medical history, and physical examination. This book outlines clinical presentations that are consistent with general medical disease. Standard orthopedic and sports medicine texts review injuries of bones, joints, and muscles, which are not discussed here.[3-7]

Diagnosis

The term *diagnosis* refers to the specific injury, illness, disease, or condition a patient has, as determined by medical examination.[2] The athletic trainer will formulate a clinical diagnosis based on the signs and symptoms, medical history, and physical examination. Often times, particularly when dealing with general medical conditions, analysis of these data results in a *differential diagnosis*, or the identification of several conditions that might have similar clinical presentations. When this occurs, the athletic trainer will typically refer the patient to a physician, who can order further laboratory or imaging studies for clarification of the diagnosis.

A disease may affect a person's ability to participate in sports or other physical activities or require that certain precautions be taken. Furthermore, *coexisting* or *comorbid conditions* (a medical condition in addition to the primary problem) can complicate recovery from an injury or illness or require treatment modifications.

Theories of Disease and Pathogenesis

Several theories explain the origin and nature of disease. The *biomedical* model of health and illness attributes the cause of disease to abnormal cell, tissue, or organ function. The abnormal function can be caused by anatomical or physiological defects or by factors such as bacteria and viruses. This book uses the biomedical model to explain pathogenesis for most conditions.

Psychosocial theories consider the psychological and social effects on illness and disease. Patients who cannot adapt cognitively or socially to a major injury may be more prone to chronic illness and may not respond to treatment as expected. In addition, emotional stress (eg, academic, financial, social, etc) can confuse the clinical presentation of an illness. Chapter Fourteen addresses psychological issues in greater detail.

Last, *genetic* factors, such as errors in DNA and RNA replication, can contribute not only to pathogenesis, but also to the effectiveness of the immune system and rate of tissue healing. Genetic and congenital disorders are commonly identified in pediatric patients (children). Where necessary, the following chapters discuss specific pediatric concerns.

Role of Athletic Trainers in Disease Prevention

The Board of Certification (BOC) identifies injury and illness prevention as a major domain of athletic training practice.[8] Table 1-1 summarizes the three stages of prevention. *Primary prevention* involves reducing risk factors, which may involve nutrition, regular exercise, and environmental hazards. *Secondary prevention* includes early detection of illness or disease and preventing or reversing the progression of disease. *Tertiary prevention* attempts to limit an established disease and restore the highest possible level of function.

Table 1-1
Stages of Disease Prevention

Stage	Goals	Interventions
Primary	Reduce risk factors	Nutrition, exercise, monitoring of environmental risks, prevention and educational programs
Secondary	Early detection, early intervention, inhibit proliferation	Regular medical checkups, self-examination, early medical treatment
Tertiary	Limit established disease	Medical treatment, supportive and restorative

Athletic trainers participate in all three stages of prevention. With respect to primary prevention, they identify risk factors, monitor the environment, and counsel athletes. Secondary prevention, such as early detection and appropriate referral, is facilitated by knowledge of clinical pathology. Tertiary prevention provides medical treatment for an injury or illness and continues through return to work or competition.

Diagnostic Reasoning and Clinical Decision Making

Diagnostic Reasoning

Medical treatment begins with diagnosis. *Diagnostic reasoning* is how a physician *differentiates* (sorts and interprets) signs and symptoms to arrive at a diagnosis. The diagnostic processes include *triage* (determining the urgency of a medical condition), medical history, physical examination, laboratory tests, and imaging studies.[9] A physician's diagnosis leads to actions such as prescription of medications, surgery, referral to medical specialists, or referral to allied health services.

Clinical Decision Making

Athletic trainers use *clinical decision making*, a process similar to diagnostic reasoning, to formulate a diagnosis (Table 1-2). Clinical decision making uses information from the medical history and physical examination to determine a differential diagnosis and the best course of action for a particular patient. Through clinical decision making, the athletic trainer's diagnosis may lead to actions such as first aid, emergency transport, treatment and rehabilitation, reassessment, modification of activity, or referral to other health care specialists. Recognizing characteristic patterns of signs and symptoms can suggest potential pathogenesis and help to determine a course of action.

Table 1-2
Clinical Decision Making vs Diagnostic Reasoning

	Clinical Decision Making	Diagnostic Reasoning
Clinician	Athletic trainer	Physician
Goals	Determine a potential diagnosis and course of action	Determine a diagnosis and course of medical treatment
Processes	History, physical exam, differential diagnosis, reassessment (evaluate progress)	History, physical exam, forming hypothesis, confirming hypothesis (with medical laboratory and imaging)
Results	Emergency transport, first aid, treatment and rehabilitation, referral to health care specialists, modify activity	Medication, surgery, referral to health care specialists

Table 1-3
Purposes of a Medical History

- Determine potential pathogenesis
- Identify coexisting conditions
- Determine the stage of the injury or illness
- Identify contraindications to treatment

Medical History

A medical history is "an account of the events" related to a patient's state of health.[9] Table 1-3 gives the purposes for the medical history. All injuries require a medical history, which is collected by interviewing the patient. The scope and extent of the interview should be appropriate to the situation. For instance, primary assessment of a traumatic injury need not include a full medical history. A person reporting vague or unusual symptoms in the athletic training room or outpatient clinic, however, needs more extensive questioning.[10] Information collected in the medical history directs the subsequent physical examination and assists clinical decision making.

Taking a Medical History

The components of the medical history are listed in Table 1-4.[9,11] Details that are potentially relevant to subsequent physical examination, treatment, or outcome are recorded in the medical record. A proper medical history focuses on the patient's issues and establishes an immediate rapport (trust) between the clinician

Table 1-4
Components of a Medical History

- Chief complaint
- Description and course of present illness
- Personal medical history
- Family medical history
- Review of systems

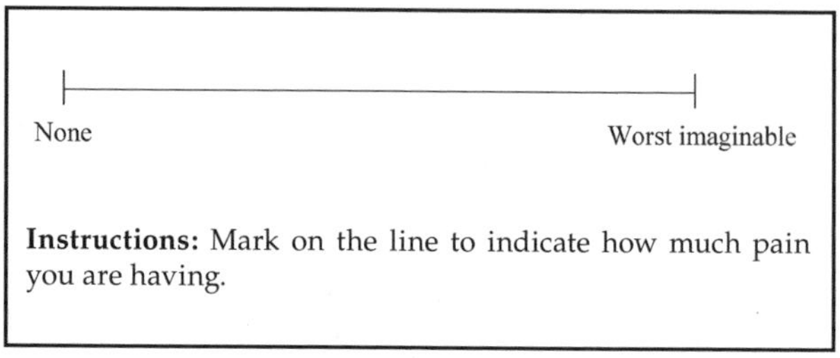

None
Worst imaginable
Instructions: Mark on the line to indicate how much pain you are having.

Figure 1-1. 100-mm visual analog scale.

and the patient.[10] Conducting a medical history requires practice to obtain complete and correct information. This information begins to build the clinical presentation.

Participants in organized athletics usually receive a *preparticipation examination*. This includes a physical screening examination, a survey of personal and family medical history, and a review of the organ-systems. This survey of an athlete's medical history can identify existing pathology that may prevent or limit participation in specific sports. This preliminary medical record should be consulted when evaluating injuries and illnesses incurred during the season. In the event that the athletic trainer is unfamiliar with the patient, such as may occur in the clinical setting, the personal and family medical history is collected during initial injury evaluation.

Chief Complaints

The *chief complaints* are the symptoms that cause a patient to seek medical attention.[9] Pain in a particular body segment is often one of the chief complaints. Some patients are also concerned with disability (inability to perform) in sport, work, or social-familial duties. The athletic trainer uses the chief complaints to guide the evaluation, to evaluate effects of injury or illness, to monitor recovery, and to focus attention on the patient's goals.

Description and Course of Present Illness

The core of the history-taking process is the history of present illness, including the patient's description of onset of symptoms, progression of symptoms since onset, and the nature of the problem. Table 1-5 lists some common questions asked during the history of the present illness. Inquiring whether the condition is "getting better, not changing, or getting worse" indicates the progression of the disease. The patient should rate their symptoms numerically using visual or verbal analog scales (Figure 1-1), which can be repeated each day to evaluate recovery.

Table 1-5
History of Present Illness

- When did your condition start?
- What makes your condition better? What makes it worse?
- Is your condition better or worse in the morning or at night?
- Is your condition better or worse with breathing, urination, eating, excitement or stress, rest, or certain body positions?
- Have you had x-rays, MRIs, or CT scans for this condition?
- What treatment have you received for this condition?
- Is your condition getting better, getting worse, or not changing either way?
- Have you ever had any condition like this before?
- Is there anything else I need to know about you or your condition?

Table 1-6
Past and Family Medical History

Heart disease	Cancer	Diabetes	High blood pressure
Stroke	Kidney disease	Liver disease	Recurrent infections
Digestive problems	Breathing problems	Headaches	Anemia
Arthritis	Nerve problems	Depression	Substance abuse

- Have you, or any immediate family member, had any of the above major health problems?
- How is your current health?
- Do you currently have any other injuries or medical conditions?
- Have you ever been admitted to a hospital?
- Have you ever had surgery?

At the conclusion of the history of present illness, the clinician should have a good idea about the patient's condition. How did it begin and how has it changed? What are the frequency, intensity, and duration of symptoms? And what makes the condition better or worse? Information from the history of present illness should guide the physical examination.

Personal and Family Medical History

The *personal medical history* and *family medical history* review the previous medical conditions or illnesses experienced by the patient and immediate family members (Table 1-6). Many patients do not consider "minor" surgeries or health problems to be relevant to their present condition, so such reports should lead to more specific questions. A coexisting condition may require modification of evaluation or treatment techniques. A family history of disease may be relevant if the clinical presentation suggests similar pathology.

Table 1-7
Review of Systems by Signs and Symptoms

General "Systemic" Signs and Symptoms	Potential Condition or System of Origin
Fever, chills, sweats	Infection, cancer; immune system
Severe night pain	Cancer; cardiovascular or gastrointestinal system
Unexplained weight change	Depression, eating disorder, infection, cancer; gastrointestinal or metabolic systems
Unusual fatigue, malaise	Depression, infection, diabetes, anemia, rheumatoid arthritis, eating disorder, cancer; endocrine system
Key System-Specific Signs and Symptoms	
Chest pain or palpitations	Cardiovascular system
Shortness of breath	Cardiovascular or pulmonary system
Dizziness, light-headedness, fainting	Medications; cardiovascular or metabolic system
Nausea, vomiting	Pregnancy, cancer, drug toxicity; gastrointestinal system
Loss of control of bowels (diarrhea)	Gastrointestinal system
Difficulty, bleeding, or pain while urinating	Infection; urogenital system
Sexual function problems	Psychological, urogenital, or neurological system
Visual disturbances	Neurological or cardiovascular system
Numbness, weakness, burning, tingling	Neurological system
Difficulty swallowing, hoarseness	Neoplasm (tumor); neurological or gastrointestinal system

Review of Systems

The *review of systems* screens for major organ-system disease by asking about specific symptoms by interview or questionnaire (Table 1-7). When any of these symptoms are present, specific questions to the respective systems are indicated. The following chapters will review these specific questions.

Table 1-8
Recent General Health Status

- Have you lost more than 5 to 10 pounds in the past month?
- What regular physical stresses does your job involve?

Sitting	Standing	Large equipment
Walking	Lifting	Small equipment
Bending	Climbing	Exposure to chemicals
Deskwork		

- Are you on a diet?
- Do you use any tobacco products?
- How much alcohol do you drink in a week?
- How many caffeinated drinks do you have in a day?

Medical Tests

Medical tests for the current condition, such as imaging studies and laboratory tests, and when those tests were performed, should be documented. In addition, medications (both prescription and nonprescription) for all current and coexisting conditions should be recorded. Many medications have side effects or require treatment precautions. Chapter Three provides a brief overview of pharmacology, and, where applicable, the individual system chapters provide information on the common medications used to treat the conditions within that system. There are several other sources that provide excellent reviews of pharmacology for athletic trainers.[12-14]

General Health Information

Other questions related to the person's health may be necessary (Table 1-8). Poor recent health may indicate *occult* (undetected) pathology or progression of a known medical condition. Sport-specific demands, work environment, or regular physical activity (or inactivity) may be related to pathogenesis and may affect treatment, *prognosis* (predicted outcome of disease), and recovery. Age, gender, race, or occupation may also be relevant to pathogenesis.[10] Important social information to collect includes regular physical stresses (eg, sitting, driving, lifting), psychoemotional stress, exposure to toxins (including smoke, alcohol, caffeine, and other drugs), and usual schedule (ie, does the person "have time" for good nutrition, medical treatment, appointments, etc).[10]

SYMPTOMS

Behavior and Characteristics

Qualities of various symptoms can reveal the nature of the disorder.[10] Table 1-9 compares several qualities of systemic (non-musculoskeletal) and musculoskeletal symptoms. Pain of systemic origin is usually constant, unchanged by movement or posture, most intense at night, and present during function of the affected system(s).

Table 1-9
General Character and Behavior of Systemic and Musculoskeletal Symptoms

Systemic	Musculoskeletal
Constant	Intermittent
No change with movement/posture	Consistent change with movement/posture
No change or worse at rest	Relief with rest
Worse at night	Relief at night
Worse with organ function	Unaffected by organ function

Table 1-10
Pain Descriptors and Possible Systemic Origin of Pathology

System	Descriptors
Vascular	Pulsing, throbbing, pounding, cramping, quivering
Neurogenic	Shooting, stabbing, drilling, sharp, cutting, pinching, pressing, pulling, burning, tingling, stinging
Musculoskeletal	Dull, sore, hurting, aching, heavy
Emotional lability (psychoemotional)	Splitting, exhausting, sickening, cruel, vicious, killing, unbearable, radiating, tight, cold, nagging

(Adapted from Melzack R. The McGill Pain Questionnaire: major properties and scoring methods. Pain. *1975;1:277-299.)*

Musculoskeletal pain is usually intermittent, changed by body position or posture, decreased at night, and is unaffected by function of the internal organ-system. Table 1-10 lists certain words patients may use to describe symptoms suggesting systemic pathology.

Anatomical location of symptoms also provides additional clues. The patient can either draw their symptom pattern on a body diagram (Figure 1-2) or simply point to their symptomatic areas. Each organ and system has a characteristic pain referral pattern, as presented in subsequent chapters. Symptoms that match these visceral (organ) patterns should prompt investigation for other signs.

Acute and Chronic Pain

The term *acute pain* describes pain of sudden onset with high intensity and relatively short duration (hours or days). *Chronic pain* appears insidiously (gradually), with lower intensity and a longer duration (weeks or months). Acute pain without trauma, chronic pain that returns in predictable cycles ("comes and goes"), or chronic pain that progresses in intensity suggest systemic pathology.

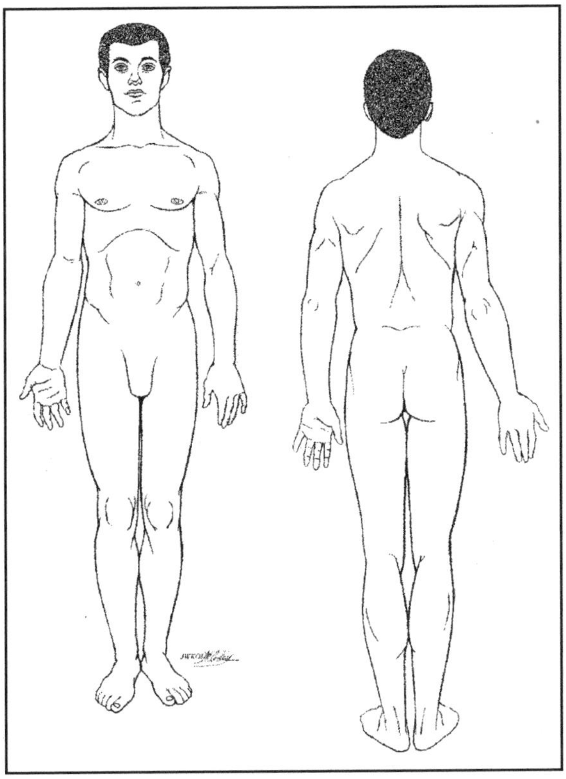

Figure 1-2. Body diagram for location of pain or other symptoms.

Local and Referred Pain

Local pain stays in a specific region or area of the body. Referred pain occurs in a region that is distant from the damaged tissue. Referred pain is more common in systemic pathology, although it can also occur with certain musculoskeletal injuries.

Constant and Intermittent Pain

Constant pain is always present, although the intensity may vary over time. Patients describe intermittent pain as something that "comes and goes." With either type, if intensity varies with certain movements or body position, an acute musculoskeletal injury may be suspected. Conversely, if intensity increases at night, with organ function (eg, digestion, breathing), or does not change at all, the pain may be systemic in origin.

Causes of Pain

Mechanical, chemical, and perceptual mechanisms cause different types of pain, although they can occur in combination with one another.

Mechanical Causes

Anatomical structures under abnormal physical loads or stress can produce pain. Most commonly, musculoskeletal injuries cause this type of pain. Pain caused by mechanical factors is intermittent, related to movement or position, and relieved by removing the offending stress. This type of pain appears only in the injured structure.

Table 1-11

Symptoms Requiring Urgent Referral to a Physician: "Red Flags"

• Constant pain	• Incapacitating pain
• Heart palpitations /flutter	• Severe dyspnea
• Fainting (syncope)	• Recurrent nausea, vomiting
• Night pain or night sweats	• Pulsating or severe cramping pain (colic)
• Difficult or painful swallowing	• Difficult or painful urination
• Visual problems	• Blood in urine
• Unexplained weight loss	• Severe or progressive dizziness
• Insomnia	• Malaise, fatigue

Chemical Causes

Biochemical substances released with tissue injury can produce pain. These substances irritate innervated tissues and cause inflammation, as reviewed in Chapter Two. Pain of chemical origin is constant, although intensity may change, and cannot be relieved by movement or position, although it may worsen with such changes. Medication addresses chemical causes and thus nearly always decreases this type of pain. Pain caused by chemical irritation is poorly localized and may refer to other locations if nerves or adjacent anatomical structures are affected.

Perceptual Causes

Pain is itself a perception, so all pain has perceptual components. A person's response to pain is affected by cultural, social, and personal experiences. It is also possible for the physical (mechanical and chemical) origin of pain to be "healed" while the perception of pain remains. If an athletic trainer recognizes this situation, he or she should report his or her observations to the supervising physician and support any subsequently prescribed treatment.

Pain-Generating Tissues

Different tissues also produce different types of pain. Skin and subcutaneous tissues generate *cutaneous* pain, localized to the area of tissue damage. *Deep somatic* pain originates in bones, nerves, muscles, tendons, ligaments, arteries, or joints. Deep somatic pain may refer or cause autonomic reactions such as sweating, pallor, nausea, and syncope. The internal organs of the cardiovascular, hematological, pulmonary, digestive, urogenital, endocrine, and reproductive systems can produce *visceral* pain. Visceral pain receptors (*nociceptors*) relay a diffuse signal that refers to associated dermatomes or may produce a deep, gnawing ache in the thorax or abdomen.

Red Flags

Certain signs and symptoms alert the athletic trainer to serious pathology (Table 1-11). These "red flags" require immediate medical attention. Some red flags are obvious emergencies (eg, loss of consciousness, breathing, or circulation).

Table 1-12
Components of the Physical Examination

• Inspection/observation	• Smell/odor	• Vital signs
• Percussion	• Palpation	• Auscultation
• Neurological exam		

Others, such as recurrent fevers, night pain, malaise, and unexplained weight loss, may be discovered during the medical history. Symptoms that are not well localized, have no incident associated with their onset, have been relentlessly worsening over time, and are unaffected by standard treatments are unlikely to be caused by a musculoskeletal condition.

Physical Examination Techniques: Differentiating Normal and Abnormal Responses

Physical examination for systemic pathology has several components (Table 1-12). The physical examination is modified according to suspected pathogenesis, the patient's symptoms, and urgency of the patient's condition.

Inspection

Inspection involves observing general appearance, eyes, skin, hair, fingernails, obvious deformities, use of assistive devices or supports, behavior, gait, and coordination. Many systemic conditions cause "classic" signs that can be readily observed.

Vital Signs

The *vital signs* are heart rate, respiration rate, blood pressure, and body temperature. Vital signs should be assessed in emergencies and when systemic symptoms (see Table 1-7) are reported. If a patient's medical history includes hypertension, cardiac pathology, recent infection, chronic illness, or cancer, vital signs should be recorded as an indicator of present health status and to provide a baseline to monitor health status throughout treatment. The common changes in vital signs that might be found with specific injuries and illnesses are discussed throughout this book.

Percussion and Palpation

Percussion (striking to cause vibration) over bones may increase the pain of a fracture or bone tumor. Percussion over the abdomen vibrates the internal organs, increasing pain if they are injured or inflamed. Percussion over the thorax can reveal differences in resonance from one side to the other which might suggest specific pathology (accumulation of fluid or punctured lung). Percussion techniques are discussed in more detail in Chapter Seven.

Superficial *palpation* (manual touch) can assess the temperature, texture, moisture, and turgidity (stiffness) of the skin and is used to examine lymph nodes and vascular pulses. Detection of abnormal masses, abdominal rigidity (see Chapter Eight), and tenderness is achieved through deep palpation.

Auscultation

Auscultation is performed with an instrument called a *stethoscope* to examine cardiac, pulmonary, vascular, abdominal, and bowel sounds. Specific auscultation techniques will be discussed in Chapters Six through Eight.

Smell

Unusual odor of the breath or perspiration suggests exhalation of metabolic substances, which can indicate disease, poisoning, or drug abuse. Foul-smelling sputum or other body fluids can indicate infection or endocrine malfunction.

Neurological Screening Exam

Any patient reporting radiating pain, sensory abnormalities, weakness, or recent head injury should receive a neurological screening examination of the cranial nerves, reflexes, sensation, and motor function.

Cranial Nerves and Reflexes

Cranial nerves control smell, vision and eye control, hearing, swallowing, facial sensation and motor control, and tongue control. Cranial nerve tests are reviewed in Chapter Thirteen.

The *deep tendon reflexes* that can be clinically tested include biceps (C5), brachioradialis (C6), triceps (C7), patella (L2-4), and ankle (S1).[15] The *Babinski sign* is an abnormal reflex that appears when the motor tracts from the brain to the limbs are disrupted, which occurs with spinal cord injury or a severe head injury.

Sensory Testing

Sensation should be tested bilaterally along dermatomal and peripheral nerve distributions. Light touch, which is transmitted to the brain through neural pathways on the sides of the spinal cord, is tested first. If sensation of light touch is impaired, sharp (or temperature) sensation and vibration tests should be performed. Sharp sensation tests the spinal cord columns opposite (contralateral) to the limb being tested and is assessed with a sharp object such as a pin. Vibration sense tests spinal cord columns on the same (ipsilateral) side and is assessed using a tuning fork.

Motor Testing

Manual muscle tests may differentiate between *myotomal* (nerve root), peripheral nerve, or muscle lesions. Injured or inflamed nerve roots produce weakness in all of the muscles that they innervate. Peripheral nerve damage affects only the few muscles supplied by that nerve, whereas traumatic muscle injuries weaken only one specific muscle. Nerve injuries do not usually cause significant pain, but do cause substantial weakness. Muscle injuries usually cause both weakness and pain. Injuries and illnesses involving the nervous system are discussed in Chapter Thirteen.

SUMMARY

Athletic trainers use clinical decision making to evaluate possible pathogenesis. This process includes taking a medical history, evaluating symptom patterns, and performing a physical examination. The medical history provides information regarding the onset, nature, and course of the condition. The physical examination tests for signs that confirm the history and reported symptoms and completes the clinical presentation. The goal of the examination process is to determine the patient's diagnosis—the medical condition with which the patient is most likely afflicted.

REFERENCES

1. National Athletic Trainers' Association. *Athletic Training Educational Competencies.* 4th ed. Dallas, TX: National Athletic Trainers' Association; 2005.
2. Hensyl WR, ed. *Stedman's Pocket Medical Dictionary.* Baltimore, MD: Williams & Wilkins; 1987.
3. Anderson MK, Hall SJ. *Sports Injury Management.* 2nd ed. Philadelphia, PA: Lippincott Williams & Wilkins; 2000.
4. Arnheim DD, Prentice WE. *Principles of Athletic Training.* 8th ed. St Louis, MO: Mosby-Year Book; 1993.
5. Hertling D, Kessler RM. *Management of Common Musculoskeletal Disorders.* 2nd ed. Philadelphia, PA: JB Lippincott Co; 1990.
6. Magee DJ. *Orthopedic Physical Assessment.* 2nd ed. Philadelphia, PA: WB Saunders Co; 1992.
7. Saunders HD, Woerman AL. *Evaluation, Treatment, and Prevention of Musculoskeletal Disorders.* Bloomington, MN: Educational Opportunities; 1985.
8. Board of Certification Inc. *BOC Role Delineation Study.* 5th ed. Omaha, NE: Board of Certification Inc; 2005.
9. DeGowin RL, Brown DD. *DeGowin's Diagnostic Examination.* 7th ed. New York, NY: McGraw-Hill; 2000.
10. Bickley LS, Szilagyi PG. *Bates' Guide to Physical Examination and History Taking.* 9th ed. Philadelphia, PA: Lippincott Williams & Wilkins; 2005.
11. Boissonnault WG, Janos SC. Screening for medical disease: physical therapy assessment and treatment principles. In: Boissonnault WG, ed. *Examination in Physical Therapy Practice: Screening for Medical Disease.* New York, NY: Churchill Livingstone; 1995:1-30.
12. Ciocca M. Medication and supplement use by athletes. *Clin Sports Med.* 2005;24(3):719-738.
13. Houglum JE, Harrelson GL, Leaver-Dunn D. *Principles of Pharmacology for Athletic Trainers.* Thorofare, NJ: SLACK Incorporated; 2005.
14. *Pharmacology for Athletic Trainers: Therapeutic Medications* [home study course]. Champaign, IL: Human Kinetics; 1997.
15. Hoppenfeld S. *Physical Examination of the Spine and Extremities.* Norwalk, CT: Appleton & Lange; 1976.

ONLINE RESOURCES

Full-text medical manuals

www.medicalstudent.com

Medline Plus (medical dictionary and encyclopedia, plus descriptions of more than 700 medical conditions)

www.medlineplus.gov

Chapter Two

Pathophysiology

Chapter Outline and Objectives

Introduction

- ❖ Explain the concept of homeostasis.
  - Homeostasis
  - Pathophysiology
- ❖ Describe cellular components and their functions.
- ❖ Describe cellular adaptations to disease.
  - The Cell
  - Tissue Healing
- ❖ Discuss the inflammatory process.
  - Inflammation
  - Infection

Cellular Physiology and Pathophysiology: Response to Cell Damage

- ❖ Explain tissue responses to disease.
- ❖ Review pathophysiology by tissue type.
  - Bone
  - Connective Tissue, Epithelium, and Endothelium
  - Muscle and Nerve
  - Specialized Cells and Tissues

This chapter addresses the following competencies from the *Athletic Training Educational Competencies, Fourth Edition*[1]:

Domain	**Cognitive**	**Psychomotor**
Acute Care of Injuries and Illnesses	18	
Orthopedic Clinical Examination and Diagnosis	1	
Pathology of Injuries and Illnesses	1–6	

INTRODUCTION

This chapter reviews normal physiology and introduces the concepts of *pathophysiology*, physiology related to disease. It will not replace formal study of normal cell structure and physiology. Basic physiology provides a basis for discussion in subsequent chapters. Many clinical and cellular pathophysiology textbooks are available for greater detail.[2-7]

Homeostasis

Homeostasis is the control of biochemical equilibrium within the body through many processes that constantly regulate fluid, chemical, and energy balance in the cells, tissues, organs, and systems.[2,8] Normal function constantly disturbs and restores this biological balance. For example, blood glucose level rises after eating a meal. In response, cells in the pancreas release insulin, a hormone that helps to move glucose from the blood into the liver and muscles. Once blood glucose levels have returned to normal, the pancreas stops releasing insulin to prevent blood glucose levels from becoming too low. These normal stimulus-response cycles are necessary to maintain health.

The healthy state can vary somewhat depending on the individual. Thus, "normal" values for chemical and functional indicators (eg, blood test results and vital signs) are usually described as a range that depends on age, gender, and other factors. In addition, these values may exceed "normal" range in response to stress to maintain organ-system function. For instance, persons living at high altitude have more red blood cells as an adaptation to the lower concentration of atmospheric oxygen. This adaptation allows the blood to hold an adequate amount of oxygen.

Pathophysiology

Many diseases disrupt homeostasis, causing deviation from the normal, balanced biochemical state. *Pathophysiology* describes the cellular mechanisms of disease and their functional systemic consequences.[2] Signs and symptoms are a result of the functional systemic consequences of pathology. Understanding the normal physiology of the body's organ-systems assists in the discussion of the effects of disease. Study of physiology begins with the basic unit of the body's tissues: the cell.

Table 2-1
Cell Structures and Their Functions

Structure	Function
Nucleus	Contains genetic material of the cell (DNA and RNA) Controls cell division and synthesis of protein
Cytoplasm	Provides internal fluid environment of the cell Supports all internal cell structures
Lysosomes	Contains catabolic enzymes within the cell Disposes cell waste and foreign substances
Mitochondria	Converts carbohydrate, protein, and fat to ATP (energy)
Cell membrane	Consists of complex semipermeable phospholipid and protein structure Provides physical border of the cell Excludes or exchanges substances between the internal and external environment of the cell

The Cell

All living cells contain many structures, including cytoplasm, a nucleus, lysosomes, mitochondria, and a cell membrane. Each structure serves a particular purpose (Table 2-1).[8]

Cells can be damaged by physical trauma, toxins, infection, genetic abnormalities, malnutrition, dehydration, hypoxia, or combinations of these factors.[2,6] Cell damage impairs one or more cell structures, which affects tissue and organ function, which in turn affects function of the associated system or systems. Cells in other tissues and organs can be affected as the effects spread to surrounding tissues, thus disrupting homeostasis. Some effects of cell damage initiate responses that attempt to limit the disease process, to initiate cell repair, and to restore homeostasis.

Once cell damage occurs, the cell either adapts or dies. Adaptation occurs if the cell can maintain function of the nucleus and begin repair.[2,6] Extreme adaptation, however, may affect the normal function of the cell, leading to subsequent problems in the tissue or organ. Cells may also respond to environmental factors by adapting before cell damage occurs.

Cells adapt in several ways.[2] First, they can shrink and become less active in response to decreased metabolic demands, a process called *atrophy*, or grow and become more active in response to increased demands, called *hypertrophy*. Atrophy is generally caused by disuse due to injury or immobilization or impaired cellular metabolism, such as malnutrition. Hypertrophy, conversely, increases cell size to meet increased metabolic or physical demands, such as weight lifting. Aging is a type of atrophic cellular adaptation caused by multiple factors, including cell damage caused by exposure to metabolic and external toxins over a lifetime.

Cells may also adapt by changing in number, type, or morphology (structure). *Hyperplasia* is an increase in the number of cells in a tissue without a change in the rate of cell division or cell function. This occurs as an adaptation to chronic increased metabolic demands, genetic abnormalities, or hormonal imbalances. *Metaplasia* is a replacement of cells of one type with another type, often in response to physical or chemical irritants. These "new" cells do not display changes in rate of division or function, but may change the relative proportion of one cell type to another within a particular tissue.

When cells adapt by changing to an abnormal cell type, increasing the rate of division, and increasing in number, the process is called *dysplasia*. Dysplasia can be caused by chronic irritation or a malfunction in DNA replication. Formation of neoplasms, or tumors, involve dysplasia. *Malignant* (severely invasive) dysplasia produces neoplasms in a process called *cancer* (rapid proliferation of undifferentiated, nonspecific cell types). Cell death, or *necrosis*, occurs when cell resources cannot meet the metabolic (ie, oxygen and energy) demands of the nucleus. A large number of dead cells impairs organ function and disables the associated body system. Cell necrosis can lead to disease or death of the organism.

Most normal cellular adapations, such as callus formation (hyperplasia) or menstruation (hyperplasia and metaplasia), are temporary physiological responses that are part of homeostasis. Other adaptations or cell damage produce general chemical and physical responses to repair tissue structure or function. An example of such a general response is inflammation, as discussed below. Other normal and abnormal effects are caused by tissue-specific adaptations, such as the hypertrophy of muscle when regularly exposed to loads or the atrophy of muscle when it loses its neural control. The general and specific effects may impair organ function, thus becoming pathology and causing signs and symptoms.

Tissue Healing

Damaged tissue is capable of healing in one of two ways. First, functional organ and tissue cells may be regenerated, essentially replacing injured tissue with normal tissue. Second, the functional cells may be replaced by connective tissue, which is a process called scarring. Scarred tissue restores structural integrity of the organ, but does not function like the original tissue. If a significant amount of scarring occurs, the function of the organ may be permanently impaired. Scarring occurs in tissues and organs that cannot regenerate their functional cells.

Regardless of method, tissue healing generally progresses in three stages: inflammatory, proliferative, and remodeling. Each stage takes a different amount of time depending on the tissue (Table 2-2). The inflammatory phase begins at the moment of tissue injury. The inflammatory phase includes hemostasis, a vascular response, and a cellular response. Hemostasis involves an immediate vasoconstriction and activation of platelets. This immediate response is an effort to control blood loss. After a period of vasoconstriction, the vessels dilate and become more permeable. This permeability allows plasma and other blood compounds to exit the vessel and enter the damaged tissue, causing edema. Some of these compounds also stimulate the cellular response. In the cellular response, various types of white blood cells move into the area to clear it of bacteria and dead cells. Some of these cells also release growth factors that stimulate cell growth and revascularization, as well as attracting cells called fibroblasts that function in the proliferative stage. The inflammatory phase typically lasts only days after injury, but can be prolonged if the source of damage is not removed.

The proliferative stage serves to close the tissue wound. Fibroblasts secrete collagen, a complex protein that binds to itself and other structures to create a scar.

Table 2-2

Cell Structures and Their Functions

Tissue	Stage	Time	Treatment or Action
Ligament	Inflammatory	48 to 72 hours	Protect; splint in approximation
	Proliferative	6 to 8 weeks	Active mobilization and activity within limits
	Remodeling	12 to 30 months	Activity as tolerated
Tendon	Inflammatory	48 to 72 hours	Protect; splint in approximation
	Proliferative	4 to 6 weeks	Active and passive mobilization within limits
	Remodeling	12 to 20 weeks	Strengthening and activity as tolerated
Muscle	Inflammatory	48 to 72 hours	Protect; gentle passive or active-assisted mobilization
	Proliferative	4 to 8 weeks	Active muscle recruitment, passive mobilization
	Remodeling	12 weeks	Strengthening and accommodation to load
Bone	Inflammatory	48 to 72 hours	Strict immobilization or surgical fixation; approximation is critical
	Proliferative	3 to 6 weeks*	Continue immobilization or fixation until union (or longer), then begin gentle range of motion (non-load bearing)
	Remodeling	6 to 24 weeks†	After consolidation, begin load-bearing activity as tolerated
Articular cartilage	Inflammatory	48 to 72 hours	Weight-bearing as tolerated; maintain muscular function
	Proliferative	6 months	Controlled weight-bearing activity to stimulate fibrocartilage
	Remodeling	2 years	Activity as tolerated
Nerve	Inflammatory	2 to 7 days	Medical evaluation; splinting may be needed to stabilize
	Proliferative	1 inch per month	Monitor; periodic sensory and motor testing
	Remodeling	Up to 1 year	Return to normal use; may need strengthening or other therapy

**Time for union, not for callus formation or consolidation. The lower extremity generally takes twice as long as the upper extremity.*

†Time for hard callus formation and consolidation; lower extremity bones generally take twice as long.

This tissue becomes vascularized and new tissue cells begin to form at the periphery of the injured region, if possible. Collagen continues to be secreted until the wound is closed, sometimes persisting for several weeks. The deposition of collagen stimulates the third stage of tissue healing: remodeling.

The remodeling stage overlaps with the proliferative stage: some tissue remodeling occurs while collagen is still being deposited to heal the damage. Remodeling involves the simultaneous breakdown and continued deposition of collagen bonds. This allows the final collagen structure to form in response to forces experienced by the tissue during this stage. The remodeling stage stops when the structure is restored, although the tissue strength often does not return to its normal, uninjured state. In tissues that are able to regenerate, remodeling involves the creation of the new tissue and restoration of organ function. The remodeling stage continues for months, until the integrity and function of the tissue and organ is restored.

Inflammation

Every tissue of the body responds to cellular injury or infection with inflammation. The inflammatory response may be limited only to the affected tissue, producing localized symptoms, or be generalized, causing "systemic" symptoms (see Table 1-7). Consequently, diseases of many organ-systems cause similar systemic signs and symptoms.

Acute Inflammation

Damaged cells release chemicals (eg, histamine, bradykinin, prostaglandins) that cause local capillaries to dilate and become more permeable. This reaction increases blood flow to the area and allows proteins and plasma fluid to enter the *interstitial space*, the space between cells.[2] Proteins in the blood interact with fibrin and begin to form a collagen clot at the damaged site. The chemicals released by the damaged cells also attract *leukocytes* from the blood. Some leukocytes act as *phagocytes* and others prolong the inflammatory response. Phagocytes dissolve and absorb damaged cell structures, invading microbes, and foreign debris.

As inflammation continues, excess interstitial fluid causes tissue pressure to rise relative to pressure in the nearby capillaries. Blood flow in the area consequently decreases, producing ischemic damage in otherwise healthy cells and increasing tissue damage. This secondary tissue damage is greatest near the site of primary cell injury.

These mechanisms cause the characteristic signs and symptoms of inflammation. *Pain* results from tissue damage (primary and secondary), the inflammatory chemicals, and ischemia. *Swelling, erythema* (redness), and *heat* are effects of increased regional blood flow and plasma fluid in the interstitial space. *Ecchymosis* (dark red, blue, or black discoloration) from red blood cells in the tissues may occur. Pain causes local muscle spasm to guard the damaged tissue, thus causing loss of movement and function. The acute phase of inflammation somewhat depends on the extent of cellular damage, but generally lasts from 48 to 72 hours.

Chronic Inflammation

Chronic inflammation, which also can occur in any tissue, is usually a result of long-term chemical irritation or mechanical stress. Chronic inflammation is destructive to the cells and tissues because the chemical action and leukocyte activity is prolonged. In addition, chronic inflammation produces more fibrin and collagen to protect the undamaged tissue or isolate the offending substance. Thus, chronic inflammation can prevent or inhibit tissue healing.

The signs and symptoms of chronic inflammation are the same as acute inflammation, but less intense. Chronic inflammation produces aching pain, pitting edema, mild to moderate muscle spasms, and increased local tissue temperature. Chronic inflammation persists until the cause of cellular damage is removed.

Infection

The response to infection is essentially a specialized inflammatory response. Cell damage caused by the infectious organism causes inflammation. In addition, activation of the immune system can also stimulate a generalized inflammatory response. This response is more widespread than occurs with a local tissue wound. Activated leukocytes in the blood affect neurons in the medulla, which causes an increase in body temperature. Involuntary shivering ("chills"), widespread vasoconstriction, and lying down and flexing the body all occur to increase body temperature to a "new" level. This process is called *fever.*

The presence of fever significantly increases metabolic demands. This causes *hyperpnea* (rapid respiration) and *tachycardia* (rapid heart rate), as well as breakdown (catabolism) of muscle and other tissues, except fat, to obtain energy. The effects of fever are unusual fatigue, *malaise* ("feeling bad"), weakness, and loss of appetite. Once the microorganism has been eliminated, the fever "breaks." To reduce body temperature, the person exhibits *diaphoresis* (sweating), *lethargy* (extreme drowsiness), and extension of the body in supine. In addition, appetite returns to replace energy stores that were drained during the course of the fever. The duration of fever depends on the virulence (aggressiveness) of the infection.

Cellular Physiology and Pathophysiology: Response to Cell Damage

Bone

Normal Morphology and Physiology

Bone provides a framework for the body, levers for muscle, and protection for internal organs (heart, lungs, kidneys, liver, spleen, brain, spinal cord). Mature bone cells are called *osteocytes,* which are produced by *osteoblasts* and resorbed by *osteoclasts.*[2] Bone tissue is being constantly resorbed and rebuilt, maintaining a balance in homeostasis. When this balance is disrupted by pathology, bone mass and density can be affected. For example, in the disease process of osteoporosis more bone is resorbed than is rebuilt, resulting in an overall decrease in bone mass and density (a sign called *osteopenia*) and, consequently, a structural weakening of the bone. There are also diseases that cause the bone to lose its mineral content, which affects the mechanical properties of bone, or cause an excess building of bone. In each of these types of conditions, the normal homeostatic process has been disrupted, which leads to deformity or injury to the affected bones.

Each bone is covered by *periosteum,* an innervated and vascular structure that provides nutrition to the cortical (compact) bone. Cancellous bone has its own blood supply and contains the bone marrow. Bone marrow is either yellow (fatty) or red.

The red marrow, a critical organ, produces blood cells.[2] In children, most bones contain red marrow, whereas adults have red marrow only in the flat bones (cranium, ribs, pelvis, vertebrae).[2] Bones articulate to form joints. Joint surfaces are covered with articular cartilage, which decreases the friction between the opposing bones. Articular cartilage is avascular, has no nervous supply, and has very few *chondrocytes* (living cartilage cells) within its tissue.

Pathological Processes

Fracture is physical damage to the structure of a bone and can occur across an entire bone, involving both cortical and cancellous bone, or occur only in the cortical bone (eg, greenstick and stress fractures). A fracture that penetrates the skin, called a compound (open) fracture, is particularly prone to infection because the bone and other deep tissues are exposed to the environment. Bone infection causes osteomyelitis, an inflammation of bone and bone marrow (see Chapter Four), which destroys normal bone cells and deforms the bone. Many genetic and metabolic abnormalities of bone, such as osteogenesis imperfecta and osteoporosis, can produce severe deformity and disability. Toxic damage, such as exposure to high-dosage radiation, is another possible source of pathology. Articular cartilage can be damaged by physical trauma (osteochondritis dissecans), inflammation (osteoarthritis, rheumatoid arthritis), or infection.

Response to Disease or Injury

Fractured bone can heal, given the appropriate environment: alignment and approximation of bone ends, stability, sterility, and nutrition.[2] In fractured bone, the inflammatory stage includes bleeding (hematoma formation) and muscle guarding.[2] The proliferative stage begins as the hematoma resolves and a fibrin clot forms; osteoblast activity increases to produce new bone cells. Fibrocartilage forms around the fracture and is then gradually replaced by a bony callus, or mass of osteocytes in various stages of formation. Once the bony callus is complete, the bone is stable and can bear weight. This process takes approximately 4 to 6 weeks in children and 8 to 12 weeks in adults.[2] The remodeling stage lasts for 1 to 2 years following the fracture as the bone remodels in response to the demands placed upon it.

Bone infections heal by a similar mechanism after the infection is eliminated, which often involves surgical resection and stabilization. Some genetic and metabolic bone disorders, such as osteogenesis imperfecta or osteoporosis (see Chapter Ten), may not allow bone to heal completely.

Articular cartilage has no blood supply. When damaged, it is either replaced by fibrocartilage, which is not as smooth, or not replaced at all. Since articular cartilage also has no nerve supply, pain does not occur unless the underlying (subchondral) bone or synovial tissue is involved. Articular cartilage injuries are relatively permanent, although function can be preserved with replacement by fibrocartilage. Articular cartilage injuries are usually accompanied by subtle joint instability and synovial (joint capsule) inflammation, a clinical syndrome known as *arthritis*. Significant damage to the articular cartilage, subchondral bone, and synovium may require surgical replacement with an artificial joint.

Connective Tissue, Epithelium, and Endothelium

Normal Morphology and Physiology

Connective tissue consists of collagen and elastin. Connective tissue attaches body structures, such as organs, bones, and muscles, to one another. A higher proportion of collagen indicates relatively greater tensile strength but less flexibility, whereas the opposite is true for a higher proportion of elastin. Connective tissue, although highly vascular and innervated, usually has only a few living cells interspersed in the tissue. There are several types of connective tissue.

Epithelium lines the interior and exterior surfaces of the body, including the skin, the gastrointestinal tract, and the pulmonary system. Epithelium provides a barrier to the external environment. *Endothelium* lines the cardiovascular system, including the heart, arteries, veins, and lymphatics. Endothelium regulates the exchange of substances, including nutrients, metabolic waste products, gases, infectious microorganisms, and toxins, between the blood and other organs. Both epithelium and endothelium have several specialized cell subtypes and exist in various cell thicknesses throughout the body. The rate of replication for these cells is very high. Thus, as a function of homeostasis, relatively "new" cells are constantly replacing "older" cells that may have been exposed to potentially toxic, infectious, or damaging substances. By constantly replacing cells that have been exposed to the environment, the body can protect itself by always presenting fresh cells as the first line of defense against potential pathogens.

Pathological Processes

Physical damage or infection cause cell damage in connective tissue. Metabolic diseases are also relatively common in connective tissue (eg, rheumatoid arthritis, gout, vasculitis), causing chronic inflammation, tissue destruction, and scarring. Epithelium and endothelium are prone to cancer and toxic damage due to their constant exposure to the environment (indirectly through the blood in the case of endothelium). Damage to epithelium or endothelium cells also causes changes in tissue permeability. Once permeability is changed, substances that normally do not enter the cell may get in or substances that normally move into the cell may be kept from doing so. This disruption in normal cellular exchange affects the function of the cell and the underlying organ, thus disrupting homeostasis.

Response to Injury or Disease

Connective, epithelial, and endothelial tissues follow the typical tissue healing stages previously outlined. Connective tissue heals with collagen only. Hence, any tissue that has elastin as a primary component loses flexibility after injury and healing. This effect may also interfere with normal organ function. For instance, scarring in the abdomen following surgery can sometimes cause a stricture, or narrowing of the intestinal passageway, thus restricting the passage of food. Similarly, scarring in the connective tissues of the thorax may restrict chest expansion or gas exchange in the lungs.

Collagen scar tissue usually provides the same tensile strength as the original connective tissue within 6 to 8 weeks, provided the optimal healing environment (nutrients and oxygen from the blood) is present and the tissue is protected from reinjury. Remodeling of the collagen tissue to arrange fiber alignment consistent with the original structure, however, may take 6 to 12 months. Since collagen aligns

Table 2-3
Muscle Cell Types, Location, and Function

Type	Body System	Function
Striated	Musculoskeletal	Movement of the bones and body through space
Cardiac	Heart	Maintain blood flow to body
Smooth	Vascular and gastrointestinal	Movement of blood and food through the respective system

along lines of consistent tissue stretch, thus providing higher tensile strength, appropriate functional demands should be placed on the tissue through this period. Again, the elastic qualities of the tissue are not restored by the remodeled collagen.

Injured epithelium and endothelium can be replaced with normal cells provided the damage does not extend through all cell layers and the genetic mechanism is not affected. The healing process takes a few days to close the wound, a few weeks to return to full strength, and several months to remodel completely. Function of the resulting scar is dependent on the extent of the injury. A larger injury, resulting in a larger scar, will have a greater impairment of tissue function. If all cell layers are damaged, the tissue is replaced by a nonfunctional collagen scar (metaplasia). If the DNA replication mechanism is affected, a cancerous lesion forms (dysplasia). Replacement of living cells with inflexible collagen not only leads to possible restrictions or obstructions, as noted above, but also causes the tissue to be nonpermeable, preventing normal cellular exchange. Cancerous changes can also cause obstructions and interfere with normal tissue function.

Muscle and Nerve

Normal Morphology and Physiology

Muscle tissue has three types: skeletal, cardiac, and smooth (Table 2-3). The principle function of muscle is contraction, which moves the skeleton, circulates the blood, or moves food through the bowels. Nerve cells transmit electrical signals that are initiated by external or internal stimuli. These signals control the movement, cognitive, and regulatory systems of the body. Nerve cells within the brain and associated structures are highly specialized, whereas the structure of nerve cells in the peripheral nervous system tend to be very similar to one another. All nerve cells contain a cell body, dendrites (projections that receive signals from other cells), and axons (projections that send signals to other cells). Chemical processes form the electrical impulses within (primarily sodium ion exchanges) and between (via neurotransmitters) cells.

Pathological Processes

Skeletal muscle is most commonly affected by physical trauma (contusion or strain) or infection (eg, tetanus), although genetic and metabolic diseases also occur (eg, muscular dystrophy, myasthenia gravis). In contrast, cardiac and smooth muscle are more commonly affected by metabolic states (such as ischemia) and infection. Toxins can also affect the various types of muscle, nervous tissue, or the neuromuscular junction, and interrupt function. Interruption of muscle function results in a loss of contraction; depending on the muscle type and location, the effect can be disabling (eg, skeletal muscle) or even fatal (eg, cardiac muscle).

Nerve cells are fragile and are easily damaged by physical trauma, toxins, infections, and metabolic imbalances. Many pathological processes directly or indirectly affect the nervous system. Thus, signs of nervous system impairment are often early indications of systemic disease. In addition, some diseases affect the biochemical mechanisms that propagate electrical impulse. In such instances, cell structure is maintained although cell function is impaired. Loss of neural function implies a loss of the ability to propagate the electrical signal; the location and type of nerve determines the functional effects of nerve injury.

Response to Injury or Disease

The response of muscle cells to damage is similar to that of connective tissue. Damaged cells and tissue are replaced by collagen tissue rather than normal contractile muscle. Depending on severity and extent of injury, a large noncontractile scar within a muscle can be disabling. If a relatively small proportion of skeletal muscle tissue is damaged, resistance training of the remaining muscle tissue can compensate for the loss of functional motor units. If a significant proportion of the smooth muscle of internal organs or cardiac muscle is damaged, however, severe impairment or complete loss of function occurs in the associated organ. Irrecoverable damage to cardiac muscle can be fatal.

Unfortunately, damage to the cell body of a nerve cell is permanent. A nerve cell can neither be replaced nor regenerated, resulting in permanent loss of the functions associated with that nerve cell. Damage to any portion of the nerve cell (dendrite, axon, or body) in the central nervous system (brain and spinal cord) is also permanent. If an axon is damaged in the peripheral nervous system, however, it can regenerate provided the myelin (a lipoprotein) sheath surrounding the axon is preserved and aligned. The axon first degenerates distal to the point of injury (a process called wallerian degeneration) and then regenerates inside the myelin sheath at a rate of approximately one-quarter inch per month.

Specialized Cells and Tissues

Normal Morphology and Physiology

Cells of the blood, gastrointestinal system, liver, kidneys, and endocrine glands are highly specialized to perform specific tasks (Table 2-4). Most of the functions are integral to larger systems or to homeostasis in general. Thus, abnormal function in one of the systems usually (eventually) affects one or more of the other systems. Pathology in these organs often produce the systemic signs reviewed in Table 1-7, which reflect the interaction of these systems clinically.

Pathological Processes

Pathology of gastrointestinal, liver, or kidney cells can be caused by infection, metabolic or genetic changes, or toxicity. Direct physical trauma, which is perhaps most common in young people and people who participate in sports, can disrupt tissues and interfere with organ function. Blood cells can also be affected by

Table 2-4
Examples of Specialized Cell Types, Location, and Function

Cell Type	Location	Function
Mucosa	Gastrointestinal	Absorb nutrients, secrete mucous for protection and enzymes for digestion
Acinar	Exocrine pancreas	Secrete digestive enzymes
Islet	Endocrine pancreas	Alpha-cells secrete glucagon, beta-cells secrete insulin
Hepatic	Liver	Secrete bile, store carbohydrate, form urea, metabolism of cholesterol, lipids, and many drugs and toxins
Renal	Kidney	Regulate fluid, form urine
Endocrine	Endocrine glands	Secrete regulatory specific hormones

infection, metabolic changes, or toxicity, and can be indirectly affected by trauma to other tissues. Substantial tissue trauma may cause a loss of large amounts of blood from the vascular system, called *hemorrhage*. Hemorrhage has serious and potentially fatal consequences as organs become progressively deprived of blood-borne nutrients and oxygen, a process known as *shock* (see Chapter Six).

The signs of shock reflect the homeostatic effort to maintain blood pressure in the vascular system and blood flow to the internal organs. These signs include pallor (pale skin) and cool ("clammy") skin as a result of peripheral vasoconstriction in an effort to preserve blood flow to the internal organs, *hypotension* (low blood pressure) as a result of low blood volume within the vascular system, and *tachycardia* (increased heart rate) in an effort to maintain blood flow to the organs of the body. Shock can also be caused by a response to heart failure (decreasing systemic blood flow) or widespread peripheral vasodilation (in response to autonomic nervous system action, systemic infection, or anaphylaxis).

Endocrine glands are rarely affected by trauma, but physical damage may occur with major injuries and diseases in surrounding organs. More commonly, genetic factors induce abnormal function or tumor development. Environmental factors also potentially affect endocrine function through toxicity. Tumors in the endocrine glands can either reduce or increase secretion of specific hormones, thus upsetting metabolic homeostasis. In addition, since hormones affect multiple organs, signs and symptoms are produced in several systems.

Response to Injury or Disease

The tissues of the gastrointestinal organs, liver, and kidneys are highly vascularized and display a typical tissue healing response in reaction to cellular damage. The inflammatory response produces clinical signs that are specific to the functions of the affected organ or organs (see Chapters Eight and Nine). Many of these cells have a limited ability to regenerate, but if chronic cell damage and inflammation persists, the damage becomes permanent and cells are replaced by scar tissue. With repeated, prolonged, or severe damage, the organs can no longer function properly, and may restrict blood flow to surrounding healthy cells, thus propagating cell damage. Examples of this type of pathology include cirrhosis of the liver, chronic renal failure, and inflammatory bowel disease.

Blood Cells

The presence of infection (*septicemia*) or a toxin in the blood causes a vigorous inflammatory response throughout the body. The high fever produced in such a condition can destroy other tissues, posing a serious threat to homeostasis and life. The blood can also be affected by genetic diseases, including sickle cell anemia (misshapen red blood cells, see Chapter Six) and leukemia (proliferation of immature blood cells, see Chapter Five). These diseases also cause a mild or moderate general inflammatory response.

Summary

Pathophysiology refers to the biological process of disease. The mechanism called homeostasis responds to the changing internal and external environment to maintain chemical, fluid, and energy balances in the body. Many pathological processes upset this equilibrium. Virtually all pathological processes can be expressed in terms of their effect on individual cells and the cellular effects on organ function. Cells can be damaged by physical, infective, metabolic, genetic, or environmental factors, causing them to either adapt or die. When enough cells die, organ functions are affected. Inflammation and infection are general responses to cell damage. Each cell and tissue type also produces specific responses. Signs and symptoms are these general and specific responses to cell damage.

References

1. National Athletic Trainers' Association. *Athletic Training Educational Competencies.* 4th ed. Dallas, TX: National Athletic Trainers' Association; 2005.
2. Gould BE. Introduction to pathophysiology. *Pathophysiology for the Health-Related Professions.* Philadelphia, PA: WB Saunders Co; 1997:3-8.
3. Majno G, Joris I, eds. *Cells, Tissues, and Disease: Principles of General Pathology.* 2nd ed. New York, NY: Oxford University Press; 2004.
4. Porth CM. *Essentials of Pathophysiology.* Philadelphia, PA: Lippincott Williams & Wilkins; 2004.
5. Sell S, Berkower I, Max EE, eds. *Immunology, Immunopathology & Immunity.* 5th ed. Stamford, CT: Appleton & Lange; 1996.
6. Shaw M, Roy CM, Bartelmo JM, et al, eds. *Pathophysiology Made Incredibly Easy.* Springhouse, PA: Springhouse Corp; 1998.
7. Underwood JCE, ed. *General and Systematic Pathology.* 4th ed. New York, NY: Churchill Livingstone; 2004.
8. Ganong WF. *Review of Medical Physiology.* 22nd ed. New York, NY: McGraw-Hill Medical; 2005.

Online Resources

Medline Plus (medical dictionary and encyclopedia, plus descriptions of more than 700 medical conditions)

www.medlineplus.gov

Online pathophysiology textbook

www.mfi.ku.dk/ppaulev/content.htm

Chapter Three

Pharmacology

Chapter Outline and Objectives

Introduction

Nomenclature

- Identify the standard nomenclature associated with pharmacology.

Classification of Drugs

- Explain the classifications of drugs.
  - Over-the-Counter
  - Prescription
  - Controlled Substances

Routes of Administration

- Explain the various routes of administration, including oral, injection, inhalation, topical, sublingual and buccal, and rectal.
  - Oral
  - Injection
  - Inhalation
  - Topical
  - Sublingual and Buccal
  - Rectal

Pharmacokinetics

- Explain the processes of pharmacokinetics and the effect of exercise on these processes.
  - Absorption
  - Distribution
  - Metabolism
  - Elimination

Pharmacodynamics

- ❖ Explain the processes of pharmacodynamics.
  - Drug Dosing
  - Drug Interactions and Adverse Reactions

Therapeutic Medications

- ❖ Discuss the routes of administration, dosage patterns, physiological effects, and side effects associated with common therapeutic medications.
  - NSAIDs
  - Corticosteroids
  - Analgesics
  - Antibiotics
  - Antihistamines
  - Decongestants
  - Bronchodilators
  - Gastrointestinal Drugs
  - Antifungals
  - Antivirals

Nutritional Supplements and Performance-Enhancing Products

- ❖ Discuss the routes of administration, dosage patterns, physiological effects, and side effects associated with select nutritional supplements and performance-enhancing substances.
- ❖ Identify supplements and drugs that might be banned by sport or workplace regulations.
  - Creatine
  - Dehydroepiandrosterone and Androstenedione
  - Androgenic-Anabolic Steroids
  - Human Growth Hormone
  - Erythropoietin

Herbal Supplements

- ❖ Discuss the intended use, side effects, and potential drug interactions associated with select herbal supplements.

Storage and Management of Medications

- ❖ Describe the federal laws and regulations related to the storage and management of medications.

Preventing and Managing Medication Poisoning

- ❖ Outline a plan for preventing and managing medication poisoning.

Drug Resources

- ❖ Identify drug information resources.

This chapter addresses the following competencies from the *Athletic Training Educational Competencies, Fourth Edition*[1]:

Domain	Cognitive	Psychomotor
Acute Care of Injuries and Illnesses		3i
Pharmacology	1–11	

Introduction

There are literally hundreds of therapeutic medications used to treat common musculoskeletal and systemic injuries and illnesses. For this reason, it is impossible for the athletic trainer to be familiar with every medication that patients may use. However, the athletic trainer must be familiar with common types of medications (antihistamines, analgesics, nonsteroidal anti-inflammatory drugs [NSAIDs], etc) and the implications that they may have on a patient's ability to participate in sports, work, or rehabilitation. The athletic trainer can also play a role in helping to improve patient compliance with medication usage.

This chapter will begin with a discussion of the foundational concepts related to pharmacology and then move to a discussion of common types of therapeutic drugs, nutritional supplements, performance-enhancing substances, and herbal medications that might be encountered by the athletic trainer in clinical practice. Subsequent chapters will discuss many of the specific drugs used to treat specific systemic diseases. A complete and thorough discussion of all concepts and physiological effects of all drugs is beyond the scope of this chapter. We recommend *Principles of Pharmacology for Athletic Trainers*[2] as a companion text for this book.

Nomenclature

Drugs are identified by one of three names: chemical, generic, or trade. The *chemical* name is rather long and refers to the chemical structure of the drug. The *generic*, or nonproprietary, name is shorter and is derived from the chemical name. The *trade* name is the recognized brand name that is assigned to a drug by the manufacturer. The trade name is proprietary and therefore cannot be used by other manufacturers. There is only one generic name for each drug, but there may be multiple trade names if the drug is marketed by more than one company. For example, ibuprofen is the generic name for both Motrin (McNeil Consumer Healthcare, Fort Washington, Pa) and Advil (Wyeth Pharmaceuticals, Madison, NJ). Any manufacturer can use the name ibuprofen to describe that particular NSAID, whereas the names Motrin and Advil can only be used by McNeil and Wyeth, respectively.

Generic names should not be confused with generic drugs. Every drug has a generic name; however, not every drug is available in a generic form. Generic drugs are copies of brand name drugs whose patents have expired. They are generally cheaper, with brand name drugs sometimes costing as much as four times that of their generic counterparts. During the patent period of a drug (approximately

20 years), only the original manufacturer may legally market that drug. A large portion of the cost associated with brand name drugs is related to the original expense of testing and retesting the drug prior to its submittal to the Food and Drug Administration (FDA) for approval. Once a drug's patent expires, other drug manufacturers can formulate and market their version (generic) of the original drug. Generic drugs must be therapeutically equivalent, meaning they must have the same chemical makeup and active ingredients as the original drug and produce the same medical effect. Since these manufacturers do not have the research expense of testing the drug, they can market their version of the drug (generic) at a much cheaper cost. Generic drugs are usually marketed using the generic name. Currently, about half of the drugs on the market are available in a generic form.

Classification of Drugs

There are three major classifications of drugs: over-the-counter (OTC), prescription, and controlled substances. Each of these classifications is discussed below.

Over-the-Counter

OTC medications do not require a prescription and are therefore also referred to as nonprescription drugs. Many OTC drugs were originally prescription drugs that have now been approved by the FDA as nonprescription drugs. These medications will typically contain less drug per dose as compared to the corresponding prescription drug. For example, naproxen sodium (Aleve [Bayer Healthcare Pharmaceuticals, Montville, NJ]) is a commonly used OTC anti-inflammatory medication and is available in 220 mg tablets. Naproxen is available by prescription, with a single tablet containing either 250 mg or 400 mg. OTC medications are typically less expensive than prescription medications and are convenient, allowing consumers to self-medicate themselves for minor conditions rather than going to see their physician.

Prescription

The purchase of prescription medications requires a written prescription from a physician or nurse practitioner and by law must be filled by a pharmacist. These medications are typically associated with a greater potential for adverse reactions and are generally prescribed for a restricted time period. Patients are only able to refill a prescription when authorized by their physician.

Controlled Substances

Drugs classified as controlled substances have a greater potential for abuse than prescription drugs. The Comprehensive Drug Abuse Prevention and Control Act of 1970, also referred to as the Controlled Substances Act, established the current categories of controlled substances, which are divided into five areas or schedules. Schedule I drugs have the highest potential for abuse while Schedule V drugs have the least potential for abuse. Table 3-1 provides examples of common drugs within each schedule category. Most narcotic pain medications are classified as Schedule III drugs. Anabolic steroids are also classified as Schedule III. The Drug Enforcement Agency (DEA) is responsible for overseeing the manufacturing, distribution, storage, and dispensing of all controlled substances.

Table 3-1
Controlled Substances

Schedule	Abuse Potential	Example Drugs
I	Greatest	Heroin, marijuana, lysergic acid diethylamide (LSD), tetrahydrocannabinol (THC)
II	↓	Amphetamines, cocaine, codeine, Demerol, methamphetamine, morphine, oxycodone plus acetaminophen (Percocet), methylphenidate (Ritalin)
III		Anabolic steroids, codeine with acetaminophen, hydrocodone with acetaminophen, propoxyphene (Darvon)
IV		Alprazolam (Xanax), diazepam (Valium), lorazepam (Ativan), phenobarbital (Luminal)
V	Least	Cough suppressants containing codeine (Robitussin A-C), antidiarrheal medication containing opium (Kapectolin PG)

Routes of Administration

There are several different routes that can be used for administering therapeutic medications. The route used is somewhat dependent on the condition to be treated, the specific drug, and whether the drug is meant to provide a systemic effect or a local effect. Oral, injection, inhalation, topical, sublingual, buccal, and rectal are all common routes for drug administration.[3] Those routes of administration that provide entry to the body by way of the alimentary canal or digestive system (ie, oral and rectal) are referred to as enteral routes. The nonenteral routes (injection, inhalation, sublingual, buccal, and topical) are referred to as parenteral routes of administration.

Oral

The oral route is the most commonly used route for administering medication. One disadvantage of the oral route is that stomach acid may completely or partially inactivate some drugs, reducing their therapeutic effectiveness. Also, medications administered orally will take longer to provide a therapeutic effect since they must first be absorbed from the stomach or intestines before they can be distributed. Some foods can interact with certain medications when ingested at the same time; therefore, it is important to read and follow all instructions printed on the medication label.

Some drugs will contain an *enteric coating* which is designed to delay the release of a medication until it reaches the small intestine. This coating is often used to protect an acid-sensitive medication or to protect the gastric mucosa by delaying the breakdown of the drug until after it has passed through the stomach. Extended-release medications may contain an enteric coating or layers of a coating designed to allow a gradual release of medication. Because the medication is released over a prolonged period of time, extended-release medications will typically contain more drug than their normal-release counterparts. Enteric-coated and extended-release medications should never be cut or crushed prior to administration.

There are a variety of dosage forms available for oral administration including tablets, caplets, capsules, syrups, and powders. Tablets, caplets, and capsules may take up to 30 minutes to provide their intended therapeutic effect since they must first be broken down or dissolved in the stomach before moving to the small intestine for absorption.[3] It is recommended that oral medications be taken with a full glass of water to help move them into the small intestines for quicker absorption.

Injection

Injections are common parenteral (non-oral) routes for drug administration and can be administered directly into the veins (intravenous [IV] drugs) or through intramuscular (IM), intra-articular, or subcutaneous tissues. IV drug administration provides an immediate systemic effect, whereas IM and subcutaneous injection provides a slower (but still faster than oral) systemic or local effect. Intra-articular injections primarily provide a local effect.

Inhalation

Inhalation is a common route of delivery for most asthma medications because it enables the medication to be delivered directly to the bronchial and lung tissues for quicker relief of symptoms (in some cases <5 minutes). Aerosol mists and dry powders are two common dosage forms of inhaled medications and are administered using metered dose inhalers (MDI) and dry powder inhalers (DPI). These dosage forms and the common asthma medications are discussed more thoroughly in Chapter Seven.

Topical

Topical medications are administered through creams, gels, lotions, sprays, drops, and transdermal patches. Creams, gels, and lotions are applied to the skin to produce a local effect and are commonly used to treat skin conditions (see Chapter Twelve). Intranasal sprays enable medications to be administered directly to the mucous membranes within the nose. Drops are used to treat ear and eye conditions. Transdermal patches should be applied to clean, dry skin with little or no hair. For prolonged use, the patch should be rotated to a different skin area periodically to avoid skin irritation. Transdermal patches should never be cut in an attempt to adjust dosage or to fit a particular area.

Sublingual and Buccal

Sublingual and buccal medications are administered under the tongue and between the cheek and gum, respectively. Drugs administered through these routes are absorbed very quickly due to the rich vascular supply of these mucosal tissues.

Rectal

The suppository is a common dosage form used to administer medication via the rectum. This route of administration is often used to administer anti-emetics for treating individuals with severe vomiting when they are unable to keep oral medications down. Some pain medications and laxatives are also administered using suppositories.

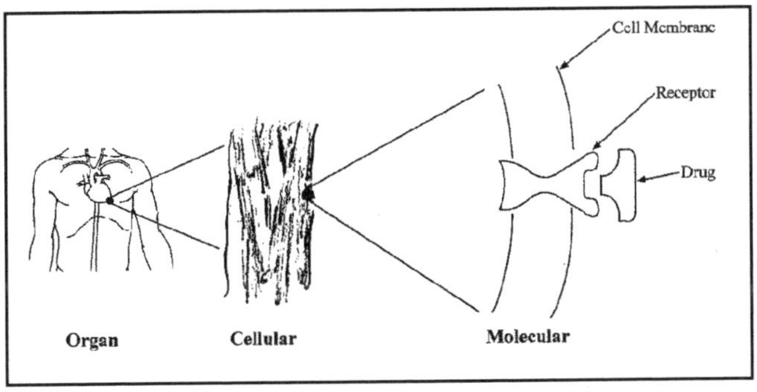

Figure 3-1. Site of action. The site of action is in specific tissues at the cellular and molecular level, often at a receptor on the cell membrane to which the drug chemically fits. (Reprinted from Houglum JE, Harrelson GL, Leaver-Dunn D. *Principles of Pharmacology for Athletic Trainers.* Thorofare, NJ: SLACK Incorporated; 2005.)

PHARMACOKINETICS

Pharmacokinetics describes the physiological processes of how the body acts on a drug and can be divided into four distinct phases: absorption, distribution, metabolism, and elimination (ADME). Each of these phases is described below.

Absorption

For a drug to produce a therapeutic effect, it must be absorbed into the bloodstream and distributed throughout the circulation to reach its site of action (Figure 3-1). Absorption of orally administered drugs occurs in the stomach and small intestine, with the majority occurring in the latter structure. The amount of drug that is actually available in the body's tissues is referred to as its *bioavailability*. The bioavailability is usually only a fraction of the dosage amount. If a drug's bioavailability is 50%, then the body will only absorb 250 mg of a 500 mg dose of medication. Bioavailability varies among drugs. For example, when comparing two commonly prescribed NSAIDs, Naproxen has a bioavailability of 95% while Voltaren (Novartis, Cambridge, Mass) has a 50% bioavailability.

A specific drug's bioavailability is affected by both the amount of drug absorbed and the rate at which it is absorbed. Gastric enzymes can affect whether a drug dissolves completely in the stomach before moving into the intestines or can inactivate a portion of a drug before it leaves the stomach. The "first pass effect" also influences the bioavailability of a drug. The first pass effect occurs if the drug is absorbed from the intestine into the liver before entering the systemic circulation. The liver serves as the main site for drug metabolism (discussed below) and may cause further inactivation of a portion of the drug. To compensate for the first pass effect, manufacturers will increase the amount of drug contained within a single oral dose. The first pass effect is only a factor when drugs are taken orally.

For absorption to occur, a drug molecule must move across one or more membranes through either simple diffusion, active transport, or passive diffusion. Passive diffusion is the most common mechanism for moving medications across membranes.[2] The lipid solubility of a drug will affect its ability to diffuse across these membranes. With *passive diffusion*, lipid soluble drugs will diffuse more quickly and easily and are capable of passing through the blood-brain barrier to affect the central nervous system. Movement of drug molecules across membranes will typically occur from the side with greatest concentration to the side with lowest concentration. When the concentration of molecules becomes equal on both sides, diffusion is stopped.

The *active transport* mechanism requires a protein to move the drug across a membrane. The protein binds to the drug molecule and transports it through the membrane. This mechanism allows selective diffusion of drug molecules in a specific direction, regardless of the concentrations on either side of the membrane. Active transport requires energy to occur. The mechanism of *facilitated diffusion* combines the processes of passive diffusion and active transport. It allows for drug selectivity through the binding of a protein; however, the drug molecule will only move from areas of high concentration to low concentration.

Exercise can delay or reduce the absorption of oral medications since blood is diverted away from the gastrointestinal tract to the working skeletal muscles. When the body absorbs less of a drug, its therapeutic effectiveness is decreased. For optimum absorption, oral medications should be taken at least 30 minutes prior to beginning exercise.

Distribution

Once absorption is complete, the drug is transported to its site of action via the circulatory system. Like absorption, a drug's distribution is also affected by its lipid solubility. Drugs with higher lipid solubility will be able to pass through more membranes providing a wider distribution, particularly with respect to the blood-brain barrier and fat cells. Lipid-soluble drugs are also capable of being stored in the body producing a longer-lasting effect, while water-soluble drugs are more easily eliminated or excreted from the body. Blood flow to an area affects the distribution of a drug to that area. For example, the vascular nature of the liver, kidney, and brain enable drug molecules to reach these structures quickly. Structures that are less vascular (bone and fat cells) will typically require more time for drug distribution.

A drug's *onset of action* is the time it takes for drug molecules to reach their site of action in sufficient quantities to produce a therapeutic effect (Figure 3-2). As the drug molecules are metabolized and excreted (discussed below), their concentration at the site of action is reduced until they are no longer able to exert a therapeutic effect. A drug's *duration of action* is that period of time when concentration levels are sufficient enough to produce a therapeutic effect (see Figure 3-2). Individual drugs differ in their onset and duration of action.

Exercise increases blood flow and therefore may increase the drug distribution rate, depending on the intended site of action. It is important to remember that blood is shunted away from some areas (stomach and intestines) in order to supply adequate blood to the working skeletal muscles.

Metabolism

Metabolism is the process by which drugs are inactivated and broken down into more water-soluble metabolites in preparation for excretion. The mechanism of metabolism is initiated by metabolic enzymes which react with the drug. The liver serves as the primary site for most drug metabolism; however, the kidneys, intestines, lungs, and brain also participate in this process.

Exercise can reduce the metabolism of some drugs, since blood is routed away from the liver and gastrointestinal tract to the working skeletal muscles. However, in most instances the time necessary for completing the metabolic break down of drugs is longer than the duration of exercise negating any overall decrease in drug metabolism.[4]

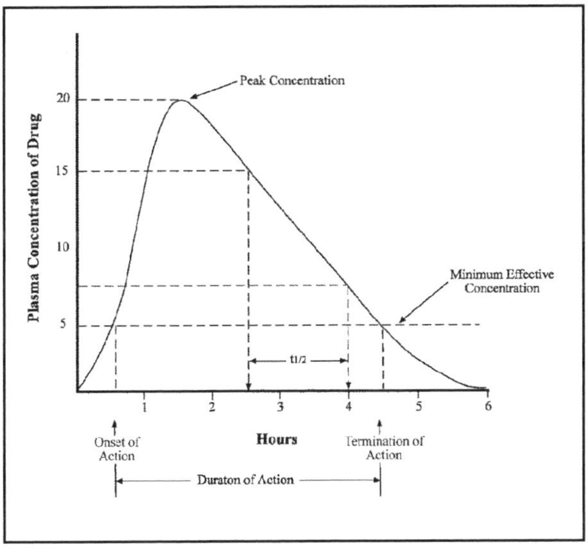

Figure 3-2. Concentration-time curve following a single oral dose of a drug. The onset of action occurs when the concentration is above the level needed to produce an effect (minimal effective concentration). Duration of action (4 hours in this example) is the time between onset and termination of action. The half-life (t½) is the time it takes for the concentration of the drug to be reduced by one half after it has reached peak concentration. In this example, t½=1½ hours; the time it takes for the concentration of the drug to decrease from 15 to 7.5. (Reprinted from Houglum JE, Harrelson GL, Leaver-Dunn D. *Principles of Pharmacology for Athletic Trainers*. Thorofare, NJ: SLACK Incorporated; 2005.)

Elimination

Elimination, or excretion, is the process by which the body rids itself of a drug. The kidneys serve as the primary site for drug excretion; however, the intestines (feces), sweat glands (perspiration), and lungs (respiration) also assist in this process. Exercise can decrease the rate of renal excretion since blood flow is directed away from the kidneys to the working skeletal muscles.

The rate at which a drug is excreted from the body is influenced by the drug's half-life. The *half-life* of a drug is the time it takes to reduce the blood concentration of the drug by 50% (see Figure 3-2). For example, if a drug has a blood concentration of 50 mg and a half-life of 2 hours, then after 2 hours, the blood concentration will be reduced to 25 mg. After 4 hours, it would be 12.5 mg, and after 8 hours it would be 6.25 mg. Drugs with greater half-lives will have greater durations of action and require less frequent dosing. Generally, lipid-soluble drugs have longer half-lives than water-soluble drugs, and will therefore stay in the body longer.

Pharmacodynamics

Pharmacodynamics describes the process of how a drug acts on the body. For a drug to produce a therapeutic effect, it must bind with a receptor, which can be a molecule on the cell membrane or within the cell, at the site of action. The relationship between a drug and a receptor is very specific, much like that between a lock and key. Any chemical change in the drug or the receptor will change this relationship. These receptors are site specific and exist within the body to regulate certain physiological mechanisms by matching with certain endogenous compounds. A drug that fits the receptor and initiates a mechanism similar to the endogenous compound is referred to as an *agonist*. A drug that fits the receptor but fails to initiate or blocks this mechanism is referred to as an *antagonist*. This process is collectively referred to as the *receptor theory of drug action*.[2]

Drug Dosing

The recommended dose of a drug is based on the potency of the drug, the therapeutic range of the drug, the patient's age, and the patient's condition. *Potency* refers to the strength of the drug. The greater the potency, the smaller the dose needed to produce a therapeutic effect. The therapeutic effectiveness of a drug is greatest when its blood concentration levels consistently stay within a certain range (therapeutic range). Dosing beyond this therapeutic range provides no additional benefit. Maintaining blood levels within the therapeutic range is referred to as *steady state* and is achieved once the blood levels from continued dosing matches the levels of excretion of a drug. In some cases, a physician may prescribe a *loading dose* of a drug, which is usually greater than the *maintenance dose* (dose needed to maintain steady state), to increase the rate at which the drug reaches its therapeutic range.

Drug Interactions and Adverse Reactions

Drug interactions can occur between two or more drugs, altering the intended effect of one or all of the drugs. Drug interactions can change how the body handles a drug or how a drug acts on the body. For example, antacids can reduce the body's ability to absorb acetaminophen from the intestine.

Drug interactions can be additive (agonistic) or inhibitive (antagonistic). *Agonistic interactions* occur when two drugs of the same type are taken together (two stimulants or two depressants). The effects of the two drugs "add" together causing an increase in the overall effect. For example, alcohol combined with an antihistamine can cause excessive drowsiness and loss of muscle coordination. *Antagonistic effects* can occur between two unrelated drugs. A common example of an antagonistic effect is antibiotics inhibiting or reducing the effectiveness of oral contraceptives.

Adverse drug reactions can range from mild side effects to severe hypersensitivity. Examples of drug side effects include the drowsiness caused by first-generation antihistamines or the loss of appetite or nausea associated with some antibiotics. Also, certain foods or herbal preparations can interact with prescription and OTC medications. Dairy products are known to decrease the absorption of tetracycline antibiotics. When herbs such as garlic, ginkgo biloba, ginseng, green tea, or grape seed are taken along with warfarin (Coumadin [Bristol Myers Squibb, New York, NY]), aspirin, or other NSAID, patients may experience increased bleeding or bruising.[2] Cases of drug hypersensitivity can range from a mild rash to anaphylactic shock. Both side effects and hypersensitivity reactions can occur immediately or be delayed.

Most allergic drug reactions are associated with NSAIDs and β-lactam (penicillins and cephalosporins) and sulfonamide antibiotics. Persons who are allergic to aspirin may experience similar reactions to other NSAIDs. Aspirin and other NSAIDs are also known to cause asthma attacks in 3% to 39% of individuals with chronic asthma.[2] Allergic reactions that produce a rash can often times be treated with topical corticosteroids to reduce the acute inflammatory reaction and an antihistamine to reduce the itching. Allergic reactions that progress to anaphylaxis are life-threatening situations requiring activation of the emergency action plan. Epinephrine is commonly used to treat an anaphylactic reaction. The epinephrine is administered subcutaneously using an EpiPen (Meridian Medical Technology, Bristol, Tenn). Table 3-2 provides step-by-step instructions for the use of an EpiPen.

Table 3-2
Use of an EpiPen

- Remove EpiPen from its case.
- Form fist around EpiPen, black tip pointing downward.
- Using your other hand, pull off the gray safety release.
- Swing (at 90-degree angle) and jab firmly into outer thigh until pen clicks.
- Continue to hold EpiPen firmly against outer thigh for approximately 10 seconds.
- Remove EpiPen from thigh and massage injection area for 10 seconds.
- Carefully place the used EpiPen (without bending the needle), needle end first, into the storage tube.

Therapeutic Medications

A large variety of prescription and nonprescription medications are used to treat musculoskeletal injuries and systemic disorders. It is impossible to discuss in detail all of the possible medications that athletic trainers may encounter in their clinical practice. This chapter does include a lengthy discussion of NSAIDs due to their widespread use (and abuse) within sports medicine. Analgesics, corticosteroids, antibiotics, antihistamines, decongestants, gastrointestinal medications, antifungals, and bronchial dilators are discussed both in this chapter and in subsequent chapters in conjunction with specific systemic disorders. Discussion of each medication will include the drug's mechanism of action, therapeutic indications, common routes for administration, availability (OTC or prescription only), and potential side effects.

NSAIDs

NSAIDs are used to treat acute and chronic inflammatory conditions like sprains, strains, tendonitis, and bursitis. Chapter Two provided a brief overview of the acute and chronic inflammatory responses and the role of chemical mediators such as prostaglandins, histamine, and bradykinin. Prostaglandins, which are potent vasodilators, are produced by arachidonic acid. They work to sensitize pain receptors to bradykinin and histamine, thereby lowering the threshold of pain and causing increased sensitivity to pain.

During the inflammatory response, arachidonic acid follows one of two pathways depending on the enzymes that are active in the damaged cells. Figure 3-3 illustrates the cyclooxygenase (COX) and lipoxygenase pathways. The lipoxygenase pathway leads to the production of leukotrienes which are often involved in the underlying inflammation associated with chronic asthma. Antileukotrienes are discussed in Chapter Seven. The COX pathway involves two separate COX enzymes (COX-1 and COX-2), with each enzyme forming a separate pathway. As shown in Figure 3-3, the COX-1 enzyme (housekeeping gene) leads to the production of prostaglandins responsible for protecting the gastrointestinal mucosa, aiding in platelet aggregation, and maintaining normal renal function. The COX-2 enzyme (inflammatory gene) leads to the production of prostaglandins responsible for inflammation, pain, fever, and wound healing.

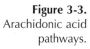

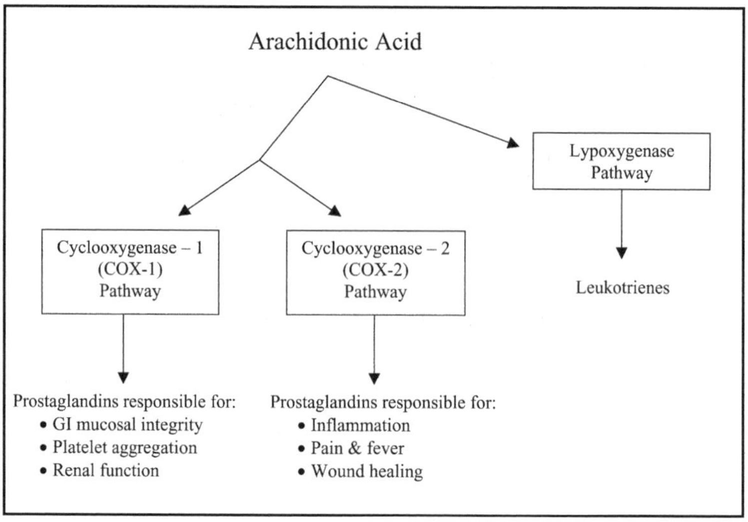

Figure 3-3. Arachidonic acid pathways.

NSAIDs work by inhibiting the COX enzyme and reducing the production of prostaglandins. Traditional NSAIDs are referred to as nonselective COX inhibitors since they block the actions along both the COX-1 and COX-2 pathways. By blocking the COX-2 enzyme, nonselective NSAIDs reduce the pain and swelling associated with inflammation. Unfortunately, they also block the COX-1 enzyme preventing the production of "good" prostaglandins that protect the stomach. As a result, gastric upset and ulcers are two side effects commonly associated with extended use of NSAIDs. Selective COX-2 inhibitors are capable of blocking the COX-2 pathway without affecting the COX-1 pathway. Celecoxib (Celebrex [Pfizer, New York, NY]) is an example of a selective COX-2 inhibitor. Until recently, there were two additional COX-2 inhibitors on the market: valdecoxib (Bextra [Pfizer]) and rofecoxib (Vioxx [Merck, Whitehouse Station, NJ]). These two drugs have been recalled by the FDA due to their suspected role in increasing the risk of myocardial infarctions (heart attacks) and strokes. The FDA has now asked the manufacturers of all OTC NSAIDs to revise their labeling to include warnings about the risk for cardiovascular events and gastrointestinal bleeding.

In addition to their role as an anti-inflammatory agent, NSAIDs are also used as an analgesic (pain reducer) and an antipyretic (fever reducer). Generally, the dosage necessary for reducing inflammation is greater than the dosage necessary for reducing pain or fever. Table 3-3 provides the recommended dosing for anti-inflammatory effects. Also, when the therapeutic goal is to treat inflammation, it is important that dosing be consistent to maintain a steady state within the therapeutic range.

NSAIDs are lipid soluble and are easily absorbed out of the stomach and intestines. Aspirin and diclofenac (Voltaren) are the only NSAIDs that are significantly affected by the first pass effect in the liver. Most NSAIDs will begin producing an effect within 15 to 30 minutes.[5] In most cases, 7 to 10 days is sufficient time to evaluate the effectiveness of a particular NSAID. If one NSAID is ineffective for a particular patient, another one should be tried. Generally, trying a NSAID from a different class will be more effective than trying another one from within the same class (salicylates, acetic acid derivative, etc). Table 3-3 provides examples of NSAIDs from within each class.

NSAIDs are associated with adverse effects involving several different organ systems. In the gastrointestinal system, NSAIDs have been reported to cause heart-

Table 3-3

Sample NSAIDs

Class	Generic (Trade) Name	Typical Anti-Inflammatory Dose	Availability
Salicylates	aspirin	650 to 975 mg, qid	OTC
Acetic acid derivatives	diclofenac (Voltaren)	50 mg, tid to qid	Rx
	etodolac (Lodine)	300 mg, bid to tid	Rx
	indomethacin (Indocin)	50 mg, bid to qid	Rx
	tolmetin (Tolectin)	200 to 600 mg, tid	Rx
Propionic acid derivatives	ibuprofen (Advil, Motrin, Nuprin)	400 to 800 mg, tid to qid	Rx, OTC
	ketoprofen (Orudis)	50 to 75 mg, tid to qid	Rx, OTC
	naproxen sodium (Aleve, Naprosyn)	275 to 550 mg, bid	Rx, OTC
Oxicam derivatives	piroxicam (Feldene)	20 mg, od	Rx
COX-2 inhibitor	celecoxib (Celebrex)	200 mg, od	Rx

bid=twice a day, od=once daily, OTC=over-the-counter, qid=four times a day, Rx=prescription, tid=three times a day.

burn, nausea, diarrhea, constipation, gastrointestinal bleeding, and ulcers.[5] Gastric irritation can be avoided by taking NSAIDs with food, milk, or antacids. The most common side effects associated with the renal system include sodium retention and edema.[5] NSAID use has also been linked to adverse effects within the hematological system. Because nonselective COX inhibitors lead to decreased platelet aggregation, these medications may cause increased bleeding in an acute injury leading to increased swelling and delayed healing.[6] Studies have shown that rheumatoid arthritis patients taking COX-2 inhibitors may have an increased risk for heart attacks and strokes. As mentioned earlier, these studies have resulted in two out of the three COX-2 inhibitors being voluntarily withdrawn. Side effects involving the central nervous system include tinnitus, sedation, and dizziness. Although not as common, allergic reactions can also occur when taking NSAIDs. Symptoms will usually present within 3 hours of taking the medication. NSAIDs should not be used by individuals with a history of sensitivity to aspirin or any other NSAIDs. They should be used with caution in patients with bleeding abnormalities, impaired renal function, or during pregnancy (especially the last trimester) or breast feeding.

Corticosteroids

Corticosteroids are used to treat asthma (see Chapter Seven), inflammatory bowel disease (see Chapter Eight), dermatological conditions (see Chapter Twelve), tendonitis, bursitis, and allergic reactions. They reduce inflammation by inhibiting the synthesis of arachidonic acid and its metabolites. Corticosteroids are

Table 3-4

Sample Corticosteroids

Generic (Trade) Name	Route of Administration	Condition Treated
budesonide (Rhinocort)	Nasal inhalation	Rhinitis
dexamethasone (Decadron)	Tablet/capsule	Asthma, chronic inflammatory conditions
	Oral inhalation	Asthma
	Nasal inhalation	Rhinitis
	Injection	Chronic inflammatory conditions
fluticasone (Flonase)	Nasal inhalation	Rhinitis
hydrocortisone (Solu-Cortef)	Injection	Chronic inflammatory conditions
hydrocortisone cream	Topical cream	Dermatological conditions
methylprednisolone (Depo-Medrol)	Injection	Chronic inflammatory conditions
triamcinolone (Azmacort)	Inhalation	Asthma

administered through oral, inhalation, injection, and topical routes. Table 3-4 provides a list of sample corticosteroids based on their route of administration and the condition treated. Side effects associated with using corticosteroids can be categorized as either general or specific to the route of administration. Common general side effects include restlessness, dizziness, sleeplessness, changes in skin color, and unusual hair growth on the face or body. Other general side effects include eye pain, nausea, vomiting, black, tarry stools, fluid retention, skin reactions, menstrual irregularities, and prolonged sore throat, fever, cold, or other signs of infection. Coughing, hoarseness, and oral candidiasis (yeast infection) are side effects specific to the oral inhalation route of administration. Local irritation can occur with nasal inhalation and joint pain and chondramalacia can result from intra-articular injections of corticosteroids.[3]

Analgesics

Analgesics are used to treat pain and are available in both OTC and prescription forms. NSAIDs, which were discussed above, are also effective in treating pain due to their effect on the COX-2 enzyme. The analgesic dosage for NSAIDs will typically be slightly less than that used for treating inflammation. Acetaminophen, one of the most widely used OTC analgesics, and narcotic analgesics are discussed next.

Acetaminophen (Tylenol)

Tylenol (McNeil Consumer Healthcare) is used to reduce effectively mild to moderate pain and fever. It is available in many different dosage forms including tablets, capsules, caplets, chewable tablets, suppositories, elixirs, and drops. A single analgesic dose will range from 325 to 1000 mg taken every 4 to 6 hours. The half-life of acetaminophen is approximately 2 hours. There are few side effects associated with the use of acetaminophen and it does not inhibit platelet aggregation like aspirin and other NSAIDs. Acetaminophen is safe to give to children suffering from colds and flus as it does not have the same risk for *Reye's syndrome* that aspirin does. The only two consistently reported adverse reactions associated with acetaminophen are increased potential for liver toxicity, particularly when combined with alcohol, and overdose. The high rate of overdose is thought to occur due to the number of combination OTC products (antihistamine, decongestant, and analgesic) on the market containing acetaminophen. Unknowingly, patients self-medicate themselves with multiple doses of acetaminophen.

Narcotics and Opiates

Both narcotics and opiates are considered controlled substances and are, therefore, available by prescription only. Drugs within these two categories are typically used to treat moderate to severe pain such as postoperative pain, pain associated with significant musculoskeletal injury, and pain associated with some cancers. These medications are known to cause drowsiness and euphoria and have a potential for abuse and addiction. Constipation is a common side effect reported with most narcotic analgesics. Serious adverse reactions are possible when these drugs are combined with alcohol.

Oxycodone (OxyContin [Purdue Pharma, Stamford, Conn]) and meperidine (Demerol [Sanofi Aventis, Bridgewater, NJ]) are just two examples of narcotics. Examples of opiates include morphine and codeine. Narcotic analgesics can be administered through oral, rectal, or injectable routes. Doses may vary between routes of administration due to adjustments that are made to account for first-pass effects in the liver. These drugs are often combined with NSAIDs to enhance the analgesic effect. Morphine is available in both oral and injectable forms. The oral dose of morphine is much larger than any other form due to its excessive first-pass effect.

Antibiotics

Antibiotics are used to treat bacterial infections; they are ineffective in treating viral infections. Most antibiotics are available for oral, IM, or IV administration. A few are also available for topical administration via ointment or drops.

There are several different methods used to classify antibiotics; this chapter will classify them according to their mechanism of action. Eight major classes of antibiotics will be discussed. These classes are grouped according to their mechanism for treating the invading bacteria.

The penicillins, cephalosporins, and carbapenems all have a β-lactam chemical structure and work to inhibit the synthesis of the bacteria's cell wall. These three classes are said to be bactericidal antibiotics because they work to kill the invading bacteria. The tetracyclines, macrolides, and aminoglycosides disrupt the normal protein synthesis within the bacteria, while the sulonamides inhibit an enzyme used to synthesize tetrahydrofolic acid within the bacteria. And finally, the fluoroquinolones disrupt DNA synthesis within the bacteria. The latter five classes of antibiotics are referred to primarily as bacteriostatic because they keep the bacteria from reproducing, allowing the immune system time to kill the bacteria. At high doses, or when used in combination with other antibiotics, these drugs can act as bactericidals.

Table 3-5 provides examples of these antibiotic classes, their therapeutic indications, and possible adverse reactions. Several general side effects associated with antibiotics are worth mentioning separately. Many antibiotics interact with oral contraceptives, decreasing their effectiveness; therefore, women taking antibiotics should be warned to use alternate methods of birth control or abstain from sexual intercourse. Also women who take antibiotics may experience vaginal yeast infections as a result of a change in the normal vaginal flora.

Physicians select antibiotics based on the mechanism of action, the specific bacteria being treated, the site of infection, and individual patient factors (eg, age, allergies). To accurately determine the bacteria involved in an infection, a culture of the infected tissue would need to be performed. However, often times, antibiotic treatment is started prior to culture results or without performing a culture. This is possible because there are many infections that are known to be caused by specific bacteria. Athletic trainers should educate their patients regarding the proper use of antibiotics and the importance of finishing their prescribed course of medication. Misuse of antibiotics has led to an increased incidence of antibiotic-resistant *Staphylococcus aureus* infections (eg, methicillin resistant *s. aureus*, or MRSA; see Chapter Twelve). The use of antibiotics is further discussed in subsequent chapters in relation to specific local and systemic infections.

Antihistamines

As discussed in Chapter Two, histamines are a chemical mediator released during the inflammatory process. There are three types of histamine receptors: H_1 which are located in the respiratory tract, H_2 which are found in the stomach, and H_3 which are in cerebrospinal fluid. H_1 antihistamines are used to treat illnesses affecting the respiratory tract (allergic rhinitis, colds, flu [Chapters Seven and Eleven]) and skin (urticaria and pruritis [Chapter Twelve]). H_2 antihistamines, referred to as H_2-blockers, are used to reduce gastric acid production and are discussed in Chapter Eight.

There are two generations of H_1 antihistamines (referred to below as just histamines without subtext number): first-generation and second-generation. The first-generation antihistamines are lipid soluble, making them capable of crossing the blood-brain barrier and affecting the central nervous system. This characteristic is what causes the side effect of drowsiness so commonly associated with these antihistamines. Commonly used OTC first-generation antihistamines include diphenhydramine (Benadryl [McNeil Consumer Healthcare]), clemastine (Tavist Allergy [Novartis]), and chlorpheniramine (Chlor-Trimeton [Schering-Plough, Kenilworth, NJ]). Second-generation antihistamines are less lipid soluble and therefore do not cause drowsiness, making them a better choice for daytime dosing, particularly in athletes and other people who perform physical work or need to be alert during working hours (eg, drivers). Common OTC second-generation antihistamines include loratadine (Claritin [Schering-Plough]) and fexofenadine (Allegra [Sanofi Aventis]).

Antihistamines are also used to counteract nausea and vomiting caused by other drugs (anesthesia or chemotherapy). Promethazine (Phenergan [Wyeth Pharmaceuticals]) is commonly used in patients who do not tolerate anesthesia well; however, it produces significant sedation as a side effect. Finally, diphenhydramine (Benadryl) is commonly used in many sleep agents (Tylenol PM [McNeil Consumer Healthcare], Simply Sleep [McNeil Consumer Healthcare]) because it produces drowsiness.

Table 3-5
Classification of Antibiotics

Classification/Examples	Mechanism of Action	Indications	Adverse Effects
Penicillins [β-lactam] amoxicillin (Amoxil) amoxicillin plus clavulanate (Augmentin)	Inhibit cell wall synthesis (bactericidal)	Urinary tract infection, respiratory tract infection, heart infection	Allergic reaction in approximately 10% of population
Cephalosporins [β-lactam] cephalexin (Keflex) ceftriaxone (Rocephin)	Inhibit cell wall synthesis (bactericidal)	Urinary tract infection, respiratory tract infection, skin and soft tissue infection	Allergic reactions (not as severe as penicillins) cross sensitivity with penicillins
Carbapenems [β-lactam] imipenem (Primaxin) meropenem (Merrem)	Inhibit cell wall synthesis (bactericidal)	Lower respiratory tract infections, urinary tract infections, skin infections, intra-abdominal and pelvic infections	Patients who have allergic reactions to other β-lactams antibiotics may also have a reaction to the carbapenems
Tetracyclines doxycycline (Vibramycin) minocycline (Minocin)	Inhibit protein synthesis (bacteriostatic)	Rocky Mountain spotted fever, Lyme disease, use alteratively when patient is allergic to drug of choice	Epigastric discomfort, nausea, vomiting, diarrhea, not recommended for patients <8 years old
Macrolides erythromycin (E-Mycin) azithromycin (Zithromax)	Inhibit protein synthesis (bacteriostatic)	GI, genital, respiratory tract, skin and soft tissue infections, use alternatively when patient is allergic to penicillin	Epigastric discomfort, nausea, vomiting
Aminoglycosides gentamicin (Garamycin) tobramycin (Nebcin) amikacin (Amikin)	Inhibit protein synthesis (both bactericidal and bacteriostatic)	Eye infections, urinary tract infections, pneumonia, upper respiratory infections	Toxicity in the ear and kidneys
Sulfonamides sulfisoxazole (Gantrisin) sulfamethoxazole (Gantanol)	Inhibit the enzyme used to synthesize tetrahydrofolic acid in bacteria (bacteriostatic)	Urinary tract and upper respiratory infections, pneumonia	Crystallization in urine, patients should increase fluid intake
Fluoroquinolones ciprofloxacin (Cipro)	Inhibit DNA synthesis (bacteriostatic)	Urinary tract, respiratory tract, prostate, GI, bone joint, and soft tissue infections	Nausea, vomiting headache, increased risk for tendon rupture and articular cartilage lesions

Decongestants

Decongestants are used to treat nasal congestion associated with allergic rhinitis and the common cold (see Chapter Eleven). These medications cause vasoconstriction of the blood vessels within the nasal passages and help to reduce swelling of the mucous membranes. Pseudoephedrine (Sudafed [McNeil Consumer Healthcare]) is the most commonly used decongestant and is available in oral form as a stand-alone decongestant or as part of a multisymptom reliever medication. Nasal decongestant sprays are also available and include tetrahydrozoline (Tyzine [Kenwood Therapeutics, Fairfield, NJ]), desoxyephedrine (Vicks Vapo Inhaler [Procter & Gamble, Cincinnati, Ohio]), phenylephrine (Neo-Synephrine 4-Hour [Bayer Healthcare Pharmaceuticals]), and oxymetazoline (Afrin 12-Hour Original [Schering-Plough], Neo-Synephrine 12-Hour [Bayer Healthcare Pharmaceuticals]). The use of nasal decongestant sprays should be limited to 3 to 5 days as they will cause rebound congestion if used longer than this. General side effects associated with decongestants include nervousness, headache, insomnia, and restlessness. Decongestants should not be used in individuals with hypertension or heart disease unless recommended by a physician. Persons with diabetes should also check with their physician before using decongestants, due to the risk in changing insulin requirements. Athletes should be made aware that certain decongestants may make them test positive on a drug test.

Bronchodilators

Bronchodilators are used by individuals with asthma to relax bronchial spasms and expand airways. Several classes of bronchodilators are prescribed by physicians including β_2-agonists, cromolyn and neocromil, glucocorticoids, and theophylline. General side effects associated with bronchodilators include tachycardia, increased blood pressure, increased blood sugar, nausea, vomiting, nervousness, restlessness, and sleeplessness. Athletes or anyone working outdoors who use theophylline should be monitored for dehydration as this drug has some diuretic properties. Bronchodilators can be administered through both oral and inhalation routes; however the inhaled drugs are able to act more quickly and are generally associated with fewer systemic side effects. Specific bronchodilators are described in Chapter Seven.

Gastrointestinal Drugs

There are a variety of medications used to treat gastrointestinal disorders including antiemetics, antidiarrheals, antacids, laxatives, proton pump inhibitors, and H_2-blockers. Table 3-6 provides examples of these types of medications and whether they are available as OTC. These medications are further discussed in Chapter Eight in conjunction with the specific disorders they treat.

Antiemetics are used to treat nausea and vomiting. These symptoms are regulated by the medulla in the brain. Nausea and vomiting occur when the vomiting center in the medulla is stimulated by one of three pathways. The neurotransmitters along these three pathways (serotonin, histamine, acetylcholine, and dopamine) are the targets for prescription antiemetics. OTC antiemetics include bismuth subsalicylate (Pepto-Bismol [Procter & Gamble]) and Emetrol (McNeil Consumer Healthcare).[7]

Antidiarrheals are used to treat the symptoms of diarrhea; however, they generally do not treat the underlying cause of the diarrhea. There are three types of

Table 3-6

Common Types of Gastrointestinal Medications

Type	Generic Name	Trade Name	Rx/OTC
Antiemetic		Emetrol	OTC
	bismuth subsalicylate	Pepto-Bismol	OTC
	dimenhydrinate	Dramamine	Rx
	prochlorperazine	Compazine	Rx
	haloperidol	Haldol	Rx
	promethazine	Phenergan	Rx
	ondansetron	Zofran	Rx
Antidiarrheals	loperamide	Imodium	OTC
	kaolin and pectin	Kaopectate	OTC
	diphenoxylate	Lomotil	Rx
	bismuth subsalicylate	Pepto-Bismol	OTC
Laxatives	methylcellulose	Citrucel (bulk-forming)	OTC
	psyllium	Metamucil (bulk-forming)	OTC
	polyethylene glycol solution	Miralax (osmotic)	OTC
	senna	Ex-Lax (stimulant)	OTC
	bisacodyl	Dulcolax (stimulant)	OTC
	docusate	Colace	OTC
PPIs	esomeprazole	Nexium	Rx
	lansoprazole	Prevacid	Rx
	omeprazole	Prilosec	Rx/OTC
	pantoprazole	Protonix	Rx
H_2 blockers	cimetidine	Tagamet	OTC
	famotidine	Pepcid	OTC
	ranitidine	Zantac	OTC
Antacids	sodium bicarbonate	Alka-Seltzer	OTC
	aluminum hydroxide and magnesium hydroxide	Maalox Tablets	OTC
	magnesium hydroxide	Milk of Magnesia	OTC
	calcium carbonate and magnesium carbonate	Mylanta Gelcaps	OTC
	aluminum hydroxide and simethicone	Mylanta Liquid	OTC
	calcium carbonate	Tums	OTC

antidiarrheals: opiods, absorbents, and bismuth subsalicylate. The opiods function by decreasing gastrointestinal motility. Examples of opiods include loperamide (Imodium [McNeil Consumer Healthcare]), diphenoxylate (Lomotil [Pfizer]), and difenoxin (Motofen [Valeant, Aliso Viejo, Calif]). Loperamide is available OTC; however, diphenoxylate and difenoxin are controlled substances due to their potential for abuse. Absorbent antidiarrheal agents function by absorbing water and other compounds to increase the viscosity of the stool. Kapectolin is an example of this type of agent. Bismuth subsalicylate (Pepto-Bismol [Procter & Gamble]) can be used to treat nonspecific diarrhea and to prevent traveler's diarrhea. When broken down in the stomach, bismuth subsalicylate is converted to salicylic acid and bismuth oxychloride, which provide both an anti-inflammatory and antibacterial effect. Since it is converted to salicylic acid, persons with allergy or sensitivity to aspirin should not take bismuth subsalicylate.[2]

Laxatives are used to treat constipation and fall into one of four categories: bulk-forming, stimulant, osmotic, and stool softeners. Common dosage forms for laxatives include tablets, liquids, enemas, and suppositories. *Bulk-forming laxatives* are made of a fiber or cellulose that swells once combined with fluid, producing a thick substance that stimulates peristalsis and pushes the intestinal content forward. To be effective, these laxatives should be taken with a full glass of water. Bulk-forming laxatives may require 12 to 72 hours to produce a result. Psyllium (Metamucil [Procter & Gamble]) and methylcellulose (Citrucel [GlaxoSmithKline, Brentford, Middlesex, UK]) are both examples of this type of laxative. *Osmotic laxatives* function to increase peristalsis by drawing water into the intestinal lumen. This type of laxative is effective in providing acute relief of constipation with onset of action times ranging from 1 hour or less up to 3 hours. Polyethylene glycol (MiraLax [Schering-Plough]) is an example of an osmotic laxative. *Stimulant laxatives* work by increasing motility of the bowels. The onset of action for this class of laxatives is generally 6 to 10 hours. These medications are also known for producing stomach cramps. Senna (Ex-Lax [Novartis]) and basacodyl (Dulcolax [Boehringer Ingelheim Consumer Healthcare, Ridgefield, Conn]) are both examples of stimulant laxatives. *Stool softeners* require 12 to 72 hours to produce a result and are therefore more effective in preventing constipation. Docusate (Colace [Roberts Pharmaceutical Corp, Eatontown, NJ]) is an example of a stool softener.

Antacids work to neutralize stomach acid and increase gastric pH. They can be used to treat peptic ulcers, heartburn, and mild cases of gastroesophageal reflux disease (GERD), although they are much less effective than *proton pump inhibitors* (PPIs) and H_2 blockers. All antacids are available as OTC medications in a variety of dosage forms including tablets, caplets, liquids, suspensions, and powders and include one or more of the following: aluminum hydroxide, magnesium hydroxide, calcium carbonate, and sodium bicarbonate. Typically, antacids are taken after meals and at bedtime and can provide relief within 5 to 15 minutes. Antacids can inhibit or reduce the absorption of other medications, therefore they should be taken at least 2 hours before or after other medications.

PPIs work to decrease acid production in the stomach. Exact dosage amounts depend on the specific condition being treated. Since stomach acid will inactivate PPIs, they commonly contain an enteric coating. Like other enteric-coated medications, PPIs should not be chewed or crushed. For optimal dosing, the makers of PPIs recommend that they be taken 30 minutes before a meal.

H_2 blockers work as antagonists to the histamine (H_2) receptors in the stomach. By blocking these receptors, H_2 blockers are able to decrease acid production in the stomach. H_2 blockers are available as OTC and are commonly use to treat mild heartburn, GERD, and peptic ulcers. Like PPIs, dosages vary depending on the condition being treated. For example, higher dosages are used when treating GERD as compared to when treating mild heartburn.

Table 3-7
Topical Antifungal Agents

Generic Name	Trade Name	Rx/OTC	Dosage Form
amphotericin B[1]	Fungizone	Rx	Cream, lotion
butenafine	Mentax	Rx	Cream
ciclopirox	Loprox	Rx	Cream, lotion
clioquinol	Clioquinol	OTC	Cream
clotrimazole	Lotrimin	OTC, Rx	Cream, lotion, solution
econazole	Spectazole	Rx	Cream
haloprogin	Halotex	Rx	Cream, solution
ketoconazole	Nizoral	Rx	Cream
miconazole	Micatin	OTC	Cream, powder, spray
naftifine	Naftin	Rx	Cream, gel
nystatin[1]	Mycostatin	Rx	Cream, ointment, powder
oxiconazole	Oxistat	Rx	Cream, lotion
sulconazole	Exelderm	Rx	Cream
terbinafine	Lamisil AT	OTC	Cream
tolnaftate	Tinactin	OTC	Cream, powder, solution, spray
triacetin[2]	Fungoid	Rx	Cream, solution, tincture
undecylenic acid	Desenex	OTC	Cream, foam, ointment, powder, soap, spray

Except where indicated, these products are effective against infections of tinea pedis, tinea cruris, and tinea corporis.
[1]*Not for tinea infections.*
[2]*Also used for onychomycosis although tolnaftate only as adjunct to systemic therapy.*
(From Houglum JE, Harrelson GL, Leaver-Dunn D. Principles of Pharmacology for Athletic Trainers. *Thorofare, NJ: SLACK Incorporated; 2005:124.)*

Antifungals

Antifungal medications are used to treat both superficial and systemic fungal infections. Athletic trainers are most likely to encounter superficial fungal infections involving the mucous membranes, skin, hair, or nails. These conditions are discussed in Chapter Twelve along with the specific antifungal medications recommended for treating each disorder.

Antifungal medications generally work as either fungicidals or fungistatics, depending on the concentration of the drug and the site of action. Fungicidals disrupt the cell membrane of the fungus thus killing the fungal cell, whereas fungistatics prevent the fungal cells from replicating, allowing the immune system to manage the infection. Most antifungal medications are administered topically for a local effect; however, some fungal infections (onychomycosis) require systemic treatment administered orally. General side effects associated with the use of oral antifungals include nausea, vomiting, abdominal pain, and headache. Topical antifungals commonly cause itching, burning, or skin irritation. Table 3-7 provides a summary of the more common OTC and prescription antifungal medications.

Antivirals

Antiviral medications can be used to treat herpes infections (see Chapters Nine and Twelve) and influenza infections (see Chapter Four). These medications are effective in preventing and reducing the duration and severity of these viruses. Acyclovir (Zovirax [GlaxoSmithKline]), valacyclovir (Valtrex [GlaxoSmithKline]), and famciclovir (Famvir [Novartis]) are three common antivirals used to treat herpes infections. These medications are only available in oral and topical forms and require a prescription. Amantadine (Symmetrel [Endo Pharmaceuticals, Chadds Ford, Pa]) and rimantadine (Flumadine [Forest Laboratories, New York, NY]) are effective in treating influenza A, while zanamivir (Relenza [GlaxoSmithKline]) can be used to treat both influenza A and B.

Nutritional Supplements and Performance-Enhancing Products

There are thousands of nutritional supplements and performance-enhancing products currently on the market, which makes it impossible for the athletic trainer to be familiar with them all. In fact, many times athletes become aware of these new types of products long before the athletic trainer does. The 1994 Dietary Supplements and Health Education Act (DSHEA) prevents the FDA from having any regulatory control over nutritional supplements. As a result, manufacturers of nutritional supplements are not required to list the ingredients on the labels of their products. This is particularly concerning for athletes who are competing at levels with banned substances and regular drug testing. There are entire textbooks that focus on nutritional supplements and performance-enhancing substances. This chapter will discuss a few of the more commonly used substances including creatine, androstenedione, anabolic steroids, human growth hormone, and erythropoietin.

Creatine

Endogenous creatine, which is formed by the amino acids arginine, glycine, and methionine, is synthesized in the liver, pancreas, and kidney and then transported to the muscles via the circulatory system. Once in the muscle cell, creatine binds with a phosphate group to form creatine phosphate. Muscles need energy to contract. As energy is produced in a contracting muscle, adenosine triphosphate (ATP) is broken down into adenosine diphosphate (ADP). Stored creatine phosphate can be used to convert ADP back into ATP. After being used for energy production, creatine phosphate is transformed to creatinine and released back into the bloodstream, where it is filtered and excreted by the kidneys.

Synthetic creatine is used therapeutically to increase strength or muscle function in patients with muscular dystrophy or amyotrophic lateral sclerosis (ALS). Athletes take creatine in the form of creatine monohydrate (CrM) to improve performance during brief, high intensity exercise that requires sudden bursts of energy (sprinting, swinging a baseball bat, jerking a weight bar, starting a new football play every minute or so). This product is ineffective in improving performance in endurance sports.

CrM is available in a variety of dosage forms including capsules, effervescent tablets, effervescent powder, dry powder, and wafers. Most common dosing patterns include a loading dose of 20 g/d for 5 to 6 days, followed by a maintenance dose of 2 to 5 g/d. It seems to be absorbed quicker when taken with glucose or other sugar source. Most doses are taken just prior to exercise. Persons taking CrM are advised to drink 6 to 8 glasses of water per day.

There are two working theories behind supplementing with CrM. First, an increased amount of creatine phosphate in the muscle helps to increase the rate at which ATP can be regenerated from ADP. Regeneration of the ATP results in decreased fatigue, allowing the muscles to work for longer periods of time. The high levels of ATP also minimize the body's dependency on glycolysis (glucose breakdown) which can lead to lactic acid build-up, muscle pain and burning, and eventual muscle inactivity. The second theory suggests that increased levels of creatine within the muscle draws fluid into the muscle cell causing an increased muscle cell volume. The increased volume produces a larger cross-sectional area which influences strength development. Following this theory, the increased cross-sectional area will allow the muscle to lift more weight, which in turn builds more muscle mass.

Most reported side effects with taking CrM have been anecdotal and include dehydration, electrolyte imbalance, heat-related illness, muscle cramping, muscle injury, kidney dysfunction, gastrointestinal upset, weight gain, and skin rash. Research has failed to link these side effects with CrM use.[8] In fact, weight gain is the only documented side effect in the research literature.[9]

Dehydroepiandrosterone and Androstenedione

Dehydroepiandrosterone (DHEA) and androstenedione are steroid hormones produced by the adrenal glands and gonads (ovaries and testicles). Endogenously, DHEA and androstenedione serve as precursors for the production of testosterone and estrogen.[10] The synthetic or exogenous versions of these substances are touted by their manufacturers as being natural steroids.

The theory behind using DHEA and androstenedione as performance enhancers is based on the fact that increased levels of testosterone are known to increase protein synthesis, muscle strength, and lean body mass. However, research has failed to show that increased levels of exogenous DHEA and androstenedione, when taken at the recommended doses, actually increase levels of testosterone. In fact, in healthy normal males, DHEA and androstenedione may lead to an increase in the production of estrogen.

Extended use of DHEA and androstenedione can lead to a decrease in high-density lipoprotein (HDL) cholesterol, which increases the risk of developing cardiovascular disease. Long-term use of these substances, particularly when taken at higher than recommended doses, may lead to serious side effects.[9] Potential side effects for males include enlarged breasts, decreased size of testicles, premature balding, enlarged prostrate, reduced sperm count, and increased aggression. Females may develop menstrual irregularities, increased masculinization, and increased hair growth.

Androgenic-Anabolic Steroids

Androgenic-anabolic steroids, a derivative of testosterone, produce both masculinizing (androgenic) and tissue building (anabolic) effects. Athletes and other individuals who take steroids do so in an effort to gain the physiological effects of increased muscle size and strength. The Anabolic Steroid Control Act of 1990

Table 3-8

Side Effects Associated With Long-Term Use of Androgenic-Anabolic Steroids

Category	Side Effects
Cosmetic	Facial and body acne, female-like breast enlargement in males, premature baldness, masculinization in females, premature closing of epiphyseal growth plates leading to limb length discrepancies, deepening of voice in females
Liver dysfunction	Jaundice, liver tumors
Cardiovascular	Increase in cholesterol, high blood pressure, stroke, heart disease
Reproductive	Reduction in testicular size, reduction of sperm production, decreased libido, impotence in males, enlargement of the prostate gland, enlargement of the clitoris
Musculoskeletal	Delay in tissue healing, tendon ruptures
Psychological	Increased aggression, possible violent behavior, depression

classifies testosterone and anabolic steroids as Schedule III drugs, making them illegal for possession or distribution without a prescription.

Androgenic-anabolic steroids are lipid-soluble hormones available for both oral and injectable routes of administration. Most of the oral products have short half-lives (several hours) and the injectable products have longer half-lives (1 to 3 days).[9]

The side effects associated with long-term use of androgenic-anabolic steroids have been well documented and can be categorized into the following areas: cosmetic, hepatic, cardiovascular, reproductive, musculoskeletal, and psychological. These side effects are summarized in Table 3-8. Athletic trainers can play a vital role in educating athletes, parents, and coaches about the side effects and health risks associated with steroid use.

Human Growth Hormone

Endogenous human growth hormone (hGH) is secreted by the pituitary and is responsible for regulating several metabolic and growth functions in the body. Clinically, hGH, also known as somatotropin, is taken to treat growth deficiencies in children; however, recently this hormone has gained attention for its alleged ability to slow aging and build strength. Research, however, has shown that hGH does increase the size of the muscle, but it does not increase strength. Many athletes and body builders take hGH for its reported effects in reducing body fat, increasing lean mass, increasing energy levels, and boosting the immune system. These changes in body composition are due in part to hGH's ability to selectively burn fats as fuel rather than carbohydrates.

As an ergogenic aid or performance enhancer, hGH is known to produce the anabolic effects of building muscle through increased amino acid uptake and protein synthesis. The hormone is administered via IM or subcutaneous injection. Unfortunately, hGH can also lead to increased growth in bone and cartilage, especially in the jaw and forehead (acromegaly). Other side effects associated with hGH use include water retention, carpal tunnel syndrome, insulin resistance and increased risk for diabetes, increased risk for osteoporosis, sexual dysfunction, enlargement of the liver and spleen, and risk of heart damage. The use of hGH is banned by the National Collegiate Athletic Association (NCAA) and the International Olympic Committee (IOC).

Erythropoietin

Produced in the kidney, the endogenous hormone erythropoietin (EPO) stimulates the production of red blood cells which increases hemoglobin levels. This increase in hemoglobin in turn increases the circulating levels of oxygen. Recombinant EPO (r-EPO) was developed to treat bone marrow disorders and certain anemias. Competitive athletes, particularly endurance athletes, are known to use r-EPO to boost the oxygen carrying capacity of their blood cells and thus gain an advantage over their opponents.

R-EPO is administered through IM or subcutaneous injection and is associated with several dangerous side effects. Increasing the number of red blood cells without also increasing plasma volume increases the viscosity of the blood. Use of r-EPO is linked with an increased potential for clotting incidents, heart attacks, and strokes. This substance is banned by the NCAA and the IOC

Herbal Supplements

Herbal supplements are taken by many individuals instead of, or in addition to, therapeutic medications to treat a variety of medical conditions. Like nutritional supplements, herbal supplements are not regulated by the FDA and therefore are not required to undergo testing or a strict drug approval process. Manufacturers of herbal supplements are allowed to make broad claims for the use of their products; however, they cannot claim that their product is effective in treating a specific disease.

Most side effects associated with herbal supplements are relatively minor; however, drug interactions with therapeutic medications could be potentially serious. Table 3-9 provides a summary of the commonly used herbal supplements along with their intended use, associated side effects, and possible drug interactions. Athletic trainers, when possible, should be aware of the herbal supplements that their patients are taking. Because many herbal supplements exhibit an antiplatelet effect, athletic trainers should specifically determine whether their patients are taking any herbal supplements before recommending the use of NSAIDs.[11]

Storage and Management of Medications

State and federal laws require that medications be kept in a locked cabinet or closet. Controlled substances must be kept separately from prescription medications, which should also be kept separate from OTC medications. Athletic trainers should conduct frequent inventories of their medications and dispose of those that have expired. Contrary to popular belief, expired medications should not be flushed

Table 3-9
Common Herbal Supplements

Herb	Indication	Side Effects	Possible Drug Interactions
St John's Wort	Depression, inflammation	GI side effects	Oral contraceptives, anticoagulants, antivirals, cardiac glycosides, immunosuppressants
Gingko	Cardiovascular and peripheral vascular disease, memory, cognitive function	Bleeding, mild GI side effects, headache, allergic skin reactions	Anticoagulants, diuretics, antiplatelet drugs, NSAIDs
Ginseng	Boost immune system, depression, chronic fatigue, GI irritation	Diarrhea, skin lesions, menopausal bleeding	MAOIs (antidepressants), anticoagulants, corticosteroids, hypoglycemic drugs
Garlic	Hypertension	Heartburn, gas, allergic reactions, dermatitis, GI symptoms	Anticoagulants, antihyperlipidemia drugs, antihypertensive drugs, protease inhibitors
Echinacea	Stimulate immune system, promote wound healing	Liver toxicity if taken longer than 8 weeks	Immunostimulants, corticosteroids, anabolic steroids

down the toilet. They should instead be disposed of in a sealed biohazard bag or container. A written log should be attached to the bag or container and should include the drug name, strength, dosage form, quantity, lot number, expiration date, and the initials of the person who completed the log.

A written log should also be used to record all medications dispensed in the athletic training facility. This medication log should include the athlete's name, date of service, reason for medication, prescription number (if prescription medication is given), physician's name, medication name, strength, dosage form, quantity, expiration date, lot number, initials of the athletic trainer, and initials of the physician.

All medications, prescription and OTC, must remain in their original containers with their original labels. Repackaging bulk medications into smaller containers for storage in an athletic training kit violates federal law. When possible, medications should be purchased in individual dose packs. Inappropriate use or mismanagement of medications can have very serious legal ramifications. Athletic trainers should be familiar with their scope of practice as well as state and federal laws related to therapeutic medications. They should also be familiar with all institution and program policies and procedures regarding the use of medications in the athletic training facility.

Table 3-10
Contacting a Poison Control Center

- Remain calm.
- Describe the patient's condition.
- Describe the medicine or other poison that was ingested.
- Note the time that the substance was ingested.
- Provide approximate age and weight of the patient.
- Provide your name and phone number.

Preventing and Managing Medication Poisoning

If taken inappropriately, many medicines and vitamins can be poisonous and are capable of causing illness or even death. If someone swallows a potential poison, he or she should be instructed not to eat or drink anything until the local poison center or physician is contacted. Do not administer ipecac syrup or force the patient to vomit unless instructed to do so by a physician or local poison center. To prevent accidental poisoning, all medications, including OTC, should be kept in their original labeled containers and stored out of sight. All medication should be taken according to the package directions or the directions of a physician. As part of an emergency action plan, athletic trainers should keep up-to-date contact information for the local poison center near the telephone. Table 3-10 outlines the steps that should be followed when contacting a poison control center.

Drug Resources

As mentioned at the beginning of this chapter, it would be virtually impossible for athletic trainers to be familiar with every drug that might be used to treat the injuries or illnesses of their patients. However, there are a variety of resources available in print, through computer software, and from the Internet that can be utilized by the athletic trainer to quickly obtain information about a medication.[12] Table 3-11 provides a sample list of resources for drug information. (Lab Exercise 3-1 provides the opportunity to use print and online resources to access drug information.) It is also recommended that the athletic trainer seek out a local pharmacist that is willing to serve as a resource for questions regarding medications.

Summary

There are a multitude of OTC and prescription medications that are taken by the athletes and patients of athletic trainers. These medications can be administered through a variety of routes including oral, sublingual, buccal, rectal, injection, inhalation, and topical, with each route influencing the drug's rate of absorption, onset of action, and duration of action. All OTC and prescription medications have the potential to produce adverse effects and many will produce drug interactions when

Table 3-11
Drug Resources

Print Resources

- *AHFS Drug Handbook*. Bethesda, MD: American Society of Health-System Pharmacists and Springhouse, PA: Lippincott Williams & Wilkins.
- *Drug Facts and Comparisons*. St Louis, MO: Facts and Comparison.
- *Physician's Desk Reference*. Montvale, NJ: Medical Economics Co, Inc.
- *PDR for Herbal Supplements*. Montvale, NJ: Thompson PDR.
- *PDR for Nonprescription Drugs and Dietary Supplements*. Montvale, NJ: Thompson PDR.
- *PDR for Nutritional Supplements*. Montvale, NJ: Thomson PDR.

Online Resources

- Drug Information Online: http://www.drugs.com
- FDA: www.fda.gov/cder/drug/default.htm
- Healthsquare: www.healthsquare.com/drugmain.htm
- Healthtouch: www.healthtouch.com/level1/p_dri.htm
- RxList: www.rxlist.com
- WebMD: http://www.webmd.com/medical_information/drug_and_herb/default.htm

combined with other medications. It is virtually impossible for athletic trainers to remember the indications, formulation, dosage, and potential side effects for all of the medications they might encounter in their clinical practice. For this reason, it is important for athletic trainers to have access to published or online drug resources that can provide this information. It is also helpful to establish a relationship with a local pharmacist who can provide resource information when needed.

Case Study

During preparticipation physical exams, you notice that Tim, one of your baseball athletes, has really bulked up over the summer. While visiting with him, he explains to you how he spent most of his summer in the weight room. He wants this year, his senior year, to be his best season ever.

Later in the semester, Tim comes into your athletic training facility complaining of shoulder pain. As he takes his shirt off for you to examine his shoulder, you notice that Tim's back is covered in severe acne. You don't remember Tim having acne before. When you question him about it, he says it started this past summer. He just figured it was due to all of the sweating he did while working out. After evaluating his shoulder, you determine that Tim has some impingement due to rotator cuff weakness, so you start him on a treatment and rehabilitation program. A few days later, while completing his shoulder exercises in the athletic training facility, Tim gets into a fight with another athlete. You've never seen Tim act this way. He has always been a very mild mannered young man. You start to worry about Tim and what might be going on with him.

Critical Thinking Questions

1. Given his clinical presentation over the course of the semester, what do you think might be influencing Tim's behavior? What signs cause you to suspect this?
2. Following the policies and procedures set forth at your institution, what would you do to follow up on your suspicions?
3. How would you address your concerns with Tim?

References

1. National Athletic Trainers' Association. *Athletic Training Educational Competencies*. 4th ed. Dallas, TX: National Athletic Trainers' Association; 2005.
2. Houglum JE, Harrelson GL, Leaver-Dunn D. *Principles of Pharmacology for Athletic Trainers*. Thorofare, NJ: SLACK Incorporated; 2005.
3. *Pharmacology for Athletic Trainers: Therapeutic Medications* [home study course]. Champaign, IL: Human Kinetics; 1997.
4. *Pharmacology for Athletic Trainers: Performance Enhancement and Social Drugs* [home study course]. Champaign, IL: Human Kinetics; 1998.
5. Biederman RE. Pharmacology in rehabilitation: nonsteroidal anti-inflammatory agents. *J Orthop Sports Phys Ther*. 2005;35(6):356-367.
6. Mautner KR. Nonsteroidal anti-inflammatory drugs and sports injuries: helpful or harmful? *Athletic Therapy Today*. 2004;9(4):48-49.
7. Flake ZA, Scalley RD, Bailey AG. Practical selection of antiemetics. *Am Fam Physician*. 2004;69(5):1169-1174.
8. Greenwood M, Kreider RB, Greenwood L, Byars A. Cramping and injury incidence in collegiate football players are reduced by creatine supplementation. *J Athletic Training*. 2003;38(3):216-219.
9. Powers ME. The safety and efficacy of creatine, ephedra, and anabolic-steroid precursors. *Athletic Therapy Today*. 2004;9(4):57-63.
10. Reents S. *Sports and Exercise Pharmacology*. Champaign, IL: Human Kinetics; 2000.
11. Martin M, Kishman M. Drug-herb interactions: are your athletes safe? *Athletic Therapy Today*. 2005;10(1):15-19.
12. Orr E. Sources of drug information for the athletic therapist. *Athletic Therapy Today*. 1998;3(2):18-23.

Online Resources

American Association of Poison Control Centers
www.aapcc.org

Food and Drug Administration Recalls and Safety Alerts
www.fda.gov

National Capital Poison Center
www.poison.org

United State Antidoping Agency
www.usantidoping.org

Lab Exercise 3-1
Use of Pharmacology Resources

Objectives

After completing this lab activity, students will be able to:

1. Access drug information (indications, dosage and administration, contraindications, side effects, etc) from both print and Internet resources.

Competencies Addressed

This lab exercise addresses the following psychomotor competencies from the NATA's *Athletic Training Educational Competencies, 4th ed*:

- Pharmacology: 1

Instructions

1. Select six drugs from the list on the next page. Select drugs from at least three different categories.
2. Using the *Physicians' Desk Reference* (PDR), find the information requested on the Drug Information Sheet (p. 62) for three of your chosen drugs.
3. Using at least two of the Internet drug resource sites listed below, find the information requested on the Drug Information Sheet (p. 62) for three of your chosen drugs.
4. Complete the Drug Information Sheet (p. 62) (may be copied for this assignment) for each selected drug.
5. Be prepared to present the requested information for three of your drug choices (from both PDR and Internet resource) to the class.

Internet Resources for Prescription Drug Information

Food and Drug Administration
www.fda.gov/cder/drug/default.htm

Healthsquare
www.healthsquare.com/drugmain.htm

Healthtouch
www.healthtouch.com/level1/p_dri.htm

RxList
www.rxlist.com

WebMD
http://www.webmd.com/medical_information/drug_and_herb/default.htm

Lab Exercise 3-1 (continued)
Use of Pharmacology Resources

Select Drug List

Anti-Inflammatories
- Anaprox—Roche
- Celebrex—Pharmacia
- Indocin—Merck
- Motrin—Pharmacia
- Naprosyn—Roche
- Relafen—GlaxoSmithKline
- Toradol—Roche
- Voltaren—Novartis

Analgesics: Non-Narcotic
- Naropin—AstraZeneca
- Ultracet—Ortho-McNeil
- Ultram—Ortho-McNeil

Analgesics: Narcotic
- Darvocet-N50—AAI Pharma
- Lortab—UCB Pharmacia
- Vicodin—Abbott
- Vicoprofen—Abbott

Muscle Relaxants
- Flexeril—McNeil Consumer
- Norflex—3M
- Skelaxin—Elan
- Soma—Med Pointe

Oral Contraceptives
- Ortho-Cyclen—Ortho
- Ortho Evra Transdermal—Ortho
- Ovrette—Wyeth
- Yasmin 28—Berlex

Bronchodilators
- Advair Diskus—GlaxoSmithKline
- Azmacont—Aventis
- Flovent—GlaxoSmithKline
- Serevent—GlaxoSmithKline
- Singulair—Merck
- Ventolin HFA—GlaxoSmithKline

Antacid
- Maalox—Novartis
- Nexium—AstraZeneca
- Pepcid—Merck

Antihistamine
- Allegra—Aventis
- Clarinex—Schering-Plough
- Claritin—Schering-Plough
- Singular—Merck
- Zyrtec—Pfizer
- Benadryl Allergy—Warner Lambert

Decongestants
- Allergra-D—Aventis
- Nasacort AQ—Aventis
- Nasarel—Ivax
- Nasonex—Schering-Plough
- Rhinocort Aqua—AstraZeneca
- Zyrtec D—Pfizer

Antitussives
- Alacol—Ballay
- Hycodan—Endo Pharmaceuticals
- Tessalon—Forest Laboratories
- Tussionex—Celltech

Expectorant
- Hycotuss Syrup—Endo Pharmaceuticals
- Vicks 44E—Procter & Gamble

Cathartics (Laxatives)
- Metamucil—Procter & Gamble
- Miralax—Schering-Plough
- Perdiem—Novartis

Antidiarrheals
- Imodium—McNeil Consumer
- Lotronex—GlaxoSmithKline
- Pepto-Bismol—Proctor & Gamble

Antiemetics
- Emend—Merck
- Kytril—Roche
- Phenergan—Wyeth

Lab Exercise 3-1 (continued)
Use of Pharmacology Resources

Drug Information Sheet

Brand Name:

Generic Name:

Drug Class:

Drug Resource Used:

Drug Uses and Indications:

Dosage and Administration:

Side Effects:

Contraindications:

Warnings/Precautions:

Adverse Reactions:

Special Instructions/Other Comments:

Chapter Four

Immune System

Chapter Outline and Objectives

Introduction

Review of Physiology and Pathogenesis

- Describe the basic physiology of the immune system.
- Review pathophysiological mechanisms of the immune system, including contributions to homeostasis.
- Describe the effect of exercise on immunology.

Signs and Symptoms

- Identify the general signs and symptoms of pathology involving the immune system.

Pain Patterns

- Identify the general pain patterns associated with pathology involving the immune system.

Medical History and Physical Examination

- Discuss medical history findings relevant to immunological pathology.
- Perform physical examination tasks relevant to the immune system.
    - Assess Body Temperature

Pathology and Pathogenesis

- Discuss the signs, symptoms, management, and medical referral guidelines for pathology involving the immune system.
    - Infections
        - Infectious Mononucleosis
        - Musculoskeletal Infections
    - Autoimmune Disorders
        - Rheumatoid Arthritis

- Chronic Fatigue and Overtraining Syndrome
- Blood-Borne Viral Diseases
    - Human Immunodeficiency Virus and Acquired Immunodeficiency Syndrome
    - Hepatitis B Virus
- Prevention of Infectious Disease
- Allergic Reactions

Pediatric Concerns

- "Childhood" Infectious Diseases
    - Chicken Pox
    - Mumps
    - Measles

This chapter addresses the following competencies from the *Athletic Training Educational Competencies, Fourth Edition*[1]:

Domain	Cognitive	Psychomotor
Medical Conditions and Disabilities	1–7, 16	
Pathology of Injuries and Illnesses	4–6	
Pharmacology	3, 11	

INTRODUCTION

Infections occur as a result of the immune response defending the body against foreign microorganisms such as viruses, bacteria, fungi, or parasites (Table 4-1). Physical, behavioral, psychological, environmental, and nutritional factors can all affect immune system function.[2] Contact with infected tissues or body fluids, contact with contaminated objects or substances, or inhaling airborne microbes are methods of person-to-person exposure to infectious organisms.[3] Athletes may be at increased risk for infection because of frequent travel, close and frequent physical contact with other individuals, sharing of facilities and equipment, and altered sleep patterns, all of which affect the immune system.[2,4]

In general, infectious organisms perpetuate themselves by passing from host to host. A *host* is a person (or animal) that harbors an infectious organism. Life cycles of some infectious organisms include a *vector,* often an insect, which transmits the disease-causing organism between two individual hosts. The vector is usually not affected itself, but can pass the infectious organism to many hosts. Infectious diseases that can pass person to person without vectors are called *contagious. Communicable* diseases can be passed from any animal to any other, and thus include vector-mediated diseases.

Table 4-1
Types of Infectious Organisms

Type	Structure	Mode of Replication	Environmental Factors
Bacteria	Simple single-celled organisms	Replicate independent of host	Do not depend on host for survival
Viruses	Noncellular genetic strands	Use host's cellular mechanisms to replicate	Cannot exist outside the biological environment of the host(s)
Parasites (protozoa)	Complex single-celled or organisms with multiple or undifferentiated cells	Replicate independent of host	Exist in the environment of the host
Fungi (mycoses)	Primitive single-celled plants, commonly yeasts and molds	Replicate by spores	Dependent on host for growth (but not necessarily for reproduction)

As previously stated, infections occur as a normal response of the immune system defending the body from foreign microoganisms. This chapter will discuss two types of infections: mononucleosis and musculoskeletal infections. System-specific infections (ie, urinary tract infections, upper respiratory infections, skin infections) are addressed in the corresponding system chapters.

Failure of the immune system to fully protect the human body can lead to several types of pathology, including the following:

- Immunodeficiency disorders, which occur when the body is unable to mount the appropriate immune responses to foreign microorganisms
- Autoimmune disorders, which occur when the body mounts an immune response against itself
- Allergic reactions, which occur when a normal immune response damages normal tissues

This chapter will discuss blood-borne viral diseases (which include immunodeficiency disorders), autoimmune disorders, chronic fatigue and overtraining syndrome, and allergic reactions.

Review of Physiology and Pathogenesis

Key components of the immune system include the thymus, spleen, lymph system, bone marrow, white blood cells, antibodies, and complement system. The thymus is located in the chest between the sternum and the heart and is responsible for producing T cells. The thymus is very active from infancy through adolescence; however, it becomes less active in the adult. The spleen is located in the upper left quadrant and functions to filter blood and lymph to remove abnormal red blood

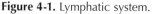

Figure 4-1. Lymphatic system.

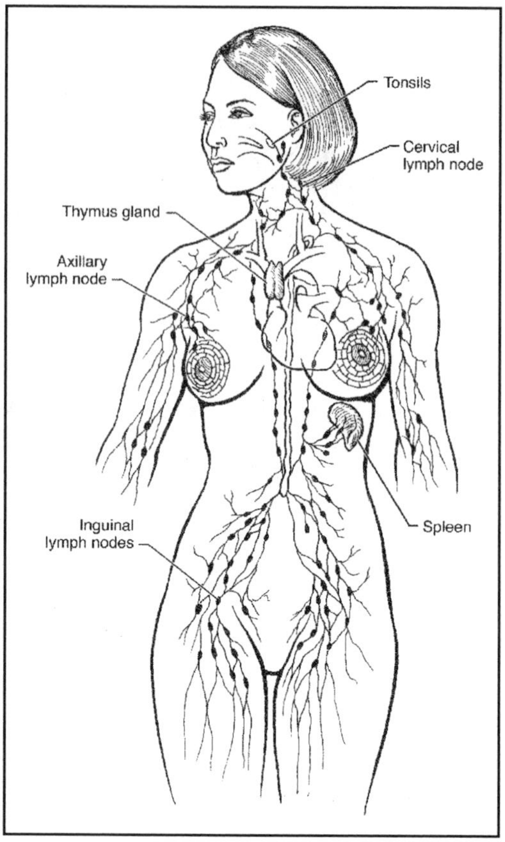

cells and to initiate an immune response against antigens through the actions of T cells and B cells. Illness and injury to the spleen are discussed in Chapter Eight.

The lymph system includes the lymph fluid, lymphatic vessels, and lymph nodes (Figure 4-1). Lymph is a clear fluid, rich in white blood cells, which circulates throughout the interstitial tissues. The lymph collects plasma and debris from the interstitial tissues and is then reabsorbed into the lymphatic vessels, which are located throughout the body alongside blood vessels. Lymphatic vessels range in size from small lymphatic capillaries to large lymphatic ducts. Like veins, lymphatic vessel walls are very thin and contain one-way valves to help move the lymph unidirectionally toward the lymph nodes and then into the thoracic duct where it is dumped back into the circulatory system. Lymph nodes are located throughout the body in clusters and function to filter the lymph fluid. The largest collection of lymph nodes occurs in the axillary, neck, groin, popliteal, supraclavicular, popliteal, abdominal, pelvic, and chest areas. Only the first three of these areas are easily palpated and are often found to be swollen and tender when someone is "fighting" an infection.

Antibodies, also called immunoglobulins and gammaglobulins, are proteins that bind to antigens to deactivate them, prevent them from moving through cell walls, or to mark them for the complement system to destroy. An *antigen* is any substance that triggers an immune response. Each type of antibody has a specific relationship with a specific antigen. The *complement system*, also made up of proteins, works cooperatively with antibodies to destroy antigens.

The bone marrow is the site for the production of red and white blood cells. The red blood cells actually mature in the bone marrow, whereas, the white blood cells

Table 4-2
Components of the Immune Response

Component	General (Nonspecific) Response	Specific (Adaptive) Response
Humoral (blood-borne)	Protein complement	Immunoglobins (antibodies)
Cell	Phagocytosis (macrophages, monocytes)	B cells, T cells

enter the bloodstream and are transported to other sites for maturation. There are many different types of white blood cells including *granulocytes* (neutrophils, eosinophils, and basophils), *lymphocytes* (T cells and B cells), and *monocytes* (macrophages). All of these white blood cells are collectively referred to as leukocytes. Regardless of the type, all *leukocytes* are produced in the bone marrow from stem cells. When cancer patients receive a bone marrow transplant, they are simply receiving stem cells. The transplanted stem cells then produce white blood cells to boost the functioning of the immune system.

The body's first line of defense is provided by the physical barriers of the skin and the mucus membranes lining the mouth, nose, digestive tract, respiratory tract, urinary tract, and reproductive tract. Any opening in the skin or mucus membranes allows an invading microorganism to enter the body.

The body's second line of defense is provided through the two immune response systems: the general (nonspecific) response and the specific (adaptive) response (Table 4-2).[5] Both of these response systems also include humoral and cell-mediated components.[6] The humoral response involves activated proteins and immunoglobins (B cell antibodies) that circulate in the bloodstream. These B cell antibodies work to neutralize microorganisms, toxins, and cancer cells or mark these antigens for destruction by the T cells. The cell-mediated component involves the activation of specific immune system cells (T cells, phagocytes, neutrophils, and macrophages) which start a chemical cascade of events to eliminate the microorganism or other tissue debris.[6] Table 4-3 lists the immune responses to the various types of invading organism.

The general response increases overall metabolism to mobilize energy sources and nutrients to meet the increased demands caused by the infection.[5] Substances released from macrophages, monocytes, and T cells in the cell-mediated general response activate protein complement in the blood, which binds to foreign particles as part of the humoral general response.[6,7] This sequence of events occurs during the fever phase in proportion to the *virulence* (aggressiveness) of the infection.[5,6]

The cell-mediated specific response involves activated T cells and B cells. The cell-mediated response is stimulated by antigens, which are proteins on the outer cell wall of the invading microbes.[6] The B cells then produce antibodies specific to the invading antigen, thus providing the humoral specific response. These antibodies cue phagocytes to recognize and destroy a foreign microbe. Vaccinations are an example of this specific immune response. The B cells "remember" antigens and secrete the appropriate antibodies when subsequently stimulated by those specific

Table 4-3
Response of the Immune System to Various Invading Organisms

Microbe	Immune Response
Bacteria or fungi	Macrophages stimulate T cells to stimulate neutrophils (general, cell-mediated) Some B cell and antibody action
Parasites	Macrophages stimulate T cells to stimulate eosinophils (general, cell-mediated) B cells, particularly if toxins produced by parasite Some humoral mechanisms
Viruses	Macrophages stimulate T cells to stimulate "killer" cells and cytotoxic T cells B cells and some humoral proteins that are effective against some viruses

antigens.[6,7] The T cells are critical to immune function since they regulate B cell activity and stimulate the general immune responses.[6]

The generalized immune response causes muscle catabolism, which releases proteins into the blood to provide extra energy (through gluconeogenesis) and supply amino acids for white blood cells to combat infection.[5] Fast-twitch muscle fibers, followed by slow twitch and ultimately cardiac muscle, are affected. Inhibition of muscle energy through both the oxidative and glycolytic pathways, impedes aerobic and strength performance. Insulin increases to enhance glucose uptake, and fat metabolism is inhibited.[5] In persons with diabetes mellitus, the lack of an insulin response prevents the uptake of glucose, therefore blood sugar levels rise. This is an important point to remember when dealing with diabetic patients who are ill or who are recovering from surgery.

During recovery from infection, strength remains limited until the metabolized muscle protein is replaced, usually in 2 to 4 weeks. Aerobic function is affected by decreases in blood volume (dehydration), hemoglobin, cardiac efficiency, and muscle mass, and may not recover for up to 3 months.[5]

Effect of Exercise on Immune Function

Prolonged, intense exercise, such as marathon training, temporarily suppresses the immune system.[8] Physical and emotional stresses are catabolic, damaging musculature and other organs, causing release of metabolic byproducts (eg, acids, "free radicals"). The immune system response to these metabolic byproducts potentially depletes resources available to fight infection if exercise is excessive.[8,9] These changes do not appear to increase the risk of infection.[2,9] Moderate exercise actually seems to have a small beneficial effect on the immune system.[9,10]

Exercise in the presence of an active infection may be contraindicated.[5] Most bacterial infections do not worsen with exercise, but viral and parasitic infections nearly always increase.[6] In addition, viruses may migrate through the bloodstream to additional organs and tissues, such as the myocardium.

Regardless of the invading organism, athletic performance nearly always decreases when an infection is present because body temperature is increased.[6] Chest pain, tightness, or palpitations during exercise with an infection requires rest from athletics until fever and other symptoms resolve.[5] Classifying an infection as bacterial or viral is impossible to determine without medical tests, so the athletic trainer should recommend rest from physical activity during fever.

Signs and Symptoms

Most infections produce pain and edema in the affected organ or system, resulting in signs and symptoms specific to that system (see Chapters Six through Thirteen).

Fever

Fever is the most common sign of infection. Fever can generally be classified as "low-grade" (less than 102°F) and "high grade" (102°F and above). While both indicate pathology, high-grade fever suggests more serious pathology. Sustained body temperature over 104°F kills brain cells and may cause irreversible cell necrosis in other organs. Fever causes other symptoms, such as arthralgia, myalgia, anorexia, fatigue, and diaphoresis.

Fatigue

Metabolic rate increases with infection. Increased energy demand from the immune response causes catabolism of muscle and other tissues as fuel, resulting in a progressive and persistent fatigue. A chronic infection that continually stimulates the immune response results in chronic fatigue.

Lymphadenitis

Swelling of the lymph nodes (lymphadenitis) indicates the presence of infection; reaction to mediators from injured tissues and antigens causes the swelling. The infection is usually in the part of the limb that is distal to the swollen lymph nodes.

Localized Pain, Redness, Heat, and Swelling

These signs occur with inflammation caused by local infection and are easily observed when superficial tissues are affected. Distinctive red streaks may appear in limbs that have a distal infection.

Unusual Muscle and Joint Pain

Infection may cause muscle or joint pain as a result of the inflammatory response to the invading organism. This type of muscle or joint pain does not change with movement and becomes progressively worse over time.

Pain Patterns

An infection produces signs and symptoms related to the involved system. Signs and symptoms may also arise in other systems that become secondarily infected.

Medical History and Physical Examination

Family and Personal History

Personal history may reveal symptoms consistent with infection, such as fever, fatigue, arthralgia, or myalgia. The course of the symptoms is important, including origin, intensity, and duration of symptoms.

Inspection and Physical Examination

Fever is the primary sign of a systemic infection. Body temperature can be evaluated using a glass, digital, or electronic oral thermometer; a tympanic thermometer; or a rectal thermometer. Normal body temperature is 37°C (98.6°F), although it may range a degree or two either way in individuals. Rectal and tympanic temperatures are approximately 0.5°C to 0.9°C (0.9°F to 1.4°F) higher than oral temperature.[11] Oral temperature fluctuates to a greater extent because it is influenced by food and drink, ambient temperature, smoking, and anything that affects mouth temperature. Body temperature also varies throughout the day. It is highest in the evening, low in the morning, and lowest while asleep. Women have a higher temperature during ovulation. Exercise also increases body temperature, as do emotionally stressful states.

Assessing Oral Temperature

Modern glass thermometers contain galinstan, an alloy (gallium, indium, and tin) that is liquid at room temperature; galinstan has replaced mercury in medical thermometers because of mercury's toxic nature. Glass thermometers must be read manually. Before using a glass thermometer, it should be "shaken down" until the liquid drops below 35.5°C (96°F). To do this, hold the end opposite the bulb tightly between your thumb and fingers and flick your wrist sharply several times. The thermometer is then inserted into the patient's mouth and placed under the tongue with the mouth closed for 3 minutes. If a high temperature is suspected, read the thermometer, reinsert it for 1 minute, and read it again. If the second temperature is higher than the first, repeat the process until the temperature reading stabilizes. To read the glass thermometer, hold the end opposite the bulb between the thumb and index finger. Roll the thermometer back and forth between the thumb and index finger until the liquid column becomes visible. The number at the end of the column is the temperature. Glass thermometers should be disinfected after each use. Digital and electronic thermometers supply a reading within 10 or 15 seconds. The electronic thermometers should be covered with a disposable latex or vinyl cover and placed under the tongue with the mouth closed. (Lab Exercise 4-1 provides the opportunity to practice assessing both oral and tympanic temperatures and to recognize the effects that beverages and exercise have on these temperatures.)

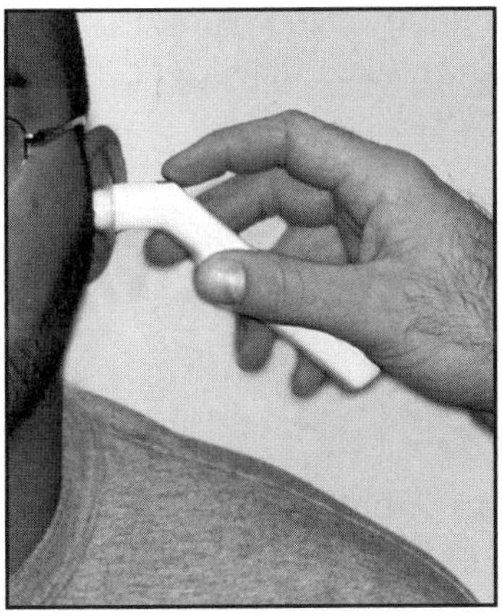

Figure 4-2. Tympanic thermometer.

Assessing Tympanic Temperature

Tympanic thermometers assess body temperature via the external auditory canal. These thermometers are battery operated and provide an easy-to-read digital display. Each model may have slightly different operational instructions; however, in general, the following steps can be followed:

- Place a disposable, protective tip on the end of the tympanic thermometer
- Turn on the thermometer
- Insert the tip of the thermometer fully into the external auditory canal and aimed at the tympanic membrane (Figure 4-2)
- Press the button to obtain a temperature reading
- Remove the thermometer after the beep
- Remove the disposable cover

Assessing Rectal Temperature

Rectal temperature can be assessed using a glass thermometer with a stubby end or using a flexible probe attached to an electronic temperature device. Instruct the patient to lie on his or her side with his or her hips flexed. Lubricate the thermometer or probe and then insert it approximately 3 cm to 4 cm (1.5 in) into the anal canal in a direction pointing toward the umbilicus.[11] The glass thermometer should be left in place for 3 minutes. The examiner should wear gloves and the thermometer should be disinfected after each use. As previously mentioned, rectal temperatures are a more accurate reflection of core temperature and will be higher than oral temperatures (0.4 to 0.5°C or 0.7 to 0.9°F).[11]

Inspection

Purulent (containing pus) drainage from a wound or body part is a sign of local infection. Likewise, erythema and edema in joints and deep body tissues indicate the presence of the inflammatory response, possibly caused by an infection.

Palpating Lymph Nodes

Lymphadenopathy (swollen lymph node) or other palpable masses within body tissues, particularly if tender, are highly suggestive of infection. As mentioned previously, the lymph node clusters in the anterior neck, axilla, and inguinal areas are most easily palpated. Swelling in the anterior neck nodes is associated with infections involving the mouth, throat, and ear, The axillary nodes drain the arm, lateral chest, and abdominal walls, while the inguinal nodes filter the lower extremities, genitalia, lower abdomen, and buttocks.

Pathology and Pathogenesis

Infections

Infectious Mononucleosis

Caused by the Epstein-Barr virus (EBV), a variant of herpes virus carried in saliva, *mononucleosis* ("Mono") is most common among persons age 15 to 25 years.[7,10] Repeated and prolonged exposure is required to induce an active infection, although an estimated 90% of Americans over age 30 show antibodies to EBV.[10,12]

Mononucleosis follows a typical course. The incubation period lasts over a month and is followed by 3 to 5 days of headache, fatigue, loss of appetite, and myalgia.[7,12] The following 1 or 2 weeks are characterized by a severe sore throat, enlargement of the tonsils, moderate fever, bilateral cervical lymphadenopathy, small red spots on the soft palate, splenomegaly in over half of all cases, and hepatomegaly in about a third of all cases.[7,10,12] Patients with these symptoms should be referred to a physician for treatment.

Treatment for mononucleosis consists of rest, hydration, analgesics, and antipyretics (medications that inhibit fever).[4,10] Rarely, corticosteroids are prescribed for symptomatic relief, but do not decrease the duration of the infection.[10] Antibiotics are not indicated unless a bacterial infection occurs concurrently.

Although the signs and symptoms rarely persist more than a month, athletic performance may be impaired for up to 3 months.[10] Mononucleosis causes splenomegaly, predisposing the spleen to rupture, primarily in males within the first 3 weeks of symptoms.[4,7,10] Thus, to protect the spleen, a minimum of 3 weeks after onset of clinical symptoms should pass before allowing return to athletics.[10] A physician should make the decision to allow return to participation, which depends largely on spleen size, absence of fever, resolution of symptoms, and normal liver function as indicated by lab tests. Return to full participation takes an additional 1 to 2 weeks and usually occurs gradually because of a tendency to become fatigued.[10]

Musculoskeletal Infections

Osteomyelitis describes infection of bone. Usually an infection in the surrounding tissue is transmitted to a bone. Open fractures, recent orthopedic surgery, and prosthetic joints also increase risk of osteomyelitis because of exposure of bone to the environment. Once a bone is infected, the blood supply becomes compromised, increasing necrosis and infection in the surrounding bone. Signs and symptoms include fever, weight loss, fatigue, and inflammation in the affected area. Definitive diagnosis usually requires x-rays or other imaging studies, with biopsy (surgical tissue harvesting) to identify the organism. Antibiotic therapy, surgical debridement, and bone grafting may be necessary to halt progression of the infection.

Septic arthrosis is the infection of a joint, which may result in destruction of synovium and cartilage, called *septic arthritis.* Immunocompromise or malnutrition increase the risk of septic arthrosis. Infectious organisms may invade a joint through wounds, the bloodstream, or surrounding tissues. The athletic trainer may encounter this condition among persons who have had a recent orthopedic surgery, a penetrating wound into a joint, or a deep subcutaneous wound. Rapid inflammation of the joint occurs, well beyond the normal postoperative inflammatory response, and extreme pain and intolerance for joint movement may be present. Fever may not occur if the infection is contained in only one joint. Medical referral for the appropriate antibiotic treatment is necessary.

Autoimmune Disorders

Rheumatoid Arthritis

Rheumatoid arthritis (RA), a chronic condition characterized by progressive degeneration of multiple joints, occurs when the immune system mistakenly perceives the synovial lining as a foreign tissue and attacks it. Bilateral inflammation of several joints, particularly the hands, feet, and ankles, and morning stiffness lasting 30 to 60 minutes are early indicators. As RA progresses, joint deformities, ruptured tendons, and disability develop. Persons with RA require lifetime medications and may undergo multiple reconstructive surgeries. Precautions, such as avoiding high loads and extremes of range of motion, are required.

Juvenile rheumatoid arthritis occurs among adolescents with a clinical presentation similar to standard RA, although the prognosis is considerably better. NSAIDs and occasionally corticosteroids are prescribed to limit synovial inflammation. Participation in athletics should be under the guidance of the treating physician and depends on the severity of the disease.

Chronic Fatigue and Overtraining Syndrome

Overtraining is excessive athletic conditioning without allowing for adequate recovery. Overtraining may result in behavioral and physical changes. Increases in cortisol in response to chronic physical stress impairs the ability to respond to hypoglycemia during and after exercise and suppresses the immune system.[13] This produces irritability, apathy, unusual fatigue, declining performance, loss of appetite, excessive thirst, and insomnia.[13,14] In addition, certain physical signs such as increases in resting heart rate, blood pressure, body temperature, or changes in body weight or bowel habits may occur.[14] Rest and a change in training routine to allow recovery between intense exercise sessions is the definitive treatment.

Blood-Borne Viral Diseases

Human Immunodeficiency Virus and Acquired Immunodeficiency Syndrome

Although no confirmed cases of *human immunodeficiency virus* (HIV) transmission have occurred in sports (two unconfirmed cases have been reported[6]), it is hypothetically possible to contract the virus through fist-fighting or other violent physical contact.[3] Hence, standard precautions (eg, using gloves, avoiding contact with body fluids) should be followed to avoid exposure to blood or other body fluids. HIV has been documented among health care workers after exposure to body fluids of infected persons. Most cases are contracted through sexual contact or sharing of IV needles.

HIV primarily impairs T cells, but also affects B cells, phagocytes, and other immune system cells, thus impairing both the specific and general responses of the cell-mediated component of the immune system. In addition, the responses of the humoral aspect of immunity are also impaired since the B cells, which mediate protein complement and immunoglobin (antibody) function, are affected. The medical result is suppression of the immune system that increases the risk of multiple opportunistic infections.

Initial signs and symptoms, which appear within a month of HIV infection, include fever, arthralgia, skin rash, and lymphadenitis throughout the body. These symptoms, which may be mistaken for influenza or other viral infection, persist for 1 to 3 weeks, then subside. The person can communicate HIV in this asymptomatic stage. Without treatment, neurological, hematological, gastrointestinal, dermatological, and pulmonary infections appear within 3 to 10 years. *Acquired immunodeficiency syndrome* (AIDS) results from HIV infection and involves the development of rare infections, such as Kaposi's sarcoma. About half of persons infected with HIV develop AIDS within 10 years.

Treatment of initial HIV infection includes a complex regimen of antiviral agents, which inhibits HIV replication and delays onset of AIDS. AIDS, once developed, is also treated with antiviral medications. Other treatments are provided depending on comorbid infections. Exercise among persons with HIV slows progression of infection and improves physical ability.[6] Currently, no cure exists for HIV infection or AIDS. HIV remains contagious for life regardless of antiviral therapy. Strict avoidance of contact with body fluids prevents communication of HIV.

Hepatitis B Virus

Hepatitis B virus (HBV) is more common, present in more body tissues and fluids, more durable outside the body, and more easily communicated than HIV. Fortunately, standard precautions prevent exposure to HBV.[15] To date, the United States has no reported cases of HBV transmission during sports, although it has occurred in other countries.[3] Vaccination against HBV is available. Health care workers should undergo the 8-month series of three injections to decrease their risk of contracting HBV.[15] Chapter Eight reviews the signs, symptoms, and treatment of hepatitis.

Prevention of Infectious Disease

Table 4-4 provides general guidelines for the prevention of infectious diseases in athletic and health care environments.[3,6,10,15,16] Position statements of various medical associations and regulations for health care facilities regarding control of infectious disease are available.[16-18]

Allergic Reactions

An *allergy* is a localized, cell-mediated immune reaction following exposure to a substance perceived by the body as toxic (an *antigen*), including certain foods, pollens, molds, and insect bites. Release of histamine and other vasodilatory and inflammatory chemical mediators from mast cells produce this reaction. Generalized allergic skin reactions are called *urticaria*, producing *wheals* (hives) that itch and may or may not drain. Mechanical, psychogenic, or physical agents can also produce urticaria.

Anaphylaxis is a systemic, massive allergic response, including smooth muscle contraction and widespread vasodilatation that produces shock. Rarely and with unknown etiology, anaphylaxis induced by physical activity ("exercise-induced anaphylaxis") can cause death. Anaphylaxis can also occur following exposure to

Table 4-4
Preventing Infectious Diseases

- Appropriate diet, recovery time between workouts, and sleep
- Individual water bottles, towels, uniform, and personal equipment
- Individual dose packaging for ointments and topical medications
- Immediate showering after participation
- Frequent laundering of uniforms
- Recognition, proper care, and protection of infectious skin lesions
- Vaccination of athletes and health care workers against preventable diseases (measles, mumps, rubella, DPT, influenza, HBV, etc)
- Prompt cleaning and covering of open wounds and body-fluid saturated uniforms
- Disinfecting soiled surfaces or equipment promptly
- Personal protective equipment and strict enforcement of hand washing and standard precautions/protocols for medical and laundry personnel
- Immunization, particularly tetanus, measles, and childhood vaccinations, should be current; may need to update immunizations when traveling to specific regions or countries
- Avoid exertion and contact with teammates during active infection
- Avoid possibly contaminated water (lakes, rivers)
- Meticulous environmental control of public areas (showers, swimming pools, weight rooms, etc)

specific antigens, most commonly insect bites, in hypersensitive persons. Avoidance of known physical triggers or allergens constitutes primary prevention. Emergency treatment to counter the histamine response, such as injectable epinephrine (EpiPen [Meridian Medical Technology, Bristol, Tenn]), may be necessary in extreme reactions (Table 3-2 provides step-by-step instruction on the use of an EpiPen). History of known allergens and reactions should be obtained during the preparticipation examination and a plan of care developed to manage accidental exposures. Athletes with known anaphylactic reactions should have epinephrine available while participating in activities where exposure is possible.

Pediatric Concerns

"Childhood" Infectious Diseases

Chicken pox (varicella virus), mumps (paramyxovirus), and measles (rubeola) are common among children, but can be contracted at any age. These conditions spread rapidly in day care centers and schools. Close physical proximity and contact, insulated environments, and sharing of food utensils and toys between children contribute to such outbreaks. While relatively harmless in otherwise healthy children, these diseases can cause severe complications among children with immunosuppression and susceptible (ie, not previously infected) adults. Thus, controlling spread of these diseases is important.

Chicken Pox

Chicken pox (varicella virus) incubates approximately 2 weeks, then causes general systemic symptoms (low-grade fever, fatigue, headache) and widespread skin vesicles that erupt, itch, and drain. The virus is most contagious immediately preceding and during vesicle formation. Chicken pox often causes epidemics in schools or other children's peer groups (eg, sports teams). Once vesicles burst, drain, and crust, the virus is no longer contagious. The lesions should not be scratched; itching may be controlled by topical antipruretics. Acetaminophen may be used to control fever, but aspirin should be avoided completely. Infection ensures lifetime immunity; adults who have not been exposed to varicella are at risk of several severe medical problems if they acquire chicken pox. A vaccine is available for children and adults to prevent chicken pox and has become a required immunization for all children enrolled in public schools.

Mumps

Mumps (a paramyxovirus) incubates 2 to 4 weeks, then causes general systemic signs and symptoms shortly before salivary and parotid glands begin to swell. This bilateral swelling causes a characteristic swollen ("chipmunk") face. Additional signs and symptoms include dysphagia, high-grade fever, and tenderness in the swollen glands. The virus is contagious (less so than chicken pox or measles) from about a week before glandular swelling through resolution. As a result of immunization programs, including use of a two-dose protocol, mumps has become relatively rare in America, with fewer than 500 cases a year reported.

Measles

Measles (rubella or German measles; Morbillivirus or 7-day measles) incubates about 2 weeks, then initiates a flu-like syndrome (fever, myalgia, malaise) followed within a week by numerous, characteristic red skin eruptions. High-grade fever (over 104°F) develops and lasts several days, after which the condition resolves. Measles is contagious from the time of infection until the rash subsides. Similar to mumps, immunization programs have reduced reported measles cases to fewer than 200 cases per year in the United States.

Summary

Infection is invasion of a tissue or organ by colonies of organisms, such as bacteria, viruses, parasites, or fungi. The immune system combats infection by using both general and organism-specific mechanisms. Infection produces signs and symptoms that are both general, including fever, myalgia, malaise, and fatigue, and specific to the affected organ or system. Contagious diseases are extremely common and affect physical performance. The majority of these conditions can be treated with rest and support of the immune system, although some require antibiotic medications or other medical care. Following relatively simple procedures can significantly reduce the risk of spreading most infectious diseases.

Case Study

During the preparticipation examination, you discover that Mark, an 18-year-old college freshman baseball player, is highly allergic to bee stings. He has known this since he was 10 years old.

Critical Thinking Questions

1. Based on Mark's history, what other questions might you ask during the preparticipation examination? What else do you need to know about Mark's history with respect to his allergy?
2. What steps will you take to prepare for Mark's participation on the college's baseball team? What specific equipment and supplies might you need? What kind of education and training might you have to provide, and to whom might you provide it? Is there anything you could potentially do to the baseball field to help prevent a bee sting?

References

1. National Athletic Trainers' Association. *Athletic Training Educational Competencies.* 4th ed. Dallas, TX: National Athletic Trainers' Association; 2005.
2. Pyne DB, Gleeson M. Effects of intensive exercise training on immunity in athletes. *Int J Sports Med.* 1998;19(Suppl):S183-S194.
3. Mast EE, Goodman RA. Prevention of infectious disease transmission in sports. *Sports Med.* 1997;24(1):1-7.
4. Hosey RG, Rodenberg RE. Training room management of medical conditions: infectious diseases. *Clin Sports Med.* 2005;24:477-506.
5. Friman G, Ilbäck N-G. Acute infection: metabolic responses, effects on performance, interaction with exercise, and myocarditis. *Int J Sports Med.* 1998;19(Suppl):S172-S182.
6. Brenner IKM, Shek PN, Shephard RJ. Infection in athletes. *Sports Med.* 1994;17(2):86-107.
7. Roberts JA. Viral illnesses and sports performance. *Sports Med.* 1986;3:296-303.
8. Nieman DC. Risk of upper respiratory tract infection in athletes: an epidemiologic and immunologic perspective. *J Athl Training.* 1997;32(4):344-349.
9. Peters EM. Exercise, immunology and upper respiratory tract infections. *Int J Sports Med.* 1997;18(Suppl 1):S69-S77.
10. Sevier TL. Infectious disease in athletes. *Med Clin North Am.* 1994;78(2):389-412.
11. Bickley LS, Szilagyi PG. *Bates' Guide to Physical Examination and History Taking.* 9th ed. Philadelphia, PA: Lippincott Williams & Wilkins; 2005.
12. Nichols AW. Nonorthopedic problems in the aquatic athlete. *Clin Sports Med.* 1999;18(2):395-411.
13. Allen DB. Effects of fitness training on endocrine systems in children and adolescents. *Adv Pediatr.* 1999;46:41-66.
14. Johnson MB, Thiese SM. A review of overtraining syndrome: recognizing the signs and symptoms. *J Athl Training.* 1992;27(4):352-354.
15. Buxton BP, Daniell JE, Buxton BHJ, Okasaki EM, Ho KW. Prevention of hepatitis B virus in athletic training. *J Athl Training.* 1994;29(2):107-112.
16. Arnold BL. A review of selected blood-borne pathogen position statements and Federal regulations. *J Athl Training.* 1995;30(2):171-176.
17. Brkich M. Infectious waste disposal plan of the high school athletic trainer. *J Athl Training.* 1995;30(3):208-209.
18. National Athletic Trainers' Association Board of Directors. Blood-borne pathogens guidelines for athletic trainers. *J Athl Training.* 1995;30(3):203-204.

Online Resources

Immunology review (book chapter)
www.ncbi.nlm.nih.gov/books/bv.fcgi?rid=mmed.chapter.137

Standard Precautions from the Centers for Disease Control and Prevention
www.cdc.gov/ncidod/dhqp/gl_isolation_standard.html

LAB EXERCISE 4-1
ASSESSMENT OF BODY TEMPERATURE

Objectives

After completing this lab activity, students should be able to assess body temperature via:

1. Oral temperature using a digital thermometer.
2. Tympanic temperature using a digital tympanic thermometer.

Competencies Addressed

This lab exercise addresses the following psychomotor competencies from the NATA's *Athletic Training Educational Competencies, 4th ed*:

- Medical Conditions and Disabilities: 4d

Equipment Needed

- Digital tympanic thermometers
- 8-ounce cups of ice water
- Stationary bicycle or treadmill

Instructions

Part 1: Following the steps outlined in the chapter, assess your partner's oral and tympanic temperature under the following four conditions:

1. Normal baseline
2. 1 minute after drinking 8 ounces of ice water
3. 2 minutes after drinking 8 ounces of ice water
4. After 20 minutes of moderate exercise (HR at 75% to 80% max)

	Baseline	1 min post ice water	2 min post ice water	After 20 min moderate exercise
Oral temperature:	_______	_______	_______	_______
Tympanic temperature:	_______	_______	_______	_______

Part 2: Prepare a two- to four-page lab report describing your methods and findings. Include a graph that illustrates your data from each of the four conditions. What implications do your findings have on your practice as an athletic trainer (your assessment of a patient's temperature in the athletic training room)?

Chapter Five

Oncology

Chapter Outline and Objectives

Introduction

Review of Physiology and Pathogenesis

- Describe the etiology and pathophysiological mechanisms of cancer.
- Explain the process of metastasis.

Risk Factors

- Discuss medical history findings and risk factors associated with cancer.

Signs and Symptoms

- Identify the signs and symptoms of cancer.
- Identify potential early warning signs of cancer.

Pain Patterns

Medical History and Physical Examination

- Identify medical history findings that are suggestive of cancer.
- Identify physical examination techniques that may be useful when cancer is suspected.

Diagnosis and Staging

- Describe the TNM System for staging cancer.
- Explain the concept of survival rates and its relation to cancer staging.

Cancer Treatment Options

- Describe the types of treatment used for cancer, including surgery, radiation, chemotherapy, and other methods.
- Explain the process of recovery from cancer.

Pathology and Pathogenesis

- Discuss the clinical presentation, treatment options, prognosis, and survival rates for common types of cancers.
  - Leukemia
  - Hodgkin's Lymphoma (Hodgkin's Disease)
  - Non-Hodgkin's Lymphoma
  - Multiple Myeloma
  - Skeletal Cancers

Pediatric Concerns

- Discuss the clinical presentation, treatment options, prognosis, and survival rates for the most common types of pediatric cancers.
  - Acute Lymphoblastic Leukemia
  - Ewing's Sarcoma

This chapter addresses the following competencies from the *Athletic Training Educational Competencies, Fourth Edition*[1]:

Domain	Cognitive	Psychomotor
Acute Care of Injuries and Illnesses	3, 4, 16	
Medical Conditions and Disabilities	1–3, 20	3, 4e
Orthopedic Clinical Examination and Diagnosis	1, 6, 16	
Pathology of Injuries and Illnesses	2, 4–6	
Risk Management and Injury Prevention	15	

INTRODUCTION

Cancer, defined as pathological cell growth and proliferation, ultimately affects one in two males and one in three females across their lifetimes.[2] At least one-third of all persons diagnosed with cancer survive at least 5 years after identification of the disease. Also, advances in cancer detection and treatment are leading to an increasing number of cancer survivors. By educating their patients about risk factors, early warning signs, and the importance of self-examination techniques, athletic trainers can play a role in both cancer prevention and early detection. Athletic trainers may also encounter patients who are recovering from cancer treatments or who are in *remission* (recovery such that no active disease is detectable); therefore, they should also be aware of the common cancer treatments, their side effects, and the precautions and contraindications relative to physical activity and rehabilitation.

This chapter will provide an overview of cancer, including the general signs and symptoms, common diagnostic procedures, staging methods, and treatment options. Additionally, this chapter will discuss several specific cancers including leukemia, Hodgkin's lymphoma, non-Hodgkin's lymphoma, multiple myeloma, and skeletal tumors. Other common system-specific cancers such as lung (see Chapter Seven); colorectal (see Chapter Eight); and breast, testicular, ovarian, and prostate (see Chapter Nine), are discussed in their associated system chapters.

Review of Physiology and Pathogenesis

Cancer is a disease of the cell and can occur in virtually any system of the body. Damaged DNA within the cell leads to rapid proliferation of abnormal cells, which causes tumors to develop. Cancers form tumors in affected organs, although not all tumors are cancerous. Benign tumors are often only abnormal accumulations of normal cells and are not usually harmful.[2,3] *Benign* tumors typically grow slowly and act like the cells in the tissue of origin. *Malignant* (cancerous) tumors, however, consist of undifferentiated, or nonspecific, cells.[3] These cells do not function like cells of the original tissue, but instead divide very rapidly due to abnormal chromosomal composition. Malignant tumors are progressive and invasive, interfering with the function of normal cells in the affected organ or system.[2,3]

The chromosomal defects associated with cancer can be inherited or acquired through exposure to environmental *carcinogens* (substances known to cause genetic mutation).[2,3] The abnormal cells do not function properly and replicate at a very high rate. Eventually, healthy, functional cells are either completely replaced by cancerous cells or the resulting tumor grows large enough to impair the organ or surrounding structures such as blood vessels or nerves.

Cancer cells may also migrate to other tissues in adjacent or associated systems through a process called *metastasis*.[2,3] Cancer metastases spread to multiple sites, most commonly the spine, lungs, and brain, subsequently causing tumors and impairment of function in those organs. This migration or spreading of the disease occurs when cancer cells enter the bloodstream or lymph system, allowing them to be transported throughout the body. Once cancer has metastasized, the *prognosis*, the most likely recovery or outcome, becomes significantly worse.

Cancers are typically named according to the organ or tissue of their origin. When cancer cells metastasize to another organ or tissue, they still look and behave like the original tumor cells. For example, when bone cancer cells metastasize to the lung and form a new tumor, this condition is referred to as metastatic bone cancer rather than lung cancer. If examined under a microscope, the new cancer cells found in the lung would be identified as bone cancer cells.

Risk Factors

Certain risk factors increase the potential for cancer to develop, including a positive family history, smoking, high-fat low-fiber diet, increased body fat, alcohol abuse, prolonged exposure to sunlight, psychoemotional stress, occupation, and gender (for certain cancers). Although an individual has no control over inherited risk factors, they can limit many of the other risk factors simply by choosing to follow a healthy diet and lifestyle.

Table 5-1

American Cancer Society's Warning Signs for Potential Cancer

- Change in bowel or bladder habits
- Unusual bleeding or discharge
- Indigestion or difficulty swallowing
- Persistent cough or hoarseness
- Non-healing wound(s)
- Thickening of tissue or lump (particularly breast)
- Change in wart or mole

Signs and Symptoms

As a result of inflammation, most cancers cause fever and pain. Many cancers may initially present with general signs and symptoms (listed below); however, the disease eventually interferes with organ function, producing system-specific signs and symptoms which are discussed in Chapters Six through Thirteen. To aid in early detection, the American Cancer Society has identified seven early warning signs of cancer (Table 5-1).

Fever

Cancer can produce a low-grade fever in response to increased metabolic activity in cancer cells and the immune system.

Fatigue

Increased demand for energy and the catabolism of muscle and other tissues causes a persistent and progressive fatigue and decreased tolerance for activity.

Lymphadenopathy

Lymphomas are cancers that originate and proliferate in the lymph nodes and lymphatic system, producing swelling in multiple lymph nodes. In addition, the lymph nodes are common sites of metastasis for many types of cancer.

Night Symptoms

Pain, diaphoresis, or other symptoms that wake a person during the night may be an early sign of cancer. Organ-systems dominated by parasympathetic control, such as gastrointestinal, hepatic-biliary, and renal-urogenital, are more active at night, and may therefore become more symptomatic when affected by cancer.

Cyclical Pain Patterns

The regular occurrence of intermittent pain cycles may reflect pathology of organ-systems that function in such a manner (eg, gastrointestinal, hepatic-biliary, and renal-urogenital). In addition, symptoms associated with certain body functions, such as digestion (following a meal), urination, or breathing, may be associated with underlying cancer in that system.

Unusual Muscle and Joint Pain

Muscle or joint pain that does not change with posture or movement and becomes progressively worse over time suggests serious underlying pathology, potentially including cancer.

Pain Patterns

An organ-system that develops cancer may produce signs and symptoms related to that system. Secondary signs and symptoms, however, commonly arise in other systems, including the lungs, bone, brain, and central nervous system once metastasis has occurred. Sometimes signs and symptoms at the sites of metastases are noticed before those of the primary system. Pain patterns associated with specific cancers are dependent on the system(s) involved and are discussed in Chapters Six through Thirteen.

Medical History and Physical Examination

Family and Personal History

Family history can be a significant risk factor for certain cancers, particularly those of the breast, ovary, and colon. Personal history may reveal presence of the warning signs and symptoms for cancer (see Table 5-1). The symptomatic course is important, including cycle (rhythm), intensity, and duration of symptoms, as well as how much time has passed since the symptoms originated.

Inspection/Palpation

Changes in appearance or size of moles and mucous membranes can indicate cancerous changes. New, growing, or tender masses; lymphadenopathy; and non-healing wounds occur with certain types of cancer. Tumors (*neoplasms*) of bone or connective tissue often become large enough to palpate. Tumors in the abdomen may also be palpable, although considerable practice and skill is necessary to discern normal abdominal anatomy from pathology (see Chapter Eight).

Physical Examination

As mentioned previously, the signs of cancer are usually associated with the tissue, organ, or system of origin or tumor site. Many of the examination procedures presented in Chapters Six through Thirteen may be used to identify functional changes in the systems as a result of cancer.

Diagnosis and Staging

Many cancers are initially identified when tumors are found during self-examination or medical imaging tests (mammogram, computed tomography [CT], magnetic resonance imaging [MRI], ultrasound, etc); however, the accurate diagnosis of cancer requires laboratory testing of sample tissue taken either during surgery or through biopsy. In most cases, once a cancer diagnosis is made, the disease is staged using the TNM System to determine treatment options and prognosis.[2] The TNM System is based on tumor size (T), involvement of lymph nodes (N), and metastasis to other organs (M).[3] In cancers that involve a tumor, the size of the mass can be estimated through diagnostic ultrasound and confirmed during surgical removal. The degree of lymph node involvement can be determined through a sentinel node biopsy. During this procedure, radioactive dye is injected into the soft tissue around the tumor. The dye is picked up by the lymphatic system allowing surgeons to identify the sentinel lymph node, or the first node that cancer cells would affect should they enter the bloodstream to travel to other parts of the body. This sentinel node is removed by the surgeon along with several other area nodes for subsequent microscopic examination. Identification of cancer cells within any of these nodes determines to what extent, if any, the nodes are involved. Medical imaging studies such as a chest x-ray, bone scan, CT scan, MRI, or positron emission tomography (PET) scan, are used to determine if the cancer has metastasized to any other organ(s). Laboratory blood work may also be performed since many cancers have specific serum tumor markers associated with them.

Once the cancer has been described by the TNM System, it is classified into one of four stages, ranging from stage I, indicating limited cellular changes that remain self-contained within the organ, to stage IV, indicating widespread cellular changes and metastasis.[2,3] Prognosis for cancer is described in terms of 5-year survival rates, or the number of patients who remain alive 5 years after diagnosis. If all patients were still alive 5 years after diagnosis, the 5-year survival rate would be 100%. If only half of the patients are still alive 5 years after diagnosis, the 5-year survival rate would be 50%. Many patients live much longer than 5 years after diagnosis for many cancers, but the 5-year survival rate is the standard measure of prognosis.

Cancer Treatment Options

Treatment options are driven somewhat by the stage of the disease and the philosophy of the oncologist (a physician who specializes in the treatment of cancer). The most common treatment options for most cancers include surgery, radiation, and chemotherapy; however, hormonal therapy and other biological treatments are also used.[2] Many cancer treatments are used in sequence or combination.

When indicated, surgery can be used to remove the tumor from the diseased tissue.[2] Even when the entire tumor can be effectively removed, radiation and chemotherapy are often still used to kill any cancer cells that might be left in the body. Depending on the type of cancer and the surgeon's and oncologist's philosophy, radiation or chemotherapy may be used first in an effort to shrink the tumor prior to surgery. Radiation and chemotherapy treatments that are given after surgery to increase the chances of a cure are referred to as adjuvant therapy.

Radiation can be focused on the particular tumor or tissue area, whereas chemotherapy has a more systemic affect. Each treatment has advantages and disadvantages. Surgery, when indicated, can provide a sure way to limit the spread of cancer, but may be disfiguring or disabling. Radiation uses high energy x-rays or other forms of radiation to attack cancer cells and prevent them from proliferating.[2] Radiation is most often delivered externally through a high-powered x-ray machine that sends radiation through the tissues, but it can also be administered internally using radioactive needles, seeds, or wires implanted in and around the target tissue. Although radiation provides a fairly localized treatment field, nearby healthy tissues can also be affected, and their function impaired. Most patients experience some degree of fatigue during the course of their radiation treatments.

Chemotherapy can be used to target specific cell types, particularly those that divide rapidly; unfortunately, it cannot distinguish normal, rapidly dividing cells from cancer cells. Therefore, chemotherapy drugs also damage healthy tissues such as bone marrow and produce many unpleasant and disabling side effects, such as nausea, fatigue, memory problems, neuropathy, and impairment of blood cell production leading to anemia, clotting delays, and immune system suppression. Because the hair, nails, and mucous membranes are made up of rapidly dividing cells, most patients undergoing chemotherapy will also typically lose their hair, experience discoloration or loss of nails, and inflammation of mucous membranes within the mouth, esophagus, and stomach.

Chemotherapy is most often administered through injection into a vein, although some forms of cancer respond well to oral doses. High-dose chemotherapy is also being used, but usually requires a bone marrow transplant afterwards. Because the high-dose chemotherapy destroys the blood-forming cells, stems cells are harvested prior to the treatment, frozen, and then thawed again after completion of treatment. The stem cells are then transplanted through infusion to help produce new blood cells.

Cancer treatment is specific to the type, extent, and severity of the disease. Research has led to other treatment options, usually used in concert with surgery, radiation, and chemotherapy. Immunotherapy attempts to stimulate the body's immune system to attack cancerous cells. Blood product transfusions may be necessary to replace blood cells lost from impairment of bone marrow. Similarly, bone marrow transplantation may be needed to restore immune function. Antiangiogenesis treatments prevent tumors from becoming vascularized; with no blood supply, the tumor cannot grow. The manipulation of a person's genes (gene therapy) to stop cancer cell division, repair faulty genes, or label cancer cells to make them more vulnerable to radiation, chemotherapy, or immune response is currently being investigated. In addition, there are cancer treatment programs that use a holistic approach to treatment, including nutritional and lifestyle modifications in addition to medical treatments.

Recovery

Return to activity during or after recovery from cancer depends on several factors, including extent and duration of the disease, patient age, type of cancer, presence of metastases and related complications, and overall health and fitness prior to onset of disease. With nearly all types of cancer, deconditioning occurs from relative inactivity during the illness, metabolic muscle wasting that accompanies severe illness, and as a side effect of medical treatments (chemotherapy, radiation, and surgery). Although many people survive cancer and return to very active lives, the recovery process is extremely individualized. The athletic trainer should consult the attending oncologist or primary care physician to obtain specific precautions or contraindications relative to rehabilitation or return of a patient to a desired level of physical activity.

PATHOLOGY AND PATHOGENESIS

Leukemia

Leukemia describes cancers of bone marrow cells and is characterized by the production of immature blood cells.[4] Abnormal white blood cells (WBC) do not respond to infection normally, so immune system function is compromised.[5] In addition, the high rate of proliferation of undeveloped WBC in the bone marrow inhibits formation of red blood cells (RBC) and platelets, thus causing anemia and clotting disorders (see Chapter Six).[5] Leukemia can be acute, producing rapid deterioration, or chronic with a slower progression.

About 35,000 people are diagnosed with leukemia each year. Leukemia, unlike most cancers, is not staged following the TNM System since the disease is known to involve the bone marrow and, in most cases, has spread to other sites at the time of diagnosis. Leukemia is classified according to the type and subtype of the disease. Survival rates vary by the type of leukemia (acute or chronic, lymphocytic or myeloid) and phase of disease (eg, chronic, accelerated, blast). Acute leukemias have a worse prognosis, with 5-year survival rates of about 33%. By contrast, treatment of some types of chronic leukemias leads to complete remission in most patients.[6]

Major signs of all leukemias are anemia, chronic recurrent infections, and abnormal bleeding from gums, nose, or in mid-menstrual cycle.[4] Additional signs and symptoms depend on other affected organs. Chronic leukemia can cause systemic signs (fatigue, weight loss, low-grade fever), dyspnea, and easy bruising. Acute leukemia produces profuse bleeding, lymphadenopathy, hepatomegaly, splenomegaly, deep bone pain, headache, high-grade fever, cranial nerve effects, and vomiting.[5,6] Unless treated, all leukemias are fatal. Chemotherapy and bone marrow transplant are the main methods of treatment.[6] Leukemia may go into remission for many years, then recur and cause death within weeks or months. Early diagnosis techniques and advances in treatment have been able to cure leukemia in many patients.

Hodgkin's Lymphoma (Hodgkin's Disease)

Hodgkin's disease is a relatively rare malignancy that develops in one or more lymph nodes during adolescence or early adulthood. Approximately 7,000 cases are diagnosed each year, and 1,400 people die of Hodgkin's disease each year.[6] Hodgkin's disease metastasizes to many lymph nodes and organs, including the spleen, liver, lungs, and bone.[5] Most commonly, the first sign is painless, large lymph nodes, palpated as firm, movable masses in the unilateral groin or neck.[4,6] Other signs and symptoms may include fever, night sweats, weight loss, fatigue, loss of appetite, and itching of the skin. General systemic signs and symptoms may also be present if the cancer has spread to other systems. In untreated, advanced stages, chronic recurrent infections and multiple symptomatic metastases occur.[5] With early recognition, Hodgkin's disease is treated with radiation and chemotherapy and has a good prognosis; the 5-year survival rate is 85% and the 15-year survival rate is 68%.

Non-Hodgkin's Lymphoma

Non-Hodgkin's lymphomas are several types of lymphatic cancer that present clinical signs and symptoms similar to Hodgkin's disease. Non-Hodgkin's lymphoma is diagnosed in 56,000 people annually and causes 19,000 deaths annually.

Non-Hodgkin's lymphoma disease is usually more widespread, aggressive, and has a worse prognosis in comparison to Hodgkin's disease. Hence, lymph node swelling, particularly if reported as persisting more than a couple of weeks, requires medical referral.

Non-Hodgkin's lymphomas can form in B cells and T cells, which have immune system functions, as well as the lymph nodes and organs with lymphatic tissue (spleen, bone marrow). If the cancer obstructs the flow of lymph, localized swelling occurs; this is most common in the abdomen, neck, and brain. Lymphoma growth may encroach on the superior vena cava, causing swelling in both arms and legs. The 5-year survival rate for all types of non-Hodgkin's lymphoma is 60%; 10-year survival is 42%.

Multiple Myeloma

Multiple myeloma is a tumor of plasma cells in the bone marrow that develops slowly, usually during middle to late adulthood. "Bone pain" in the back, pelvis, or ribs, either as an intermittent mild ache or as sudden excruciating pain, are usual first symptoms. X-rays show characteristic "punched-out bone" lesions.[4] Pathological fractures and skeletal deformities may occur, producing neurological signs, symptoms, and impairment. Systemic signs and signs of anemia occur if blood cell production is impaired by the diseased bone marrow. Degeneration of bone leads to metabolic imbalances, including hypercalcemia (high levels of calcium in the blood), hyperuricemia (high levels of uric acid in the blood), dehydration (from vomiting and frequent urination), and renal impairment. Treatment includes anti-inflammatories, analgesics, chemotherapy, and bone marrow transplantation. Notoriously difficult to treat, less than 10% of patients with multiple myeloma survive 10 years after diagnosis.

Skeletal Cancers

Bone cancers are relatively rare, with a total of 6,700 cases per year diagnosed and 1,200 deaths annually; primary bone cancer accounts for 0.2% of all cancers. There are many types of bone cancer, and some are more severe than others. Five-year survival for all types of bone cancer is 88% if detected in early stages but decreases to less than 10% for advanced disease.

Osteoid Osteoma/Osteoblastoma

These benign, but painful bone tumors may impair joint motion or impinge nerves or blood vessels as they grow. Most prevalent before age 30, a recurrent dull, aching pain that increases at night and nearly completely disappears with anti-inflammatory use suggest osteoid osteoma (<2 cm) or osteoblastoma (>2 cm). Soft tissue swelling and deformity may also be visible depending on the location. These benign tumors have been reported to occur more frequently in men than women and most commonly involve the femur or tibia. Treatment is by surgical excision and bony stabilization, if needed.[7] After postoperative healing and rehabilitation, return to full unlimited activity can be anticipated.

Osteochondroma and *chondroblastoma* are two additional types of benign bone tumors, both of which present similarly to osteoid osteoma and osteoblastoma. An osteochondroma is made up of cartilage and bone and is most commonly seen near the epiphyseal plates in the shoulder or knee. These tumors present as hard, immobile masses that may or may not be symptomatic; however, the adjacent soft tissue may become sore. Chondroblastomas occur within the epiphysis and are most commonly seen in the shoulder, hip, or knee. Symptoms are similar to those of osteochondromas. The diagnoses for both chondroblastomas and osteochondromas are made through x-rays, CT scans, or MRIs. Treatment for both types of tumors involve surgical excision and bone grafting when necessary. Generally recovery is complete, but can be prolonged if large sections of bone are involved.

Osteosarcoma and Chondrosarcoma

These malignant tumors occur in the metaphysis of long bones and articular cartilage, respectively.[8] Osteosarcoma is most common among adolescent and young adult males, whereas chondrosarcoma presents more often among middle-aged adults.[7,8] Osteosarcoma has an affinity for the rapidly growing epiphysis, often in the distal femur, and causes pain, swelling, and joint impairment without a history of injury. Pathological fracture may also occur if the bone is sufficiently weakened. Metastases to the lungs and brain occur early in osteosarcoma and are associated with a worse prognosis.

In contrast, chondrosarcoma progresses more slowly and is less likely to metastasize. Clinical signs are few, with a gradually increasing tender bone mass as the most frequent sign. Surgery is an integral part of the treatment for bone tumors; however, chemotherapy is commonly used prior to surgery in an effort to shrink the tumor. Prognosis is considerably better than that of osteosarcoma. Recent advances in diagnosis and treatment continue to increase the survival rates for both tumors.

Pediatric Concerns

Acute Lymphoblastic Leukemia

Acute lymphoblastic leukemia (ALL) is the most common form of childhood leukemia. ALL appears most often in early childhood (under 5 years of age).[5] Signs and symptoms follow those outlined for acute leukemia above. Bone pain in the chest or tibia is also common. Clinical presentation of ALL is initially suggestive of acute infection, with high-grade fever and rapid physical collapse. ALL is a medical emergency, but timely treatment leads to a 75% 5-year survival rate.

Ewing's Sarcoma

Ewing's sarcoma can affect any part of the bone, usually appearing in the lower extremity. This is the most common malignancy in children, with most cases diagnosed before the age of 20 years.[8] Non-traumatic pain of the affected region is the main symptom, accompanied by limb swelling and a low-grade fever.[7] A tender mass may be palpable over the bone in more advanced stages. Neurologic signs and symptoms occur if the tumor impinges a nerve. Like other bone cancers, treatment consists of radiation, chemotherapy, and surgery, including wide-scale tissue resection or amputation as necessary to remove all cancerous cells.[7] Between 50% and 70% of children with Ewing's sarcoma survive at least 5 years, with better prognosis for earlier diagnosis and lack of metastases. Ewing's sarcoma is detectable by routine x-ray. Any child or adolescent with unexplained, vague limb or joint pain should be promptly referred for appropriate diagnostic testing.

Summary

Cancer is pathological proliferation of undifferentiated cells that forms malignant tumors, that in time may impair normal organ-system function. Cancer produces signs and symptoms of both general illness and specific to a particular system, presenting a clinical picture of chronic or acute severe illness. Athletic trainers should be aware of risk factors and early warning signs for cancer. In addition, they should be aware of potential precautions for physical activity for persons recovering from cancer. Education of students, athletes, and patients with respect to warning signs and self-examination techniques may help them detect cancer in earlier stages, thereby increasing probability and duration of survival.

Case Study

Casey is a 15-year-old male soccer athlete who plays on the varsity soccer team at your school and on an elite soccer team outside of school. He is complaining of medial knee pain (5/10) in his left leg. He doesn't remember any particular injury, but rather remembers that his knee just started aching about 2 or 3 weeks ago and has been hurting ever since. He explains that his knee aches all the time, but the pain is worse at night. Initially he didn't think anything of the knee pain since he had played in two tournaments that weekend, one with his high school team and another one with his elite team. He just thought that maybe he had overdone it.

As you begin your physical exam, you notice some mild swelling along the medial aspect of the knee. On palpation, you find him to be tender over the distal medial femoral condyle; however, all other palpation findings are negative. Range of motion is slightly limited in the left knee with the following measurements: R knee flexion=130 degrees, L knee flexion=118 degrees. Although his history does not indicate ligamentous injury, you decide to perform a thorough physical exam that includes valgus, varus, lachman, and McMurray tests. All of these tests are also negative. Your evaluation fails to yield any clues as to the cause of Casey's knee pain, and you are concerned that his pain worsens at night. You decide to refer Casey to Dr. Smith, a local orthopedist, to see what he might find.

A few hours after his doctor's appointment, Casey and his mother show up at your office. After looking at his x-rays, Dr. Smith is concerned that Casey might have a bone tumor. He has or ordered an MRI and would like for Casey to see Dr. Jones, a local oncologist for consultation and further tests.

Critical Thinking Questions

1. Casey and his mother have many questions for you. First, what causes bone tumors and are there different kinds of bone tumors? If he does have a bone tumor, does that mean he has cancer? Also, what does this mean for Casey's soccer career?
2. Casey's mother also asks what kinds of tests that you think Dr. Jones is likely to have done? What will these tests be looking for?

References

1. National Athletic Trainers' Association. *Athletic Training Educational Competencies.* 4th ed. Dallas, TX: National Athletic Trainers' Association; 2005.
2. Caudell KA. Alterations in cell growth and replication: neoplasia. In: Porth CM, ed. *Essentials of Pathophysiology: Concepts of Altered Health States.* 6th ed. Philadelphia, PA: Lippincott Williams & Wilkins; 2002:64-83.
3. Damjanov I. Neoplasia. In: Damjanov I, ed. *Pathology for the Health-Related Professions.* 2nd ed. Philadelphia, PA: WB Saunders Co; 2000:71-98.
4. Damjanov I. The hematopoietic and lymphoid systems. In: Damjanov I, ed. *Pathology for the Health-Related Professions.* 2nd ed. Philadelphia, PA: WB Saunders Co; 2000:209-240.
5. Gould BE. Cardiovascular and lymphatic disorders. *Pathophysiology for the Health-Related Professions.* Philadelphia, PA: WB Saunders Co; 1997:159-212.
6. Caudell KA, Gaspard KJ. Alterations in white blood cells. In: Porth CM, ed. *Essentials of Pathophysiology: Concepts of Altered Health States.* 6th ed. Philadelphia, PA: Lippincott Williams & Wilkins; 2002:191-205.
7. Gunta KE. Alterations in the skeletal system: trauma, infection, and developmental disorders. In: Porth CM, ed. *Essentials of Pathophysiology: Concepts of Altered Health States.* Philadelphia, PA: Lippincott Williams & Wilkins; 2002:789-813.
8. Damjanov I. Bones and joints. In: Damjanov I, ed. *Pathology for the Health-Related Professions.* 2nd ed. Philadelphia, PA: WB Saunders Co; 2000:439-462.

Online Resources

American Cancer Society
www.cancer.org

Leukemia and Lymphoma Society
www.leukemia.org

Musculoskeletal Tumor Society
http://msts.org

National Cancer Institute
www.cancer.gov

Chapter Six

Cardiovascular and Hematological Systems

Chapter Outline and Objectives

Introduction

Review of Physiology and Pathogenesis

- ❖ Describe basic cardiovascular and hematological anatomy and function.
- ❖ Explain the pathophysiological mechanisms of the cardiovascular and hematological systems.
- ❖ Describe the response of the cardiovascular and hematological systems to exercise.
- ❖ Identify the minimum cardiovascular screening components that should be included in a preparticipation physical exam.

Signs and Symptoms

- ❖ Identify signs and symptoms of common cardiovascular and hematological pathology.

Pain Patterns

Medical History and Physical Examination

- ❖ Discuss medical history results that are relevant to cardiovascular and hematological pathology.
- ❖ Perform physical examination tasks relevant to the cardiovascular and hematological systems.
    - Heart Rate
    - Respiration Rate
    - Blood Pressure
    - Auscultation
    - Palpation

Pathology and Pathogenesis

- Describe signs, symptoms, treatment, and return-to-play criteria for cardiac conditions.
  - Sudden Cardiac Death
  - Hypertrophic Cardiomyopathy
  - Coronary Artery Anomalies
  - Disorders of the Myocardium and Coronary Artery Disease
  - Valve Disorders
  - Cardiac Conduction Disorders
  - Marfan Syndrome
  - Commotio Cordis
  - Hypertension
- Describe signs, symptoms, treatment, and return-to-play criteria for disorders of the blood.
  - Anemia
  - Sickle Cell Disease and Sickle Cell Trait
  - Hemophilia
- Describe signs, symptoms, treatment, and return-to-play criteria for vascular disorders.
  - Trauma
  - Occlusion Syndromes
  - Thoracic Outlet Syndrome
  - Deep Vein Thrombosis and Pulmonary Embolism
  - Aneurysm
  - Headaches

Pediatric Concerns

- Describe signs, symptoms, treatment, and return-to-play criteria for pediatric cardiovascular conditions.
  - Pediatric Chest Pain
  - Congenital Heart Conditions

This chapter addresses the following competencies from the *Athletic Training Educational Competencies, Fourth Edition*[1]:

Domain	Cognitive	Psychomotor
Acute Care of Injuries and Illnesses	4, 7, 8, 10, 11, 16, 30	
Health Care Administration	1	
Medical Conditions and Disabilities	1–3, 10, 11	4a, 4b
Orthopedic Clinical Examination and Diagnosis	1, 6, 16	
Pathology of Injuries and Illnesses	3–6	
Risk Management and Injury Prevention	2, 6, 7	

Introduction

The incidence of cardiovascular disease has declined in the United States over the past 20 years, but heart disease and stroke remain among the leading causes of death.[2] Through ambitious public health education, the prevalence of many cardiovascular risk factors such as smoking, high blood pressure (BP), high cholesterol, and diabetes have been significantly reduced. The American College of Sports Medicine (ACSM) and the American Heart Association (AHA) recommend that all persons who exercise regularly be routinely evaluated for signs of potential cardiovascular disease.[3] This is particularly important for physically active people over the age of 35 years, for whom coronary artery disease (CAD) is the leading cause of exercise-associated death.[3-8] Unfortunately, cardiovascular abnormalities in the younger population often initially present as sudden cardiac death (SCD). Cardiovascular events cause most of the on-the-field sudden deaths among athletes.[4,5,9] For this reason, one of the primary purposes of the preparticipation physical examination is to identify athletes who may be at risk for a cardiac incident.[7,9]

Although most athletic trainers work with a relatively healthy and active population, some athletic training practice settings include patients from a wide range of ages and disease states. Regardless of the practice setting, athletic trainers should be familiar with the signs and symptoms of cardiovascular disease and the common cardiovascular and hematological abnormalities. Additionally, since athletic trainers are often the first health care professional to see the patient, particularly in the sports settings, they must be able to perform a basic cardiovascular assessment.

Review of Physiology and Pathogenesis

The cardiovascular system consists of the heart, blood, and blood vessels, including arteries, veins, and capillaries. The heart (Figure 6-1), a four-chambered organ made of special muscle called *myocardium*, pumps blood throughout the body. Muscular septa, or walls, separate the left and right atria in the superior part of the heart, and separate the left and right ventricles, which lie inferior to the respective atrium. A sac of connective tissue, called the *endocardium*, encloses the entire heart. Tissue called *pericardium* attaches the endocardium (and therefore the heart) to the thorax. Potential pathology affecting the myocardium includes heart failure, cardiomyopathy, congenital defects, trauma, and ischemia (a loss of blood supply). The endocardium and pericardium are subject to infection, and edema can form in between these tissues.

Arteries, veins, and capillaries circulate blood to and from the heart (Figure 6-2). The walls of arteries and veins have three layers: an inner layer (tunica intima) of endothelium, a middle layer (tunica media) of elastic fibers and smooth muscle, and an outer layer (tunica adventitia) of connective tissue. The relative thickness of these layers, as well as the proportion of elastic fibers or smooth muscle, depends on the vessel type and location in the body. Capillary walls are very thin and contain a single layer, the tunica interna.

Arteries, which carry oxygenated blood from the heart, are classified as either muscular or elastic. Arteries with a large portion of muscle can regulate blood flow to specific organs. The major arteries of the trunk are elastic to accommodate sudden pressure increases during heart contraction. This elasticity also maintains unidirectional blood flow during heart relaxation.

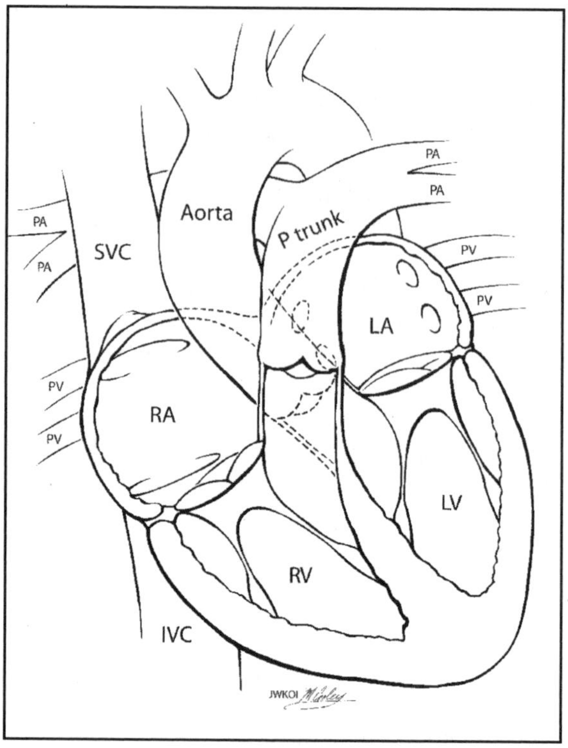

Figure 6-1. Structure of the heart. IVC=inferior vena cava, LA=left atrium, LV=left ventricle, P trunk=pulmonary trunk, RA=right atrium, RV=right ventricle, SVC=superior vena cava.

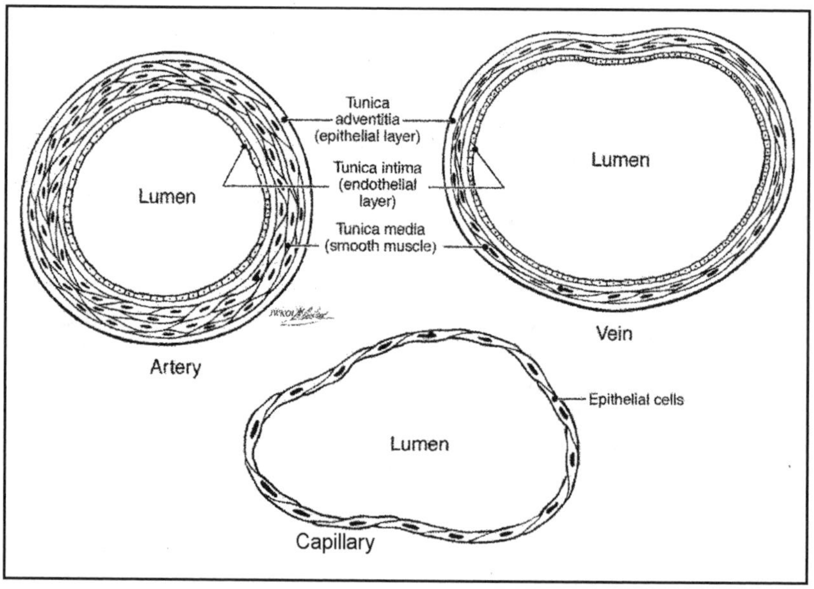

Figure 6-2. Cross-section of a typical artery, vein, and capillary.

Veins, which return blood to the heart, have very little muscle. Blood flow back to the heart is supported by skeletal muscle contraction, which creates pressure in veins. Lower pressures in the thorax (during inspiration) also draw blood toward the heart. In addition, valves in the veins prevent back flow of blood.

Capillaries connect arteries to veins through networks of tiny vessels referred to as capillary beds. The actual exchange of gases, nutrients, hormones, and other materials take place in these capillary beds.

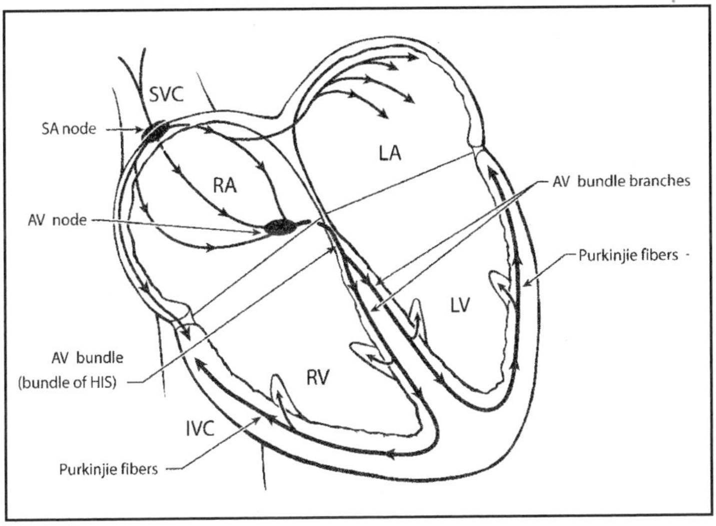

Figure 6-3. Cardiac conduction system. AV=atrioventricular, IVC=inferior vena cava, LA=left atrium, LV=left ventricle, P trunk=pulmonary trunk, RA=right atrium, RV=right ventricle, SA=sinoatrial, SVC=superior vena cava.

Heart muscle requires oxygen and other nutrients, as all living tissues do. The *coronary arteries* branch from the base of the aorta to supply the entire myocardium. The left coronary artery is larger than the right and thus supplies a greater proportion of the heart. Congenital deformities of the coronary arteries pose a threat during vigorous exercise. Pathology affecting the rest of the vascular system includes obstructive diseases, peripheral vascular disease, abnormal vasomotor responses, congenital vessel malformations, and aneurysms.

The heart has an intrinsic electrical conduction system that functions independently from the nervous system. The heartbeat begins as an electrical discharge, which causes a wave of muscular contraction. First, the sinoatrial (SA) node depolarizes (electrically discharges) and spreads electricity through pathways in the atria, causing them to contract. When depolarization reaches the atrioventricular (AV) node, it propagates into the ventricular walls, by way of the AV bundle (Bundle of His), bundle branches, and Purkinje fibers as shown in Figure 6-3. The contraction of the ventricles pumps blood into the aorta and pulmonary arteries. Pathology affecting this conduction system changes the rhythm, pattern, or effectiveness of contraction.

The heart's contraction circulates blood to every cell in the body. *Diastole* refers to the period when the atria and the ventricles are both relaxed, as opposed to *systole*, the contraction phase. During diastole, blood flows into and through the atria to the ventricles. At least 70% of ventricular filling occurs during this phase.

Atrial contraction (atrial systole) precedes ventricular contraction (ventricular systole). Atrial contraction begins after SA node depolarization. As atrial pressure increases (Figure 6-4a), blood is forced down into the ventricles. During ventricular contraction, the mitral valve closes off the left atria and the aortic valve opens to allow blood to be pumped into the aortic artery. Simultaneously, the tricuspid valve closes off the right atria and the pulmonary valve opens to allow blood to flow into the pulmonary artery (Figure 6-4b). As the ventricles relax, the aortic and pulmonary valves close, and the next cardiac contraction begins. The amount of blood pumped into the aorta during a single ventricular contraction is the *stroke volume*. Stroke volume multiplied by heart rate (beats per minute) yields *cardiac output*, which is the volume of blood pumped per minute. Due to its role in providing circulation to the entire body by way of the aorta, the left ventricle is larger than the right ventricle.

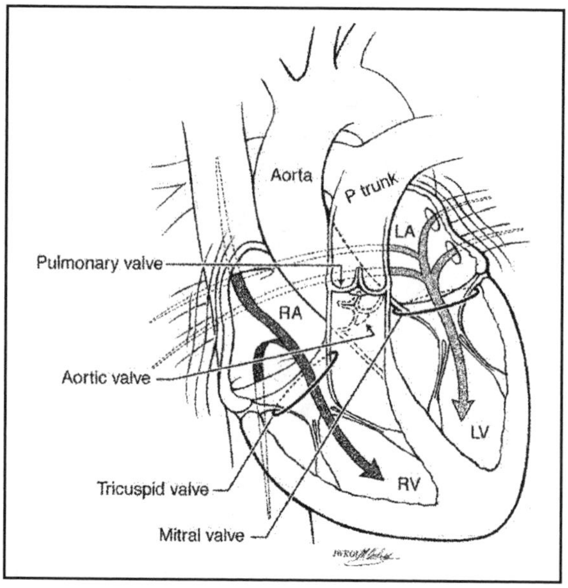

Figure 6-4a. Schematic of heart valves during ventricular diastole. LA=left atrium, LV=left ventricle, P trunk=pulmonary trunk, RA=right atrium, RV=right ventricle.

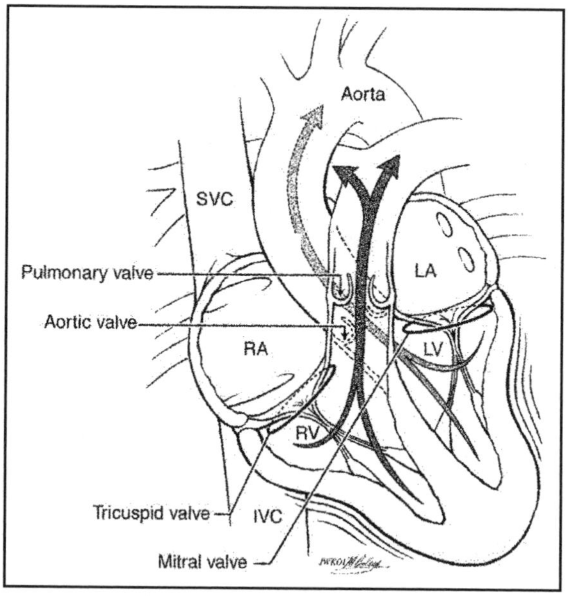

Figure 6-4b. Schematic of heart valves during ventricular systole. IVC=inferior vena cava, LA=left atrium, LV=left ventricle, RA=right atrium, RV=right ventricle, SVC=superior vena cava.

Table 6-1 lists the basic blood cells, their functions, and their normal values as measured through a complete blood count (CBC). Most blood cells form in the red bone marrow of the long bones and flat bones. Production of red blood cells (RBCs) is stimulated by the hormone erythropoietin, which is released by the kidney. RBCs are biconcave in shape, which provides a greater surface area to transport oxygen to the tissues. The number of RBCs in the blood determines its viscosity. Increased numbers of RBCs can increase the viscosity of the blood, causing the heart to have to work harder and increasing the risk for blood clots. As mentioned in Chapter Three, blood doping and the use of erythropoietin as a performance enhancer can lead to increased blood viscosity. Many diseases and pathological states affect the production and function of RBCs and platelets. Leukocytes (white blood cells) play a critical role in the body's defense system and were discussed in Chapter Four.

Table 6-1
Blood Cells and Their Functions

Cell Type	Function	Normal Levels
Red blood cells (erythrocytes)	Transport oxygen, remove carbon dioxide	3.6 to 6.1 million/µL*
White blood cells (leukocytes)	Phagocytosis, mediate immune system response	4000 to 11,000/µL
Platelets (thrombocytes)	Clotting	150,000 to 440,000/µL

**Normal values vary slightly by gender, patient population, and laboratory.*

Table 6-2
Basic Factors Affecting Blood Pressure

Factor	Effect on BP	Mechanism
Decreased blood volume	Decrease	Inadequate fluid within vascular system to maintain pressure
Widespread vasodilation	Decrease	Systemic capacity exceeds fluid volume
Increased extracellular fluid	Increase	Higher BP needed to diffuse nutrients against the increased pressure gradient in capillaries
Renal failure	Increase	Higher BP needed to diffuse fluids against the increased pressure gradient in kidney capillaries

Blood pressure, or BP, the pressure of the blood against the arterial walls, maintains perfusion of oxygen into the organs. Maintenance of BP within a certain range is crucial. If BP falls too low, the brain suffers from lack of oxygen. Conversely, over time high BP will damage capillaries. Table 6-2 summarizes some basic factors and mechanisms that affect BP.

Responses and Adaptations to Exercise

Exercising muscles require much more oxygen than muscles at rest. Heart rate and respiration rate both increase significantly once exercise begins, which produces stress on the heart. Regular aerobic exercise increases left ventricular mass and volume, and leads to increases in heart rate and stroke volume, which in turn produce greater cardiac output.[10] These changes are adaptations to the increased cardiac demand, greater venous return, and increased oxygen demand from the body that result from aerobic exercise.[11] Resistance exercise also increases the muscle mass of the left ventricle to adapt to increased resistance to blood flow. Oxygen demand, however, does not increase with resistance training, so the volume of the left ventricle does not change significantly.[11]

Preparticipation Screening

Appropriate preparticipation screening can identify persons who may be at risk for a cardiac event.[3,10] In 1996, the AHA published a set of minimal components that should be included in a preparticipation screening examination.[10,12,13] These same components have recently been recommended by the 36th Bethesda Conference in its published document, "Task Force 1: Preparticipation Screening and Diagnosis of Cardiovascular Disease in Athletes."[14] Each of the task force reports provide medical guidance for persons who have cardiac conditions but wish to participate in sports. The full report is available at the American College of Cardiology Web site (www.acc.org).

The 12 AHA components fall into three categories: family medical history, personal medical history, and physical examination (Table 6-3). Preparticipation screening is often done with simple questionnaires, such as the Physical Activity Readiness Questionnaire or the Health/Fitness Facility Preparticipation Screening Questionnaire.[3] Most of these forms contain questions that cover the AHA's family and personal history components. Positive responses to these questions, particularly if these symptoms have ever interrupted a workout, may identify up to 50% of at-risk athletes.[4,6] Medical examination during preparticipation screening should include auscultation of the heart and lungs and resting BP.[7] If any abnormalities are suspected, follow-up medical testing by electrocardiogram (ECG), echocardiogram, electron-beam computed tomography (CT) scanning, cardiac magnetic resonance imaging (MRI) coronary artery angiography, or exercise testing may be required to rule out potential causes for SCD.[15]

An ECG detects electric activity of the heart and is used to identify pathology of the heart's electrical system. The ECG traceline has several waves; each subsequent wave is identified by the letters P, Q, R, S, and T (Figure 6-5). Each wave represents a specific heart action. The P wave is atrial depolarization; the QRS segment is ventricular depolarization, which hides atrial repolarization; and the T wave is ventricular repolarization. The interval from P to R represents the propogation of depolarization from the SA node in the atria through the AV node. The interval from Q to T represents the ventricular depolarization-repolarization cycle. By examining the ECG, many diseases can be identified.

There is some controversy as to whether preparticipation screening should include ECGs, echocardiograms, or blood testing. The ECG is an affordable test and is useful in identifying individuals with ventricular arrhythmias and long QT syndrome; however, the ECG is known to produce a large number of false-positive test results. These results can lead to undue mental stress and financial burden on the individual and his or her family. The echocardiogram is very useful in identifying thickening of the left ventricular wall caused by hypertrophic cardiomyopathy. Unfortunately, echocardiograms are cost prohibitive for screening entire sports programs, particularly given the rarity of many of the causes of SCD. Blood tests that can screen for sickle cell trait (SCT) are inexpensive and very reliable. Athletic trainers should discuss the use of these cardiovascular screening tests with their

Table 6-3

American Heart Association Minimal Components for Preparticipation Physical Exams

Family Medical History

- Premature death of a relative
- Living relative under age 50 diagnosed with heart disease or other known cardiac conditions (ie, hypertrophic cardiomyopathy, long QT syndrome, Marfan syndrome, or clinically important arrythmias)

Personal History

- Heart murmur
- Hypertension
- Unusual fatigue
- Exertional syncope (fainting)
- Excessive exertional dyspnea
- Exertional chest pain

Physical Exam

- Resting heart rate
- Blood pressure
- Auscultation of the heart in supine and standing
- Assessment of femoral pulses
- Observation for signs of Marfan syndrome

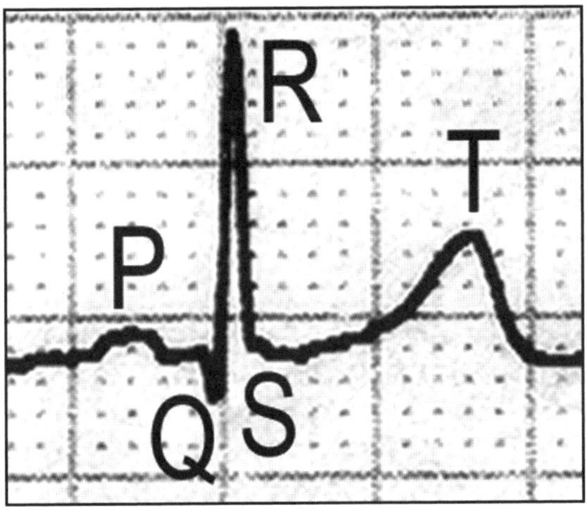

Figure 6-5. The normal electrocardiogram traceline.

team physicians. The decision to include these tests in the standard preparticipation physical exam is both a philosophical and financial one. Since many of the potential causes of SCD are known to occur within specific populations (ie, SCT in African Americans), it may be prudent to make these decisions based on the physical characteristics and/or ethnic background of the patients to be screened.

Signs and Symptoms

Chest Pain (Angina)

Chest pain is the principal symptom of cardiac pathology; this pain originates from the myocardium when it is deprived of oxygen (myocardial ischemia). Anything that damages or causes inflammation in the myocardium can produce cardiac pain; angina also occurs when the heart increases the amount of work it is doing but its blood supply is inadequate to meet the demand. Cardiac pain occurs over the left chest and radiates to the left neck, shoulder, or arm. The pain may be described as pressure in the chest that worsens with physical exertion. Autonomic system responses, such as diaphoresis or pallor, that appear with angina are signs of an impending cardiac emergency.

Dyspnea

Shortness of breath (*dyspnea*) occurs when cardiac output decreases. Most cardiac problems affect the ability of the heart to pump blood to the body. As blood flow from the heart decreases, less oxygen is available to the body. To compensate for the falling oxygen level, the respiration rate increases to draw in more air. As a result, the patient feels short of breath. The dyspnea improves with rest, which reduces oxygen demand, and worsens with activity, which increases oxygen demand. Cardiac-related dyspnea is unaffected by posture or body position, whereas sitting generally relieves dyspnea caused by pulmonary disorders.

Fatigue

When cardiac output decreases, the cells of the body adapt by lowering their metabolic demand for energy and oxygen. The effect is a reduction in the body's capability to perform work, a state called *fatigue*. The person may also notice becoming easily fatigued by his or her routine physical activities, which is a symptom of the heart's inability to keep up with the increased tissue demand for oxygen during those activities. This type of fatigue, associated with heart failure, gets progressively worse over the course of the day.

Palpitations

A palpitation is the sensation of "skipped beats" or the heart "fluttering" uncomfortably. Disturbance of the electrical activity that controls the heartbeat (*arrhythmia*) causes cardiac contractions of excessive pace or strength; these irregular contractions are felt as palpitations. Palpitations accompanied by chest pain, dyspnea, fatigue, or light-headedness suggest a cardiac condition.

Syncope

Syncope, or fainting, is a complete loss of consciousness and postural tone resulting from a sudden reduction in the brain's blood supply. Reduction in blood flow results in reduced oxygen, and the brain will shut down suddenly when its oxygen supply falls too low. Syncope indicates serious arrhythmia or heart disease and requires emergency medical care. There are three primary causes of syncope.

The first cause is sudden peripheral vasodilation, known as orthostatic syncope. A rapid perfusion of the extremities decreases blood to the brain because there is not enough blood in the system to fill all of the body's vessels to their capacity at the same time. Widespread vasodilation in the extremities thus causes a drop in BP, which leads to syncope.

The second cause of syncope is increased intracranial pressure. The increased pressure in the cranium exceeds the pressure in the incoming blood vessels and thus prevents adequate blood flow to the brain. The most common cause of increased intracranial pressure is intracranial bleeding from a head injury.

The third cause of syncope is an acute reduction in cardiac output, called heart failure. As discussed with dyspnea and fatigue, a decrease in cardiac output decreases the oxygen being delivered to the body. A sudden drop in cardiac output, usually caused by a medical emergency such as a heart attack (myocardial infarction [MI]), deprives the brain of oxygen and syncope occurs.

Claudication

Claudication, meaning impaired gait, occurs when the blood flow to a lower limb is blocked. Consequently, oxygen does not reach the muscles in sufficient quantity to meet its metabolic demands. The result is muscular ischemia, leading to pain and decrease in function. Claudication produces cramping, aching, and unusual fatigue in the affected limb. The specific vascular disorders that lead to claudication are discussed later in this chapter.

Skin and Nail Temperature, Color, and Appearance

Vasomotor disorders can cause the skin to become notably cool ("clammy"), from vasoconstriction, or hot, from vasodilation. The skin or nails may also change color, ranging from very pale (vasoconstriction, low BP) to bright red (vasodilation, hypertension [HTN]) to blue or purple (lack of oxygen in the affected tissue). Patients who are in shock or experiencing a severe cardiac event often have pale, clammy skin as a result of decreased BP and decreased blood flow to the skin. Some cardiovascular disorders cause ulcers or lesions on the skin, usually a sign of chronic tissue ischemia (lack of blood), and "clubbing" (rounding) of the fingertips and nails (Figure 6-6).

Edema

Edema, the abnormal accumulation of fluid in the interstitial spaces, occurs with chronic cardiac conditions or obstruction of veins or lymph vessels. In both conditions, fluid in the blood is forced from the vessels into the surrounding tissues. Edema is caused by an increase in capillary pressure, a decrease in capillary osmotic pressure, an increase in capillary permeability, or venous or lymphatic obstruction. Heart failure increases capillary pressure. Cardiac failure causes generalized edema, whereas edema from vascular occlusion occurs only in the part of the limb that is distal to the obstruction.

Pain Patterns

Cardiac

As noted above, inflammation of the heart tissues produces chest pain and can produce referred pain along the pathways of the spinal nerves C3 through T4. Thus,

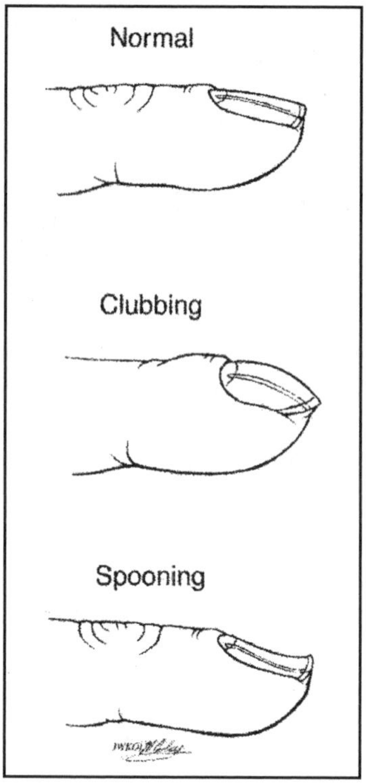

Figure 6-6. Clubbing and spooning of the fingernails.

pain of cardiac origin can occur anywhere from the neck or throat to the medial side of the arm. As classically described, a "crushing" or pressure sensation begins in the chest and radiates predominantly into the left arm (Figure 6-7).

Vascular

Vascular pain, described as a tearing, sharp, or throbbing sensation, occurs locally in the region of the affected vessel. Symptoms may appear in other tissues that are supplied by the vessel if their blood supply decreases.

Medical History and Physical Examination

Family and Personal History

A history of SCD under age 40 in immediate family may indicate an inheritable cardiac condition.[7] A personal history of physical inactivity, smoking, HTN, high blood lipids, obesity, diabetes, Marfan syndrome, or connective tissue disorders increases the risk of cardiovascular pathology.[2-4] Retrospective studies of sudden death among athletes have shown that many of the victims had reported a positive family history of cardiovascular disease and about 20% of them had cardiovascular signs or symptoms, such as exertional angina, dyspnea, syncope, unusual fatigue, palpitations, a known heart murmur, or increased BP, before their fatal event.[4-7,9,16] A personal or family history of SCT or sickle cell disease is also associated with an increased risk of sudden death during exertion.

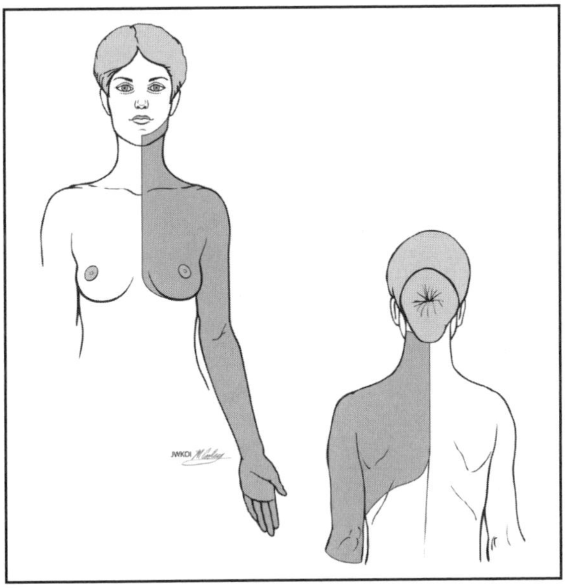

Figure 6-7. Cardiac pain pattern.

Symptoms

Pain of cardiac origin is either acute (sudden and severe) and constant or subacute (insidious and moderate) and recurrent. This pain is described as a crushing pressure in the chest. Chest pain associated with exertion also suggests cardiac pathology.[17,18] Pain associated with pathology of the pericardium becomes worse in supine and improves when sitting.[17] The radiating chest and arm pain called angina is a hallmark of ischemic cardiac pathology. Up to 30% of people with sudden angina at rest have a MI (heart attack) within 3 months. Unexplained syncope, palpitations, or dyspnea, particularly with chest pain or during exertion, requires a referral for medical examination.[7]

Symptoms of vascular pathology include cramping, heaviness, weakness, swelling, pulsing, fatigue, or cold or cyanotic extremities. These symptoms invariably worsen with exertion and are relieved by rest.[19-23]

Inspection

Certain physical characteristics are associated with cardiovascular conditions. Individuals with Marfan syndrome present with the distinct stigmata of physical characteristics (Table 6-4) that should be screened for during the preparticipation physical exam and during any evaluation involving cardiovascular symptoms. A lack of the normal thoracic kyphosis, or a deformed (pectus carinatum or pectus excavatum) or displaced sternum, may be a sign of a congenital heart abnormality.[24] Any notable deformity of the chest wall in a child should be examined by a physician.

Heart Rate

Heart rate, the number of heart beats per minute (bpm), can be palpated over the heart apex, at pulse-pressure sites (brachial, femoral, radial, posterior tibial, or dorsal pedis arteries), or at the carotid artery (Figure 6-8). When assessing heart rate, the rate (bpm), rhythm (regular vs irregular), and character (strong vs weak)

Table 6-4 Signs of Marfan Syndrome
• Tall, thin body type
• Arm span longer than height
• Disproportionately long legs
• Thoracic spine kyphosis
• Sternum deformity (pectus carnitum, pectus excavatum)
• Hyperlaxity in joints
• Visual problems
• Overlap of the thumb and fifth digit when wrapping the fingers around the wrist
Any two signs warrants medical referral for cardiac screening.

Figure 6-8. Location of pulse sites.

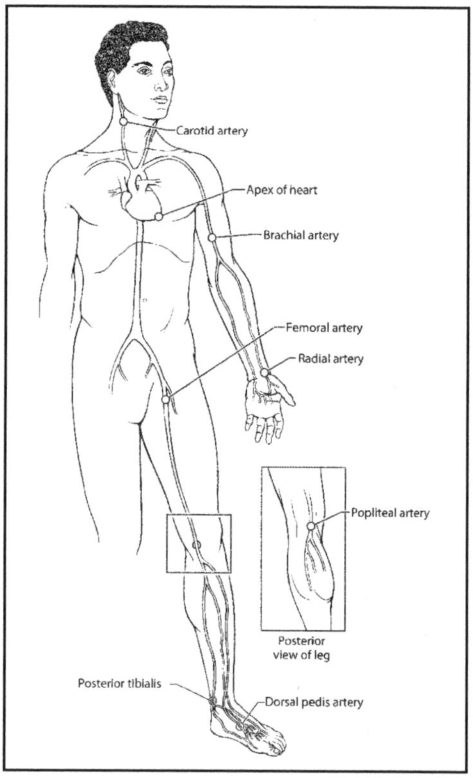

should be reported (eg, "120 bpm, regular and weak"). The normal heart beat is regular and strong. A weak or irregular ("skipping beats") pulse indicates a potential cardiac emergency.

"Normal" heart rate in adults ranges between 70 and 100 bpm. Heart rate gradually decreases during childhood until it reaches its adult value. Newborns have a heart rate ranging between 90 and 180 bpm. Children between 1 and 6 years of age have a heart rate between 70 and 140 bpm. Preadolescents between 10 and 14 years of age have a normal heart rate between 55 and 115 bpm. Adolescents' heart rate is approximately the same as adults.

A slow heart rate is called bradycardia and a high heart rate is termed tachycardia. Resting bradycardia (<60 bpm) occurs as an adaptation among trained persons and is not generally an indication of pathology.[4,5] A resting heart rate above 100 beats per minute (tachycardia) should be investigated by a physician

Table 6-5 describes the method for assessing heart rate. (Lab Exercise 6-1 provides the opportunity to practice the assessment of vital signs, including heart rate.) The radial artery is the most common site for assessing a patient's heart rate. The pulse should be palpated using the pads of the second and third fingers. There are several counting methods that can be used, depending on the characteristics of the pulse. If the rate and rhythm feel normal, the pulse can be counted for 15 seconds and the result multiplied by 4.[24] Other methods include counting for 10 seconds and multiplying by 6 or 30 seconds and multiplying by 2. Each of these "short-cut" methods is associated with some degree of error. Therefore, if the pulse rate is unusually fast or slow, the beats should be counted for a full 60 seconds. If the rhythm is irregular, the pulse should be assessed by auscultation, as the attempt to count the beats may be inaccurate.

Respiration Rate

The respiration rate for adults is normally 10 to 15 breaths per minute and can be easily evaluated at the same time as heart rate or BP. Similar to heart rate, respiration rate decreases during childhood. Infants have a respiration rate of 30 to 60 breaths per minute, young children between 20 and 40 breaths per minute, and older children between 15 and 25 breaths per minute. Respiration at rest should be regular, moderate in depth, and require little effort. Forced or difficult respiration, obvious dyspnea, or rapid, shallow breaths are abnormal.

Table 6-5 describes the assessment of respiration rate. When assessing a patient's respiration rate, observe the chest or stomach rise and fall with each breath, noting rate, rhythm, depth, effort, and odor. As with heart rate, respirations can be counted for 15 or 30 seconds and the result multiplied by 4 or 2, respectively. If rhythm or rate is abnormal, the respirations should be counted for a full 60 seconds. The following statement is an example of an abnormal respiration rate: "Respiration rate is 22, irregular, shallow, labored, with no odor." Some individuals will unintentionally alter their breathing pattern when they know they are being observed. For this reason, the athletic trainer should not announce that he or she is counting respirations. The respiration rate can be assessed while it appears that the athletic trainer is taking the pulse.

Blood Pressure

BP measures the pressure inside the arteries during systole and diastole. BP is usually measured at the brachial artery using a stethoscope (Figure 6-9) and a sphygmomanometer.[4,9,16] Table 6-6 outlines the steps which should be followed when measuring BP. The sounds used to determine systolic and diastolic BPs are referred to as Korotkoff sounds. The ease at which you hear these sounds can be influenced by a variety of factors including the quality of the stethoscope and the placement of the stethoscope diaphragm or bell over the brachial artery (Figure 6-10). Also, the stethoscope ear pieces should be placed in the ear at a slightly forward angle. Raising the patient's arm up above his or her head before and while you inflate the cuff may be helpful in increasing the intensity of the Korotkoff sounds. Also, you can have the patient make a fist several times after you have inflated the cuff, but before you begin the deflation process.[24]

Table 6-5

Assessment of Heart Rate and Respiration Rate

Heart Rate

Step 1.	Sit or stand facing your patient.
Step 2.	Use your non-watch-bearing hand to grasp the patient's wrist, as if you are shaking hands (patient's right wrist with your right hand or patient's left wrist with your left hand).
Step 3.	Compress the radial artery with your index and middle fingers.
Step 4.	Note whether the pulse is regular or irregular: **Regular**—evenly spaced beats, may vary slightly with respiration **Regularly irregular**—regular pattern overall with "skipped" beats **Irregularly irregular**—chaotic, no real pattern, difficult to measure accurately
Step 5.	Count the pulse for 15 seconds and multiply by 4.
Step 6.	Count for a full minute if the pulse is irregular.
Step 7.	Record the rate and rhythm.
Step 8.	**Interpretation:** Normal: between 60 and 100 beats/minute Tachycardia: a pulse greater than 100 beats/minute; tachycardia is a normal response to stress or exercise Bradycardia: a pulse less than 60 beats/minute; athletes tend to be bradycardic at rest due to their level of conditioning

Respiration Rate

Step 1.	Best done immediately after taking the patient's pulse, while still grasping the patient's wrist.
Step 2.	Do **not** announce that you are measuring respirations.
Step 3.	Without letting go of the patient's wrist, begin to observe the patient's breathing. Is it normal or labored?
Step 4.	Count breaths for 1 full minute to yield the breaths/minute.
Step 5.	**Interpretation:** Normal: resting respiratory rates between 14 to 20 breaths/minute Tachypnea: rapid respiration over 20 breaths/minute

Figure 6-9. Stethoscope.

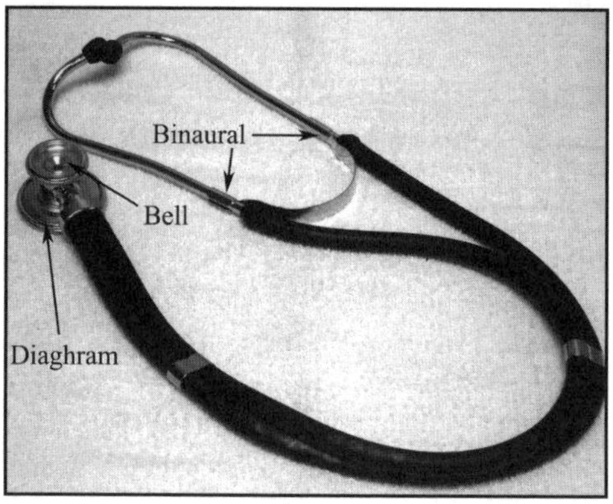

Table 6-6
Assessment of Blood Pressure

Step 1.	Position the patient so the antecubital crease is level with the heart.
Step 2.	Support the patient's arm with your arm or rest the arm on a table with the elbow slightly flexed.
Step 3.	Center the bladder of the cuff over the brachial artery, with the lower edge of the cuff resting approximately 2.5 cm or two finger widths above the antecubital crease.
Step 4.	Palpate the brachial artery in the area of the antecubital crease.
Step 5.	Place the bell of the stethoscope over the brachial artery (Figure 6-10).
Step 6.	Inflate the cuff to approximately 200 mmHg **or** rapidly inflate the cuff until the radial pulse disappears and add 30 mmHg to the value obtained. This latter method can avoid unnecessary discomfort for the patient. (If using the latter method, deflate the cuff and wait 15 to 30 seconds before actually measuring the blood pressure.)
Step 7.	Release the pressure slowly at a rate of 2 to 3 mmHg per second.
Step 8.	The level at which you consistently hear beats is the systolic pressure (read to the nearest 2 mmHg).
Step 9.	Continue to lower the pressure until the sounds muffle and disappear. This is the diastolic pressure (also read to the nearest 2 mmHg).
Step 10.	Quickly deflate the cuff to zero.
Step 11.	Record the blood pressure as systolic over diastolic (eg, 120/70).

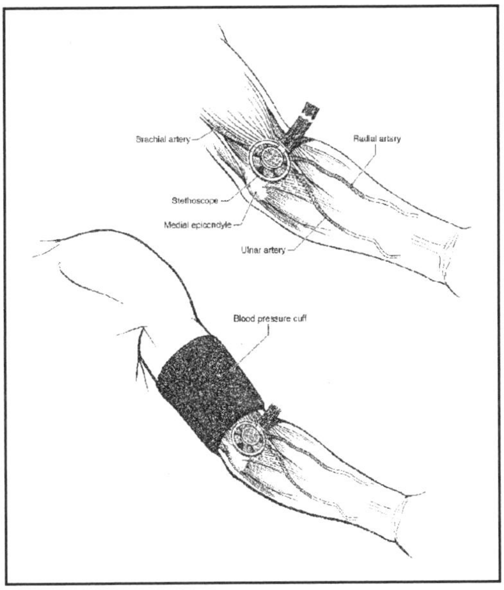

Figure 6-10. Stethoscope placement during blood pressure assessment.

Proper selection of cuff size is important for accuracy in BP readings. Using a standard cuff on an obese patient or an athlete with a large upper arm will result in a false measurement of HTN. By the same token, using a standard cuff on a thin arm may result in false measures of hypotension. Large, pediatric, and thigh-size BP cuffs should be used when necessary.

Normally, systolic BP ranges from 100 to 140 mmHg and diastolic BP ranges from 70 to 90 mmHg. Infants and very young children have lower BP; for example, at birth, systolic pressure is around 70 mmHg and a BP of 120/80 in a 10 year old suggests HTN. BP varies in children by body size (height and weight) in addition to age, making interpretation difficult, but BP in young children should be considerably lower than adult values. BP reaches adult levels in late adolescence. BP equal to or greater than 140/90 on consecutive days indicates HTN (high BP) and needs further medical evaluation. Large differences in systolic BP (>15 mmHg) between lying, sitting, and standing suggests possible orthostatic hypotension, which may be caused by dehydration or loss of blood.

Auscultation

Auscultation involves using a stethoscope to listen to internal body sounds. Cardiac auscultation allows you to listen to heart sounds.[4,5,9,16,17,24,25] The athletic trainer's role with auscultation is to identify abnormal heart sounds rather than diagnose cardiac pathology. The ability to recognize abnormal sounds requires practice in listening to normal sounds. There are numerous Web sites that provide examples of normal and abnormal heart sounds. Several of these resources are provided at the end of this chapter.

The normal, rhythmic "lub-dub" heart sounds is produced by the heart valves closing. The first sound, S1 ("lub"), corresponds to the closing of the mitral and tricuspid valves with ventricular systole. The second sound, S2 ("dub"), corresponds to the aortic and pulmonary valves closing after ventricular systole. Abnormal cardiac sounds include "extra" heart sounds (S3 and S4), muffled heart sounds, murmurs, or rubbing or hissing sounds caused by valve deformities. These sounds are produced by the turbulence of blood flowing through narrowed or incompletely closed heart valves.

Cardiac auscultation is performed over four distinct listening zones which correspond to the location of the four heart valves (Figure 6-11). The aortic listening zone (A) is located just to the right of the sternum in the second intercostal space. Moving just left of the sternum, the pulmonary listening zone (P) is located in the left, second intercostal space. Palpating down the left sternal border, the tricuspid zone (T) is located in the left, fourth or fifth intercostal space. The mitral listening zone (M) corresponds to the apex of the heart and is located in the left, fifth intercostal space in line with the midclavicle. Auscultation should be performed with the patient in three different positions: supine, left sidelying, and sitting (Figures 6-12a through 6-12c). Table 6-7 outlines the step-by-step procedures for performing cardiac auscultation. (Lab Exercise 6-2 provides the opportunity to practice cardiac auscultation.)

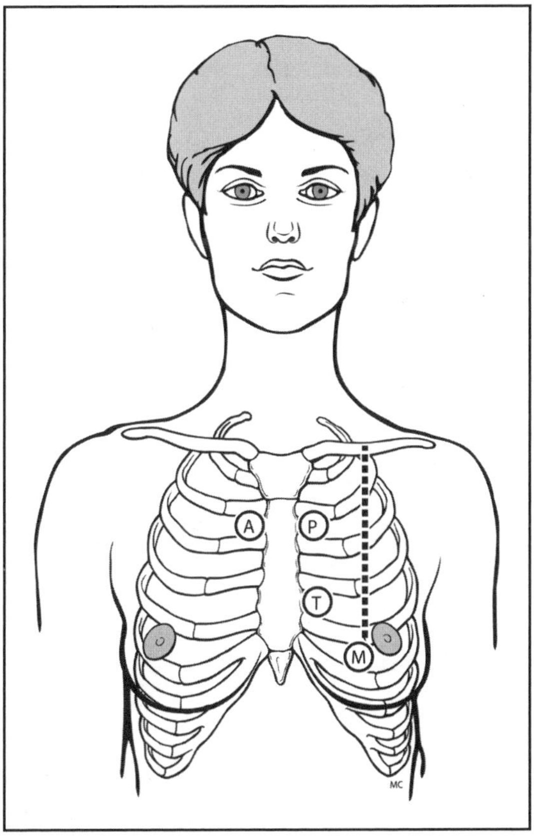

Figure 6-11. Cardiac auscultation listening zones.

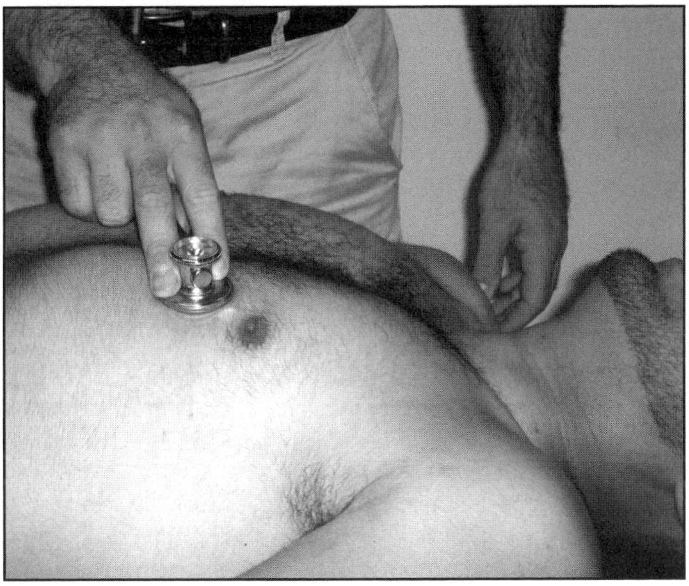

Figure 6-12a. Patient positioning for cardiac auscultation: supine.

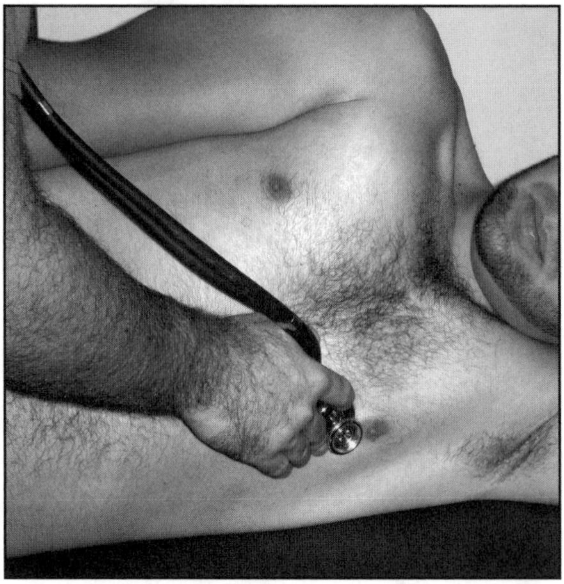

Figure 6-12b. Patient positioning for cardiac auscultation: sidelying.

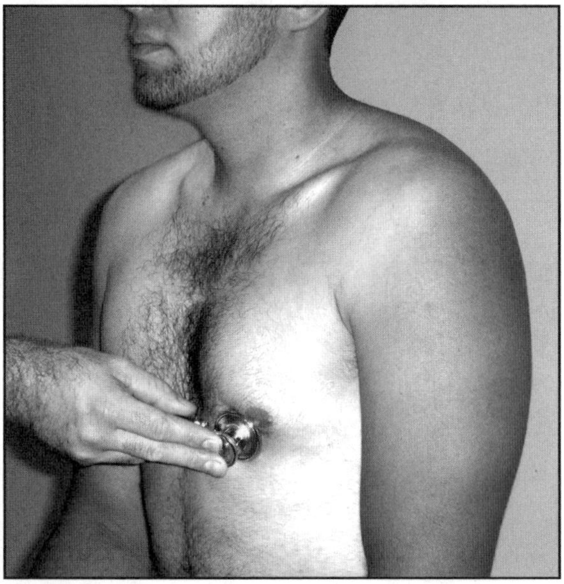

Figure 6-12c. Patient positioning for cardiac auscultation: sitting.

Many stethoscopes include both a diaphragm and a bell. The diaphragm is better suited for hearing the normal S1 and S2 sounds as well as aortic murmurs. The bell is more sensitive to the high-pitched S3 and S4 sounds as well as some mitral valve disorders.

Ausculation can also be used to examine the major vessels, such as the abdominal aorta, brachial arteries, and femoral arteries. Normally, the sound of the heartbeat may be faintly detectable, accompanied by intermittent rushing sounds created by blood flowing through the vessel. Abnormal vascular sounds, called *bruits*, include loud clicks, pounding, or continuous rather than intermittent rushing sounds. The turbulent blood flow in arteries that have been pathologically narrowed (atherosclerosis) or deformed (aneurysm) cause bruits.

Table 6-7
Cardiac Auscultation

Step 1.	Position patient in supine, males without shirt (see Figure 6-12a), females wearing sports bra.
Step 2.	Instruct the subject to breathe as normally as possible.
Step 3.	Locate the aortic listening zone (A) at the superior right sternal border in second intercostal space (as shown in Figure 6-11).
Step 4.	Carefully listen for the S1 and S2 ("lub-dub") heart sounds during several cardiac contraction cycles. Also listen for additional sounds (S3 and S4) or abnormal sounds (murmurs, rubs, etc).
Step 5.	Move the stethoscope sequentially to auscultate the remaining three zones: Pulmonary valve (P) at the superior left sternal border at second intercostal space Tricuspid valve (T) at the inferior left sternal border at fourth or fifth intercostal space Mitral valve (M) at fifth intercostal space in midclavicular line An alternate technique can be used which starts with M (the apex of the heart) and moves sequentially through T, P, and A.
Step 6.	If no abnormal sounds are heard in supine, have the patient lie on his or her left side (see Figure 6-12b) and again auscultate the four listening zones. This position moves the apex of the heart closer to the chest wall, making mitral valve disorders more distinguishable.
Step 7.	If left sidelying auscultation is normal, have the patient sit, lean forward, exhale completely, and hold his or her breath (ie, not inhale) (see Figure 6-12c). Again, listen to several heart cycles at each zone. Instruct the patient to breath between zones.
Step 8.	With the patient sitting, instruct him or her to hold his or her breath and bear down as if he or she was going to empty his or her bowels (Valsalva maneuver). Auscultate the heart apex (M). A "clicking" sound during this maneuver suggests potential mitral valve prolapse.

Palpation

Arterial pulses can be palpated where major arteries are close to the skin (see Figure 6-8). Pulses may be absent or diminished in vascular occlusion syndromes. Aneurysms may be palpated as a "throbbing mass" on the affected artery. A palpable abdominal pulse wider than the normal aortic pulsation that extends 2 inches to either side of midline may indicate an aortic aneurysm.

Pathology and Pathogenesis

Sudden Cardiac Death

Exercise-induced death is relatively rare, ranging from 1 fatality in 50,000 to 200,000 males and 1 fatality in 200,000 to 769,000 females of high school or collegiate age.[6,9,11,16,26] Although SCD can occur in any sport, it has been reported most frequently in basketball and football.[27] Nontraumatic SCD usually presents symptoms

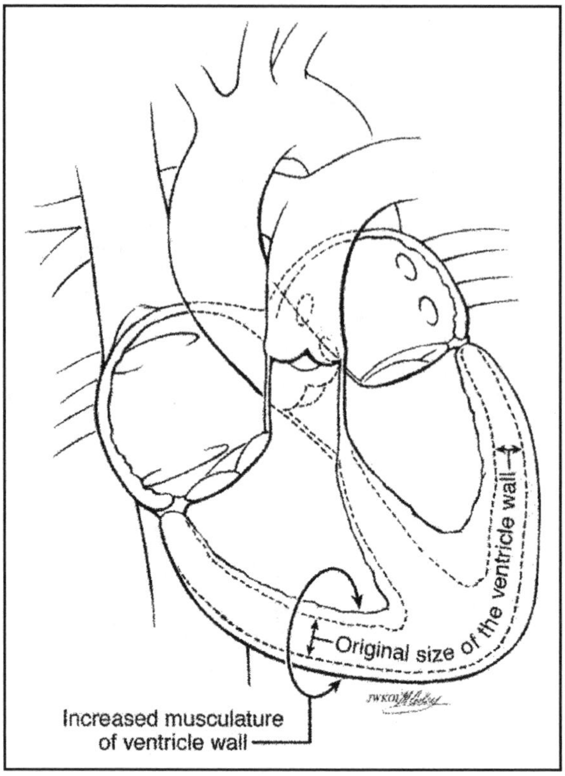

Figure 6-13. Cardiac hypertrophy.

within 1 hour of the onset of exercise or sports participation or shortly after the cessation of exercise. The most common causes of SCD in athletes are hypertrophic cardiomyopathy, congenital coronary artery anomalies, electrical and conduction abnormalities, or acquired myocarditis.[2-8,10,11,16,26] Some contributing factors in SCD include high-intensity exercise, electrolyte imbalances (a consequence of dehydration), high body temperature (from exercise in extreme heat and humidity), sudden cessation of intense physical activity (causing vasodilation and falling BP, similar to shock),[4,7,11,16] and the use of performance-enhancing substances or dietary supplements.[14] Other less common causes of SCD include aortic rupture (Marfan syndrome), commotio cordis, aortic stenosis, congenital cerebrovascular deformities, pulmonary disease, peripheral embolism, and drug abuse.[4-6,9-11,16]

Hypertrophic Cardiomyopathy

Three types of cardiac hypertrophy, or enlargement of the heart (Figure 6-13), are recognized: general cardiac hypertrophy (both ventricles), left ventricular hypertrophy, and right ventricular hypertrophy. General cardiac hypertrophy occurs in highly fit persons as an adaptation to strenuous aerobic exercise and is not considered pathological; this so-called "athlete's heart" does not reduce the size of the left ventricle cavity.[26,28,29] By contrast, pathological enlargement of the heart is called hypertrophic cardiomyopathy (HCM) and is associated with an asymmetrical enlargement of the left ventricular cavity. In this inherited condition, abnormal myocardial fibers form asymmetrical (ie, left or right) hypertrophy of the myocardium, which causes ventricular obstruction and arrhythmia. Eventually, hypertrophic cardiomyopathy leads to heart failure, ischemic myocardial damage, or fatal arrhythmia as the tissue propagates and interferes with the heart's muscle function, vascular supply, or electrical system, respectively.[2]

Hypertrophic cardiomyopathy is the leading cause of SCD in young, competitive athletes.[28] An estimated 1 in 500 young adults display signs of potential hypertrophic cardiomyopathy; not all of these people, however, have cardiac pathology.[4-7,9,16] Identifying which are most at risk for a catastrophic event during sports is the challenge. Most people with hypertrophic cardiomyopathy have a family history of sudden death under age 50 or a personal history of unexplained episodes of syncope, angina, or dyspnea.[4,7,26] A heart murmur that increases with a Valsalva maneuver (see Table 6-7) is sometimes auscultated at the lower left sternal border, medial to the apex of the heart.[11,26,30] Definitive diagnosis requires echocardiography.[5,9,26] A left ventricular wall thickness of 15 mm or more results in the clinical diagnosis of HCM.[31,32]

Hypertrophic cardiomyopathy is treated through medications (β blockers) and activity restriction; however, surgery is sometimes required.[33] Risk of arrhythmia increases as cardiac demand increases. β blockers decrease heart rate and the force of cardiac contractions, which decreases the risk of arrhythmia. β blockers also lead to exercise fatigue and decreased athletic performance; therefore, noncompliance with these medications is often a problem with competitive athletes.

The 36th Bethesda Conference classified sports for making return-to-play decisions in individuals who have a cardiovascular abnormality. Table 6-8 describes the classification system which is based on the level of intensity and the potential for bodily collision. The 36th Bethesda Conference recommends that an athlete with HCM be restricted from most competitive sports with the exception of Class IA, or low intensity, sports. Ironically, some athletes and their parents may choose to ignore a physician's recommendation and risk a fatal cardiac event with continued participation. Under these circumstances, athletic trainers and physicians must counsel the athlete and parents of the potential risk in order for them to make an informed decision.[14,16]

Coronary Artery Anomalies

Congenital coronary artery anomalies are the second leading cause of SCD in young athletes.[10,34] The most common type of coronary artery anomaly involves the left main coronary artery being abnormally positioned such that it runs between the aortic and pulmonary trunks (Figure 6-14). As the aortic and pulmonary trunks expand during exercise, they compress the left main coronary artery leading to ischemia of the myocardium and, eventually, fatal arrhythmias.

Unfortunately, patients with coronary artery anomalies may not experience symptoms prior to SCD. Resting and exercise ECGs are typically normal. Therefore, individuals who experience exertional syncope should be referred to a physician for follow-up. The 36th Bethesda Conference recommends that athletes who are diagnosed with coronary artery anomalies be restricted from all competitive sports.[34]

Disorders of the Myocardium and Coronary Artery Disease

Heart Failure

When cardiac output decreases because of an insufficient heart pump mechanism, the resulting condition is called *heart failure*. Several types of heart failure are

Table 6-8

Sport Classification (36th Bethesda Conference, 2005)

	Class A ($<40\%$ $MaxO_2$)	Class B (40% to 70% $MaxO_2$)	Class C ($>70\%$ $MaxO_2$)
I. Low (<20% MVC)	Billiards, bowling, cricket, curling, golf, riflery	Baseball, softball, fencing, table tennis, volleyball	Badminton,cross-country skiing, field, hockey, orienteering, race walking, squash/racquetball, running (long distance), soccer, tennis
II. Moderate (20% to 50% MVC)	Archery, auto racing, diving, equestrian, motorcycling	Football, field events in track (jumping), figure skating, rugby, rodeoing, surfing, running (sprint), synchronized swimming	Basketball, ice hockey, cross-country skiing, lacrosse, running (middle distance), swimming, team handball
III. High (>50% MVC)	Bobsledding/luge, field events in track (throwing), martial arts, gymnastics, sailing, water skiing, sport climbing, weightlifting, surfing	Body building, downhill skiing, skateboarding, snowboarding, wrestling	Boxing, canoeing/kayaking, cycling, decathlon, rowing, speedskating, triathlon

$MaxO_2$=maximum volume of oxygen (aerobic capacity), MVC=maximum voluntary contraction.

identified by the side of the heart that is affected (left or right) and whether the failure is acute or chronic. Acute heart failure is immediately life threatening whereas chronic heart failure causes gradual but progressive failures in the body's organ-systems. Table 6-9 summarizes the respective effects of these conditions.

Cor pulmonale is the term used for right heart failure as a consequence of pulmonary disease.[35] The pulmonary disease increases pressure in the pulmonary vascular system. The increased pressure increases the workload on the right ventricle, which pumps blood through the pulmonary artery to the lungs. If the pressure rises high enough, such as occurs with a complete vascular occlusion in the lung, the right ventricle cannot push the blood into the lungs—which is acute right-sided heart failure. Signs and symptoms of cor pulmonale are similar to those of right heart failure plus signs of pulmonary disease (see Chapter Seven).

Myocardial Ischemia

Myocardial ischemia occurs when the oxygen needed by the myocardium exceeds the oxygen in the blood delivered by the coronary arteries. This ischemic state causes angina (chest pain). In addition to angina, ischemic disorders affect-

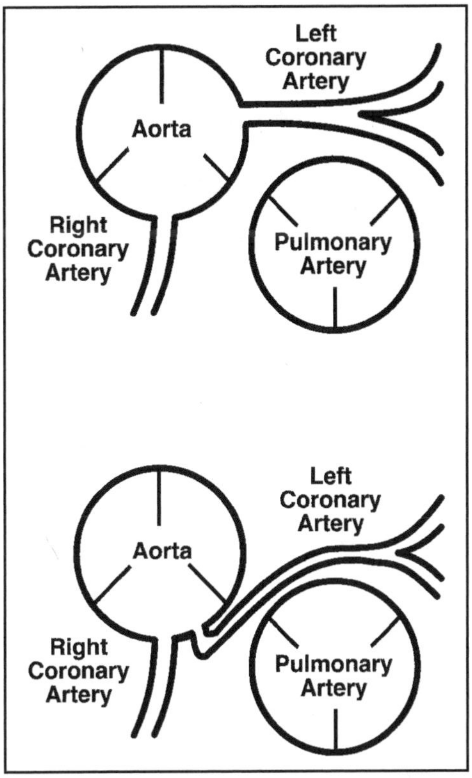

Figure 6-14. Coronary artery anomaly. The top shows a normal anterior coronary artery. The bottom depicts an abnormal course of the anterior coronary artery, running between the aorta and the pulmonary artery.

Table 6-9

Types of Heart Failure, Mechanism, and Signs

Location	**Mechanism**	**Signs**
Acute left	Failure to deliver blood to the body Pulmonary edema Typical pathology: myocardial infarction	Dyspnea, pink frothy pulmonary edema and sputum, cyanosis hypotension
Chronic left	Failure to deliver blood to the body Pulmonary edema Typical pathology: cardiomyopathy	Dyspnea with exertion and during sleep, unusual fatigue, tachycardia, cool skin, cyanosis, pulmonary edema
Acute right	Usually with pulmonary embolism Failure to deliver blood to lungs Systemic edema Typical pathology: acute cor pulmonale (pulmonary embolism)	Cool skin, hypotension, cyanosis
Chronic right	Failure to deliver blood to lungs Systemic edema Typical pathology: chronic pulmonary disease	Dyspnea, fatigue, abdominal discomfort, decreased appetite, peripheral edema

ing the myocardium usually exhibit typical cardiac signs and symptoms: unusual fatigue, dyspnea, dizziness, and syncope.[4,5,9,11] In a cardiac emergency, the vital signs (heart rate, respiration rate, BP) change rapidly.

Anything that limits myocardial blood supply causes angina. For example, if CAD obstructs the coronary arteries, the associated myocardium becomes ischemic and dies, a condition called myocardial infarction, or MI. A significant proportion of MIs are caused by moderate to heavy activity, such as manual labor or athletics.[6] CAD, including arteriosclerosis, comprises the majority of cardiac deaths among physically active persons over 35 years of age.[9,11] For this reason, angina accompanied by other cardiac signs and symptoms, particularly changes in vital signs, warrants activation of the emergency action plan and immediate referral.

Arrhythmogenic Right Ventricular Dysplasia

Arrhythmogenic right ventricular dysplasia (ARVD) is fatty infiltration (penetration) and fibrosis of the myocardium of the right ventricle.[7,11] ARVD has a genetic component and produces ventricular tachycardia or life-threatening ventricular arrhythmia.[7,11,32] Persons with ARVD may have a history of cardiac signs and symptoms upon exertion and should be excluded from participation in most sports.[11]

Valve Disorders

The heart valves can be affected by congenital deformities or acquired disease. Two deformities are stenosis (narrowing) that restricts blood flow through the valve (Figure 6-15) and structural malformations that do not allow the valve to close completely. Valve disorders cause murmurs from turbulent blood flow through the deformed valve on auscultation. Heart valve disorders are often present with other cardiac or systemic diseases. Infection can also damage the heart valves, particularly in children.

Generally, people who have valve disorders with normal heart rate and rhythm, normal heart size, and normal cardiac function are not excluded from participating in sports or other physical activity.[36] Decisions related to the participation of people who have more severe valve deformities that cause electrical (arrhythmia) or structural changes (hypertrophy) or affect heart function depend on the severity of the disorder and the person's chosen activity.[36]

Mitral valve prolapse (MVP) is the most common valve disorder. MVP is a deformity of the mitral valve leaflets that prevents it from closing completely. The leaflets bulge back into the left atrium during ventricular systole.[32] As a result, blood flows back into the left atrium, decreasing the flow of blood into the aorta (see Figure 6-15). This backflow varies depending on the severity of the deformity. For many people, MVP causes no functional problem. MVP is usually first detected during cardiac auscultation and may be heard as a mid-systolic click or a mitral regurgitation murmur. The condition can be further diagnosed through an echocardiogram. Persons with MVP but without syncope, family history of sudden death, arrhythmia, substantial back flow, or a previous cardiac-related event can participate in sports without restriction.[14]

Cardiac Conduction Disorders

Conduction disorders, problems with the heart's electrical system, result in arrhythmia. Benign atrial arrhythmia occurs in some highly fit persons as a result of exercise-induced resting bradycardia.[4] Pathological arrhythmia is produced by

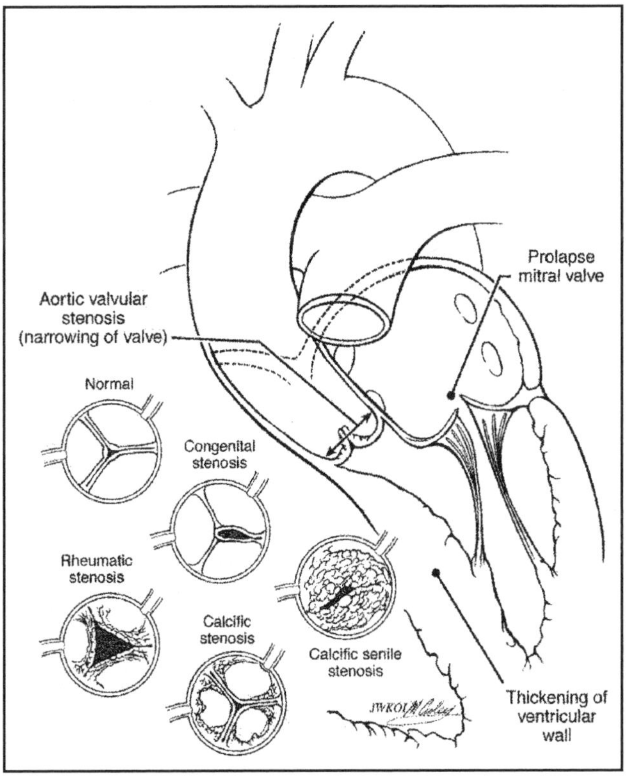

Figure 6-15. Common valvular disorders.

abnormal or blocked conduction pathways, leading to ventricular fibrillation and acute heart failure.[7,37] Arrhythmias are diagnosed by ECG.

Most people with a clinically significant arrhythmia have exertional palpitations or exertional syncope.[7,37] Syncope during exercise is highly suggestive of significant cardiac arrhythmia.[38] Patients with symptomatic arrhythmia should be excluded from sports competition or heavy physical activity for at least 6 months and cleared by ECG before returning.[37] Qualification for sports depends on the type and severity of the arrhythmia.[38]

Paroxysmal Supraventricular Tachycardia

An intermittently occurring very rapid heart rate at rest, exceeding 150 bpm, is called paroxysmal supraventricular tachycardia (PSVT). The etiology of PSVT is a defect in the discharge pattern of the SA node, atria, or AV node that causes a drastic increase in heart rate. This condition is most common in children and may also be observed in adolescents. An attack of PSVT is usually accompanied by palpitations, anxiety, dyspnea, chest pain or tightness, and possible syncope. Physical examination reveals a very rapid, but regular and strong, heart rate. The heart rate returns to normal between attacks. An ECG monitor may have to be worn for 24 hours or longer to detect this syndrome because the ECG trace is normal between attacks.

PSVT may last for several minutes or several hours and is generally not dangerous or life threatening. Use of nicotine, caffeine, alcohol, or drugs may precipitate an attack, but not necessarily. Mild PSVT may spontaneously remit and require no treatment. A longer attack may be interrupted by the patient performing a Valsalva maneuver, holding the breath and pushing with the abdominal muscles as if having a bowel movement. The increased pressure stimulates pressure receptors in the blood vessels, which creates an autonomic signal to decrease heart rate. A strong cough may have the same effect. Electrical shock, medications, or surgery to disrupt the electrical pathway or implant a pacemaker may be necessary in extreme cases.

Long Q-T Syndrome

The Q-T interval is the time it takes for the ventricles to depolarize and repolarize. About 1 in 10,000 people inherit a condition in which the Q-T interval is longer than normal.[10] This increase in the depolarization-repolarization cycle interferes with the heart's contraction and can lead to a fatal ventricular tachycardia when heart rate increases, as occurs with exercise.[32] Many people are asymptomatic until the arrhythmia occurs, but others will have a history of exertional syncope. Approximately 30% will have a family history of SCD or actual diagnosis of long Q-T syndrome.[10] Diagnosis can be made by ECG before or after symptoms appear. A person with long Q-T syndrome requires medication to control heart rate, avoidance of physically stressful activity, including sports, and sometimes a pacemaker. β blockers are the most commonly prescribed medications for long Q-T syndrome.

Wolfe-Parkinson-White Syndrome

This syndrome involves an accessory conduction pathway between the atria and ventricles.[32] The accessory pathway conducts more rapidly than the AV node, and the result is that one of the ventricles depolarizes just slightly before the other. Atrial fibrillation may occur when a premature atrial depolarization stimulates the additional pathway, which conducts the depolarization in reverse to the atria. This condition causes the depolarization to circulate in a loop between the atria and additional pathway, one stimulating the other, resulting in atrial fibrillation. Less common but more ominous, the premature atrial depolarization may bypass the AV node into the ventricles, which creates a depolarization that goes back to the atria through the additional pathway, and then down the AV node to the ventricles again. The result is a loop of depolarization that causes ventricular fibrillation, which is fatal unless defibrillation occurs within minutes. The presence of exertional syncope or cardiac symptoms increase the risk for ventricular fibrillation. These individuals should undergo a 12-lead ECG, exercise testing, and an echocardiogram to rule out other cardiovascular abnormalities. The syndrome is treated with medication to limit heart rate and surgery to obliterate the additional conduction pathway. Surgery is necessary for individuals that have multiple accessory pathways or demonstrate ventricular rates greater than 240 bpm. Athletes may continue participation in all sports if they have no history of palpitations or structural abnormalities and they do not present with tachycardia.

Marfan Syndrome

Marfan syndrome is an inherited connective tissue disorder associated with increased risk for SCD.[32] Most individuals (80% to 90%) with Marfan syndrome develop potentially fatal deformities in the aorta.[11,34,39,40] The clinical diagnosis of Marfan syndrome is based on the distinct and easily recognizable physical characteristics presented in Table 6-4.[32] Definitive diagnosis can be made through echocardiographic measurement of aortic root dimension. The 36th Bethesda Conference recommended that athletes with Marfan syndrome can participate in competitive sports (Class IA or IIA only) if "they do not have one or more of the following: (1)

aortic root dilation, (2) moderate to severe mitral regurgitation, or (3) family history of dissection or sudden death in a Marfan relative."[41]

Commotio Cordis

Sudden blows to the chest that occur during the vulnerable phase of cardiac repolarization can induce a severe ventricular arrhythmia called *commotio cordis*.[32,42] Commotio cordis was associated with 130 deaths during the time period of 1998 to 2001, with the average age of victims being 13 years. This life-threatening condition can occur in any sport. It has been reported most frequently in baseball, softball, ice hockey, football, and lacrosse due to sudden physical contact or projectiles (balls or hockey pucks).[42]

Life-saving efforts should focus on immediate application of an automatic external defibrillator (AED). Commotio cordis has a very low rate of resuscitation (15%), unless defibrillation by an AED[43] occurs within 2 minutes of onset.[10,11]

The National Athletic Trainers' Association (NATA) has published an official statement on commotio cordis which includes suggestions for preventing this condition.[44] The NATA recommends that coaches and officials be trained in first aid, cardiopulmonary resuscitation (CPR), and the use of AEDs. Also, emergency action plans should be in place to ensure immediate access to an AED and advanced life support. Coaches should make sure that all protective equipment fits properly and that young athletes are instructed on the proper techniques for avoiding blows to the chest. For example, young baseball and softball athletes should be instructed to turn away from an inside pitch rather than turn into it.

Hypertension

HTN is defined as a consecutive resting BP greater than 140/90 on two or more occasions.[45-47] Optimal BP is less than 120/80 mmHg. Prehypertension is defined as a systolic pressure of 120 to 139 mmHg with a diastolic pressure of 80 to 90 mmHg. People with prehypertension are at risk for developing HTN. Prehypertension is not considered a pathological state, but is used to identify people at risk for development of HTN. Persons with prehypertension should be counseled to make modifications in their diet, to participate in regular exercise, and to avoid sodium and alcohol. The pathological condition of HTN is currently categorized into two stages. Stage I HTN is defined as a systolic BP of 140 to 159 mmHg or diastolic BP of 90 to 99 mmHg. Stage II HTN is defined as systolic BP of 160 mmHg or greater or diastolic BP of 100 mmHg or greater.[46]

Primary ("essential") arterial HTN often has unknown pathogenesis, but genetic and environmental factors contribute (eg, urban living, diet, obesity, chronic stress, smoking) to the condition. Secondary HTN is the result of another medical condition, most often a renal, hormonal, or metabolic disorder.[35]

Many persons with HTN are asymptomatic, although some experience frequent occipital headaches and epistaxis (nosebleed). A headache occurs when diastolic pressure exceeds 120 mmHg. HTN headaches are usually mild, present upon waking, and are relieved by mild activity.[48] Extreme BP responses during exercise (systolic pressure of 240 mmHg or greater) may be a sign of severe cardiovascular pathology.[49]

Long-term complications of HTN include heart disease, stroke, retinal damage, renal failure, and peripheral vascular disease.[35] The constant high pressure in the vessels eventually damages those vessels and the associated tissues. In addition, the left ventricle becomes hypertrophied as an adaptation to the increased work of pumping blood in the highly pressurized system. Left ventricular hypertrophy, if HTN remains unaddressed, increases the risk of ischemic heart damage, arrhythmia, and heart failure.

Persons with mild to moderate HTN without associated organ damage or heart disease need not be restricted from participating in sports, but should be reevaluated every 2 to 4 months to ensure that their HTN remains controlled. Severe HTN requires avoidance of strenuous sports that require high-load muscle contraction (eg, power lifting, gymnastics, snow skiing, cycling) until it is controlled by lifestyle or medication and organ damage has been assessed.[46]

A variety of medications are used to manage HTN. Acetylcholinesterase (ACE) inhibitors and calcium channel blockers that are prescribed for HTN have no particular precautions relative to exercise restrictions. Patients taking diuretics to limit plasma volume, thus reducing BP, need to be monitored during activity for dehydration. These patients may also require potassium supplementation to avoid hypokalemia (low potassium levels), which can decrease blood flow to muscles and cause serious muscle damage during intense exercise.[47] β blockers limit maximum heart rates, so heart rate should be monitored during exercise.[45]

Regular aerobic exercise at 60% to 70% of maximum heart rate has been shown to decrease resting BP, particularly for patients with mild HTN.[45,46] All patients with controlled HTN should participate in a regular exercise program under the guidance of their physician.[47]

Disorders of the Blood

Anemia

Anemia is described as a hemoglobin level or RBC volume (hematocrit) lower than the levels or volumes of 95% of persons of the same age. For adults, this means hemoglobin levels of less than 13 g/100 dL in men and less than 11.5 g/100 dL in women.[50,51] Since the hemoglobin in RBC carries oxygen, anemia limits work capacity because it limits the amount of oxygen that is available.[52] Therefore, anemia affects physical performance.[51]

Primary risk factors for anemia include malnutrition and chronic disease. Other risk factors are intense physical training (destroys RBC), prolonged use of analgesics (impairs RBC formation), family history, heavy menstruation (depletes RBC),[51] and medical treatments such as chemotherapy and radiation (destroys RBC). Anemia produces pallor, swollen tongue, spooning (thin, concave) nails (see Figure 6-6), scaly lips with fissures at the edges, fatigue, and impaired attention.[51]

Dilutional anemia, also known as "sports anemia" or "psuedoanemia," is common among highly fit individuals. Exercise increases blood plasma volume but does not affect RBC production. In these individuals, blood tests may show anemia because the RBC count looks low relative to blood volume. Dilutional anemia produces no symptoms and does not affect performance because the total number of RBC is normal, so the amount of oxygen being delivered is unaffected.[51,53]

Most studies indicate that exercise neither causes nor exacerbates true anemia.[51] Chronic blood loss in physically active women, most often through a combination of menstruation, increased stress, intense exercise, and oral contraceptives, will lead to lab tests showing low blood iron. Low iron levels are not equivalent to anemia, but can lead to anemia if uncorrected because hemoglobin requires iron. Mild iron deficiency alone will not affect physical performance.[51]

Sickle Cell Disease and Sickle Cell Trait

Sickle cell disease is an inherited condition that produces abnormally shaped RBC that inhibit the binding of oxygen[54] and can lead to life-threatening events. Individuals who inherit two genes of sickle hemoglobin (one from each parent) are said to have sickle cell disease or sickle cell anemia. The result, like all true anemias, is decreased oxygen delivery. Due to the extreme deficiency in oxygen delivery, these individuals will rarely participate in competitive or recreational sports. Individuals who inherit one gene of sickle hemoglobin and one normal gene are said to have SCT. Between 8% and 10% of African Americans carry the genetic SCT, and about 1% develop sickle cell anemia.[54]

The relative risk of sudden death is 27 times higher among persons of African descent who carry the SCT than among persons of African descent without the trait, and 40 times higher than the risk in other races.[11] Sudden death in persons with SCT is usually caused by emboli, since sickled cells tend to clot easily, or by sickle cell crisis, which leads to widespread vascular occlusion, organ infarction, shock, and death. Warning signs for sickle cell crisis include severe muscle cramping in the legs, buttocks, and low back; tachycardia; hypotension; hyperventilation; and loss of consciousness. Risk for sickle cell crisis is greater during exercise in hot and high altitude environments. Unfortunately, the clinical presentation of sickle cell crisis can mimic that of heat illness or cardiac arrest. Knowledge of an individual's SCT status can help in the differentiation of sickle cell crisis.

SCT is also a risk factor for acute exertional rhabdomyolysis, which is a sudden metabolic breakdown of skeletal muscle that usually occurs during vigorous exercise in hot, humid weather.[11,55-57] In this condition, myoglobin (a muscle protein) and enzymes from the damaged muscle enter the bloodstream. Acute renal failure, shock, and death may result as the proteins and enzymes block the glomeruli, the functional unit of the kidneys.[57]

Effective management of sickle cell crisis requires early recognition and immediate referral. Preventative efforts should focus on gradual acclimatization to hot or high altitude environments and proper hydration.

Hemophilia

Hemophilia is a genetic disorder that impairs the ability of the blood to clot.[58] Several types of hemophilia exist. The types depend on the clotting factors that are deficient (Table 6-10). Most of the types are extremely rare. Some types of hemophilia, such as types A and B, are more common and lead to prolonged, severe blood loss with even minor injuries, and are therefore dangerous for competitive athletes. The general recommendation for persons with the severe types of hemophilia is to avoid collision sports and some contact sports, thus decreasing the risk of injury.[59] Furthermore, replacement of blood clotting factors is recommended to prevent severe hemorrhaging during sports participation.[58] Prolonged bleeding also means that persons with hemophilia may take longer than expected to recover from injuries.[59]

Vascular Disorders

Trauma

Repeated blunt trauma, particularly in the hand and fingers from catching a ball, can damage the capillaries and arterioles, producing ischemia distal to the

Table 6-10

Types of Bleeding Disorders Caused by Deficiencies in Clotting Factors

Clotting Factor	Disorders	Characteristics	Treatment
VIII	Hemophilia A	X-linked recessive trait: affects men, very rarely affects women 80% of all hemophilia cases	Desmopressin acetate (DDAVP) to stimulate release of clotting factors from blood vessel walls Factor VIII infusion at the first sign of bleeding Plasma and plasma concentrates More severe cases may require prophylactic Factor VIII
IX	Hemophilia B (Christmas disease)	X-linked recessive trait Second most common type of hemophilia	Factor IX infusion at the first sign of bleeding Plasma and plasma concentrates
von Willebrand	von Willebrand disease	Autosomal dominant trait, affects 1% to 2% of the population Abnormal von Willebrand protein affects platelet function	DDAVP to stimulate release of clotting factors, including von Willebrand, from blood vessel walls
I (fibrinogen)	Afibrinogenesis Hypofibrinogenesis Dysfibrinogenesis	Autosomal recessive trait Very rare: only 200 known cases	Cryoprecipitate Plasma
II (prothrombin)	Hypoprothrombinemia Dysprothrombinemia	Autosomal recessive trait, or acquired from severe vitamin K deficiency or liver disease Inherited condition is very rare: only 30 known cases	Plasma Prothrombin complex concentrates (PCCs)
V	Parahemophilia Owren's disease	Autosomal recessive trait Very rare: only 150 known cases	Factor V accelerates thrombin activity; deficiency slows clot formation Plasma, only useful when bleeding because Factor V breaks down very quickly

continued

Table 6-10 (continued)

Types of Bleeding Disorders Caused by Deficiencies in Clotting Factors

Clotting Factor	Disorders	Characteristics	Treatment
VII (proconvertin)	Factor VII deficiency	Autosomal recessive trait, extremely rare Is also rarely acquired when using Coumadin, an anticoagulant	Plasma, only useful when bleeding because Factor VII breaks down very quickly
X (Stuart-Prower)	Factor X deficiency	Autosomal recessive trait Extremely rare: only 50 known cases reported	Plasma, only useful when bleeding because Factor X breaks down very quickly PCCs for bleeding episodes
XI	Hemophilia C, plasma thromboplastic antecedent, Rosenthal syndrome	Autosomal recessive trait Very rare: only 200 known cases Usually discovered with excessive bleeding during surgery	Plasma Fresh frozen Factor X concentrate Fibrin glue to create a clot during surgery DDAVP
XII (Hageman)	Factor XII deficiency	Autosomal recessive trait, very rare Does not cause excessive bleeding	Typically, no treatment is required
XIII (fibrin stabilizing factor)	Factor XIII deficiency	Autosomal recessive trait, exceptionally rare Clot forms, but is very weak because Factor XIII cross-links fibrin Very severe bleeding	Plasma Cryoprecipitate Fresh frozen Factor XIII concentrate

injury.[22,60] Symptoms occur in the affected region and include hypersensitivity to cold, numbness, and pallor.[22,60] This condition is treated with rest, padding, and avoidance of cold. Medications to produce vasodilation may also be required.[60]

Occlusion Syndromes

Occlusion of arteries can be caused by mechanical pressure, inflammation, or blood clots. Common sites of occlusion include the subclavian, axillary, popliteal, and femoral arteries.[20,23] Chronic arterial occlusion produces intermittent muscle cramps, diminished distal pulses, bruits upon auscultation, dystrophic (yellow, scaly) skin and nails, ulcerations of the skin, and loss of hair in a distal area. Acute arterial occlusion produces the "five P's": pain, pallor, pulselessness, paresthesia, and paralysis distal to the occlusion. There are several occlusion syndromes common in physically active populations.

Thoracic Outlet Syndrome

Thoracic outlet syndrome is when the subclavian or axillary artery becomes occluded between scalene muscles, between the clavicle and first rib, or by the pectoralis minor tendon near the coracoid process. The patient's history usually reveals repetitive strenuous overhead activity or prolonged postures involving scapular protraction (eg, deskwork). Symptoms include diffuse arm aching that increases with exertion, paresthesia that increases at night, easy fatigability of the limb, and intermittent swelling of the limb.[23] Clinical signs vary, but distal temperature changes and cyanosis are common. In addition, diminished distal (radial) pulse during clinical tests, such as Adson's test, military bracing, Allen's test, or repeated clenching of the fist with the hand overhead, may be positive.[61,62]

Other occlusion syndromes can also occur. Acute (traumatic) or exertional compartment syndromes can occlude an artery in the affected compartment. Compartment syndrome of the anterior compartment of the lower leg produces weak dorsiflexion, numbness of the first web space (between toes 1 and 2), and weak or absent dorsal pedis pulse. Buerger's disease (thrombangitis obliterans) is a condition associated with tobacco use, producing segmental inflammation and occlusion of arterioles and resulting in signs of occlusion simultaneously in the upper and lower extremities that subside with cessation of tobacco use.[20]

Deep Vein Thrombosis and Pulmonary Embolism

Deep vein thrombosis (DVT) and pulmonary embolism (PE) can occur after casting or other immobilization, after surgery, or in a hypercoaguable state that may be the result of an inherited abnormality, a disease, or the use of oral contraceptives.[63] As blood pools in large veins, the cells clot together to form a mass called a *thrombus,* usually resulting in venous swelling called *thrombophlebitis.* The presence of a thrombus in a vein is called *thrombosis.* A thrombus that has broken free and is moving through the circulation is called an *embolus.*

The classically described signs and symptoms of DVT in the lower extremity are: severe calf tenderness, distended veins, distal edema, and pain with passive dorsiflexion (Homan's sign). Fewer than one-third of the patients who have DVT, however, actually exhibit these symptoms.[64] Diagnosis is made by Doppler ultrasound, which uses high-frequency sound waves to measure blood flow velocity; abnormally slow blood flow in a vein indicates occlusion. To prevent DVT, particularly for patients with immobilized or casted lower extremities, walking or active

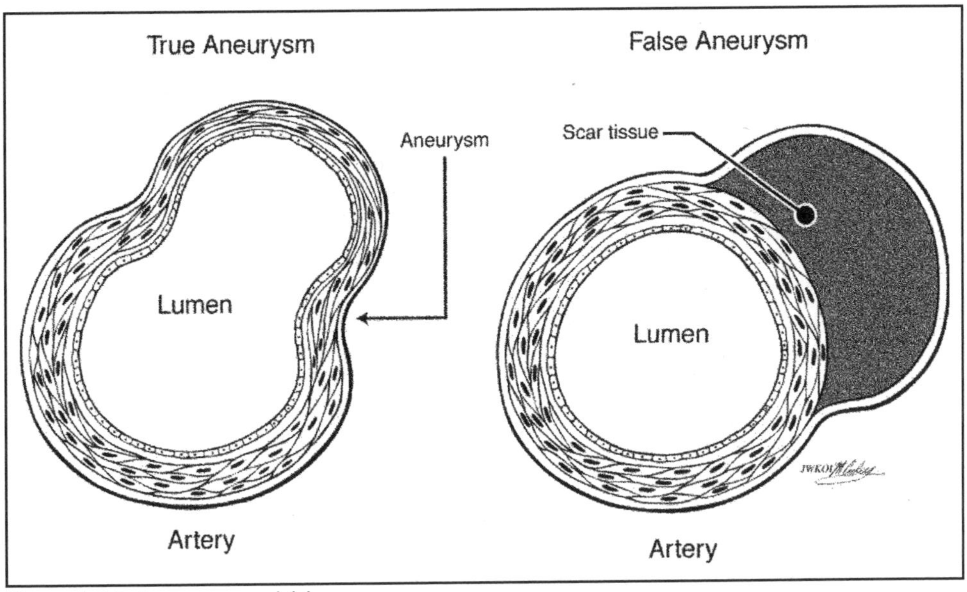

Figure 6-16. Aneurysm and false aneurysm.

range of motion exercises should be performed several times a day. If such activity is not possible, treatments such as medication (anticoagulants) and intermittent compression may be used.[64] Compression stockings are also often used to prevent DVT.

PE occurs when an embolus travels to a lung, blocks a blood vessel and the blood flow to a portion of the lung, and can cause necrosis of lung tissue.[65] This condition presents with chest pain, dyspnea, cough, hemoptysis (bloody sputum with cough), diaphoresis, anxiety, and hyperpnea (over 20 breaths per minute). A PE is a medical emergency because, if it affects a large lung segment, it can produce syncope, shock, and death.[65] Most cases will resolve if treated appropriately with hospitalization and anticoagulants. In some cases, anticoagulant medications may be taken for up to 3 months after the occurrence of the PE.[63,65]

Aneurysm

An aneurysm is a weakness in the wall of a blood vessel, usually a result of arteriosclerosis or infection, which causes a local dilation of all layers of the vessel wall (Figure 6-16).[20,66] Aneurysms produce pulsing pain, auscultated bruits, and asymmetrical distal pulses. Aneurysms are susceptible to rupture, which may cause severe internal hemorrhage, shock, and death if untreated. Common sites at which aneurysms develop include the aorta (common in Marfan syndrome), the iliac artery, the subclavian artery, and cerebral arteries.

A *false aneurysm* can occur after trauma in sports or other physical activity. In a false aneurysm, the wall of the vessel tears and causes a hematoma that subsequently develops into a fibrous scar (see Figure 6-13). The interior diameter (lumen) of the vessel is unchanged, and blood flow is unaffected.[20] Symptoms are caused by the bulging scar compressing nearby anatomical structures, such as nerves or other vessels. History typically includes a local traumatic injury that has not resolved as expected. A painful, pulsatile mass is often palpable at the site of the false aneurysm, but pulses distal to the injury are normal.[19,20] Rest is usually all that is needed, although occasionally surgical excision is required.

Headaches

Headaches can be caused by several neurovascular problems. A *migraine headache* causes intense throbbing pain, usually unilaterally, with associated symptoms of nausea, vomiting, photophobia (aversion to light), and phonophobia (aversion to sound).[48] Many who suffer migraines have a positive family history. The causes and mechanisms of migraine headaches are poorly understood, but may be related to alterations in the neurotransmitter serotonin, inflammatory effects on the trigeminal nerve complex, and hormonal variations.

A *cluster headache* is an intense, gnawing pain that is deep and non-throbbing in nature, occurring unilaterally around one eye. Lacrimation (tearing), rhinorrhea ("runny nose") or nasal congestion, diaphoresis, unilateral pupillary constriction (miosis), ptosis (drooping eyelid), and psychomotor agitation may also be present as a result of trigeminal nerve and parasympathetic involvement.[67] A cluster headache episode lasts up to 45 minutes and may recur on a daily basis; the defining characteristic is the recurrence of the headache across several days followed by a long period with no headache.[48] Common exacerbating factors include psychoemotional stress and alcohol or tobacco use. Similar to migraines, the etiology and pathophysiology of cluster headaches are not well understood, but may be related to neurovascular, hormonal, or autonomic nervous system abnormalities.

A *toxic vascular headache* presents diffuse, throbbing, severe pain over the entire crown of the head; this type of headache is never unilateral.[48] Etiology includes infection (usually accompanied by fever), caffeine abuse or withdrawal, alcohol abuse or withdrawal (hangover), hypoxia, hypoglycemia (low blood sugar), and metabolic disorders.[48]

Persons with vascular headaches are awake and alert, have no fever, and demonstrate a negative neurological examination (see Chapters One and Thirteen).[48] Treatment consists of rest in a quiet, dark room and prescription medication if the headaches are recurrent and disabling. If other systemic signs occur simultaneously with a severe headache, emergency medical attention is required.

Pediatric Concerns

Pediatric Chest Pain

Chest pain in a child is rarely due to cardiac pathology. Chest pain is usually attributable to a musculoskeletal condition or a specific traumatic event.[17] Asthma, depression, anxiety disorders, hyperventilation, autoimmune disease, anemia, school or family stress, or physical abuse may also cause chest pain. Children with a family history of heart disease who have chest pain, however, should be referred for medical examination.[17]

Congenital Heart Conditions

The most common congenital heart problems are septal wall defects and vascular anomalies. These disorders are often detected and surgically corrected during infancy, but subtle cases occasionally go undetected.[7] Some children with congenital heart conditions have a history of frequent illnesses, delayed growth, intolerance to activity, malaise, and other chronic disease signs. Signs of potential cardiac pathology include digital clubbing, cyanosis, syncope, fatigue, dyspnea, and auscultated pericardial rub, murmurs, or clicks.[17]

Most congenital heart conditions are not adversely affected by exercise and do not prevent participation in sports.[68] Some exceptions are hypertrophic cardiomyopathy, congenital coronary artery anomalies, cardiac complications of Marfan syndrome, myocarditis, and major heart-vascular malformations.[34] Each child who has a heart condition should be considered individually. Physical activity should be restricted only to the extent that it is medically necessary. In general, baseline and annual exercise testing with ECG and BP monitoring should be conducted to ascertain progression of disease as the child matures.[34] Again, the 36th Bethesda Conference guidelines should be consulted when making decisions regarding sports participation

Summary

The hallmark of cardiac pathology is chest pain, or *angina*, which often refers into the left upper arm, anterior throat, face, jaw, or posterior chest wall. Other symptoms associated with cardiac pathology include dyspnea, unusual fatigue, palpitations, and syncope. Clinical signs include cyanosis; edema; diaphoresis; clubbing of fingers and toes; dystrophic (yellow, scaly) nails; changes in rate, rhythm, or character of heartbeat; auscultated murmurs; and changes in BP. Symptoms of vascular pathology include changes in skin temperature, numbness, cramping, or pain with activity and limb fatigue during activity. Associated signs are localized skin pallor or cyanosis; distal edema; changes in rate, rhythm, or character of distal pulses; dilated or distended veins; and palpable pulsatile masses.

A thorough preparticipation physical exam can play an important role in identifying individuals who might have a potentially serious cardiovascular condition. When planning these exams, athletic trainers should ensure that the AHA minimal components are included in both the history and physical exam portions of the screening. Athletic trainers should also be diligent in following up on all potential cardiovascular conditions identified through the preparticipation physical exam.

Case Study

Tiffany, 16-year-old African American female basketball athlete, is carried into your athletic training facility by her coaches. The coaches explain that they were conducting conditioning drills outside on the track when Tiffany fainted. She had been complaining throughout the drills, but this was natural for Tiffany. When she fainted, they knew that they needed to bring her to you. She is conscious now and complaining of dizziness, chest pains, and shortness of breath.

As you begin your physical exam, you find that her pulse is 98, weak, and irregular; BP is 150/80; respirations are 24, rapid, shallow, and labored.

As you question her further, Tiffany tells you that she fainted once before when she was in middle school. She said it happened during basketball practice. Her mother took her to the doctor, but he didn't find anything wrong with her.

Critical Thinking Questions

1. Based on Tiffany's complaints and your initial physical exam, what conditions would you include in your differential diagnosis? Why?
2. What steps will you take in managing Tiffany's condition?
3. What are the potential risks for Tiffany?

References

1. National Athletic Trainers' Association. *Athletic Training Educational Competencies.* 4th ed. Dallas, TX: National Athletic Trainers' Association; 2005.
2. NIH Consensus Development Panel on Physical Activity and Cardiovascular Health. Physical activity and cardiovascular health. *J Am Med Assoc.* 1996;276(3):241-246.
3. American College of Sports Medicine and American Heart Association. Recommendations for cardiovascular screening, staffing, and emergency policies at health/fitness facilities. *Med Sci Sports Exerc.* 1998;30(6):1009-1018.
4. Franklin BA, Fletcher GF, Gordon NF, Noakes TD, Ades PA, Balady GJ. Cardiovascular evaluation of the athlete: issues regarding performance, screening and sudden cardiac death. *Sports Med.* 1997;24(2):97-119.
5. O'Connor FG, Kugler JP, Oriscello RG. Sudden death in young athletes: screening for the needle in a haystack. *Am Fam Physician.* 1998;57(11):2763-2770.
6. Thompson PD. The cardiovascular complications of vigorous physical activity. *Arch Intern Med.* 1996;156:2297-2302.
7. Basilico FC. Cardiovascular disease in athletes. *Am J Sports Med.* 1999;27(1):108-121.
8. Thompson PD, Balady GJ, Chaitman BR, Clark LT, Levine BD, Myerburg RJ. 36th Bethesda conference task force 6: coronary artery disease. *J Am Coll Cardiol.* 2005;45(8):1348-1353.
9. Maron BJ. Risk profiles and cardiovascular preparticipation screening of competitive athletes. *Cardiol Clin.* 1997;15(3):473-483.
10. Koester MC. A review of sudden cardiac death in young athletes and strategies for preparticipation cardiovascular screening. *J Athletic Training.* 2001;36(2):197-204.
11. Futterman LG, Myerburg R. Sudden death in athletes: an update. *Sports Med.* 1998;26(5):335-350.
12. Maron BJ, Thompson PD, Puffer JC, et al. Cardiovascular preparticipation screening of competitive athletes: a statement for health professionals from the Sudden Death Committee (clinical cardiology) and Congenital Cardiac Defects Committee (cardiovascular disease in the young), American Heart Association. *Circulation.* 1996;94(4):850-856.
13. Lyznicki JM, Nielsen NH, Schneider JF. Cardiovascular screening of student athletes. *Am Family Physician.* 2000;62(4):765-774.
14. Estes NAM, III, Kloner R. 36th Bethesda conference task force 9: drugs and performance-enhancing substances. *J Am Coll Cardiol.* 2005;45:1368-1369.
15. Terry GC, Kyle JM, Ellis JM, Cantwell J, Courson R, Medlin R. Sudden cardiac arrest in athletic medicine. *J Athletic Training.* 2001;36(2):205-209.
16. Maron BJ. Cardiovascular risks to young persons on the athletic field. *Ann Intern Med.* 1998;129(5):379-386.
17. Anzai AK. Adolescent chest pain. *Am Fam Physician.* 1996;53(5):1682-1690.
18. VanCamp SP. Sudden death. *Clin Sports Med.* 1992;11(2):273-289.
19. Bandy WD, Stong L, Roberts T, Dyer R. False aneurysm-a complication following an inversion ankle sprain: a case report. *J Orthop Sports Phys Ther.* 1996;23(4):272-279.
20. Cohn SL, Taylor WC. Vascular problems of the lower extremity in athletes. *Clin Sports Med.* 1990;9(2):449-470.
21. Karas SE. Thoracic outlet syndrome. *Clin Sports Med.* 1990;9(2):297-310.
22. Rettig AC. Neurovascular injuries in the wrists and hands of athletes. *Clin Sports Med.* 1990;9(2):389-417.
23. Sotta RR. Vascular problems in the proximal upper extremity. *Clin Sports Med.* 1990;9(2):379-388.
24. Bickley LS, Szilagyi PG. *Bates' Guide to Physical Examination and History Taking.* 9th ed. Philadelphia, PA: Lippincott Williams & Wilkins; 2005.
25. DeGowin RL, Brown DD. *DeGowin's Diagnostic Examination.* 7th ed. New York, NY: McGraw-Hill; 2000.

26. Smith AN, Bell GW. Hypertrophic cardiomyopathy and its inherent danger in athletics. *Athletic Training.* 1991;26(4):319-323.
27. Maron BJ, Zipes DP. 36th Bethesda Conference Introduction: recommendations for competitive athletes with cardiovascular abnormalities---general considerations. *J Am Coll Cardiol.* 2005;45:1318-1321).
28. Maron BJ. Hypertrophic cardiomyopathy: practical steps for preventing sudden death. *Physician Sportsmed.* 2002;30(1):19-24.
29. Puffer JC. The athletic heart syndrome: ruling out cardiac pathology. *Physician Sportsmed.* 2002;30(7):41-47.
30. Bryan G, Ward A, Rippe JM. Athletic heart syndrome. *Clin Sports Med.* 1992;11(2):259-272.
31. Maron BJ, Douglas PS, Graham TP, Nishimura RA, Thompson PD. 36th Bethesda conference: preparticipation screening and diagnosis of cardiovascular disease in athletes. *J Am Coll Cardiol.* 2005;45(8):1322-1326.
32. Mason PK, Mounsey JP. Common issues in sports cardiology. *Clin Sports Med.* 2005;24(3):463-476.
33. Miles WM, Zipes DP. Myocardial and pericardial disease. In: Andreoli TE, Carpenter CCJ, Plum F, Smith LH Jr, eds. *Cecil Essentials of Medicine.* 2nd ed. Philadelphia, PA: WB Saunders Co; 1990:105-112.
34. Graham TP, Driscoll DJ, Gersony WM, Newburger JW, Rocchini A, Towbin JA. 36th Bethesda conference task force 2: congenital heart disease. *J Am Coll Cardiol.* 2005;45(8):1326-1333.
35. Gould BE. Cardiovascular and lymphatic disorders. *Pathophysiology for the Health-Related Professions.* Philadelphia, PA: WB Saunders Co; 1997:159-212.
36. Bonow RO, Cheitlin MD, Crawford MH, Douglas PS. 36th Bethesda conference task force 3: valvular heart disease. *J Am Coll Cardiol.* 2005;45(8):1334-1340.
37. Garson AJ. Arrhythmias and sudden cardiac death in elite athletes. *Periatr Med Chir.* 1998;20:101-103.
38. Zipes DP, Ackerman MJ, Estes NAM, III, Grant AO, Myerburg RJ, Van Hare G. 36th Bethesda conference task force 7: arrhythmias. *J Am Coll Cardiol.* 2005;45(8):1354-1365.
39. Herbert PN, Hricik D. Inherited disorders of connective tissue. In: Andreoli TE, Carpenter CCJ, Plum F, Smith LHJ, eds. *Cecil Essentials of Medicine.* 2nd ed. Philadelphia, PA: WB Saunders Co; 1990:444-445.
40. McKeag DB. Preparticipation screening of the potential athlete. *Clin Sports Med.* 1989;8(3):373-397.
41. Maron BJ, Ackerman MJ, Nishimura RA, Pyeritz RE, Towbin JA, Udelson JE. 36th Bethesda conference task force 4: HCM and other cardiomyopathies, mitral valve prolapse, myocarditis, and Marfan syndrome. *J Am Coll Cardiol.* 2005;45(8):1340-1345.
42. Maron BJ, Estes NAM, III, Link MS. 36th Bethesda conference task force 11: commotio cordis. *J Am Coll Cardiol.* 2005;45:1371-1373.
43. Cantwell JD. Automatic external defibrillators in the sports arena: the right place, the right time. *Physician Sportsmed.* 1998;26(12)(12):33-34, 76 (passim).
44. National Athletic Trainers' Association. *Official Statement from the National Athletic Trainers' Association on Commotio Cordis.* Dallas, TX: National Athletic Trainers' Association Web site; 2004.
45. Tanji JL. Exercise and the hypertensive athlete. *Clin Sports Med.* 1992;11(2):291-302.
46. Kaplan NM, Gidding SS. 36th Bethesda conference task force 5: systemic hypertension. *J Am Coll Cardiol.* 2005;45(8):1346-1348.
47. Chintanadilok J, Lowenthal DT. Exercise in treating hypertension: tailoring therapies for active patients. *Physician Sportsmed.* 2002;30(3)(3):11-23, 50 (passim).
48. Dimeff RJ. Headaches in athletes. *Clin Sports Med.* 1992;11(2):339-349.
49. Palatini P. Exaggerated blood pressure response to exercise: pathophysiologic mechanisms and clinical relevance. *J Sports Med Phys Fitness.* 1998;38(1):1-9.
50. Frenkel EP. Anemias. In: Beers MH, Berkow R, eds. *The Merck Manual of Diagnosis and Therapy.* 17th ed. Whitehouse Station, NJ: Merck Research Laboratories; 1999:849-883.
51. Raunikar RA, Sabio H. Anemia in the adolescent athlete. *Am J Dis Child.* 1992;146:1201-1205.
52. Chatard J, Mujika I, Guy C, Lacour J. Anaemia and iron deficiency in athletes: practical recommendations for treatment. *Sports Med.* 1999;27(4):229-240.
53. Nichols AW. Nonorthopedic problems in the aquatic athlete. *Clin Sports Med.* 1999;18(2):395-411.
54. Jones JD, Kleiner DM. Awareness and identification of athletes with sickle cell disorders at historically black colleges and universities. *J Athl Training.* 1996;31(3):220-222.

55. Browne RJ, Gillespie CA. Sickle cell trait: a risk factor for life-threatening rhabdomyolysis. *Physician Sportsmed.* 1993;21(6)(6):80-88.
56. Cleary MA. Sickle cell trait and exertional rhabdomyolysis. *Athl Ther Today.* 2003;8(5):66-67.
57. Harrelson GL, Fincher AL, Robinson JB. Acute exertional rhabdomyolysis and its relationship to sickle cell trait. *J Athl Training.* 1995;30(4):309-312.
58. Fiala KA, Ritenour DM. Medical care for athletes with hemophilia. *Athl Ther Today.* 2004;9(2):16-19.
59. Buzzard BM. Sports and hemophilia: antagonist or protagonist. *Clin Orthop.* 1996;328:25-30.
60. Nuber GW, McCarthy WJ, Yao JS, Schafer MF, Suker JR. Arterial abnormalities of the hand in athletes. *Am J Sports Med.* 1990;18(5):520-523.
61. Hoppenfeld S. *Physical Examination of the Spine and Extremities.* Norwalk, CT: Appleton & Lange; 1976.
62. Magee DJ. *Orthopedic Physical Assessment.* 2nd ed. Philadelphia, PA: WB Saunders Co; 1992.
63. Harmon KG, Roush MB. Pulmonary embolism: sifting the risk factors. *Physician Sportsmed.* 1998;26(12):53-56.
64. Nesheiwat F, Sergi AR. Deep venous thrombosis and pulmonary embolism following cast immobilization of the lower extremity. *J Foot Ankle Surg.* 1996;35(6):590-594.
65. Alexander JK. Pulmonary embolism. In: Beers MH, Berkow R, eds. *The Merck Manual of Diagnosis and Therapy.* 17th ed. Whitehouse Station, NJ: Merck Research Laboratories; 1999:593-601.
66. Hallett JWJ. Diseases of the aorta and its branches. In: Beers MH, Berkow R, eds. *The Merck Manual of Diagnosis and Therapy.* 17th ed. Whitehouse Station, NJ: Merck Research Laboratories; 1999:1776-1784.
67. Garten CE. Headaches and athletes. *Athl Ther Today.* 2005;10(3):28-29.
68. Committee on Sports and Fitness. Medical conditions affecting sports participation. *Pediatrics.* 2001;107(5):1205-1209.

Online Resources

Heart Sounds

Auscultation Assistant
    www.med.ucla.edu/wilkes/intro.html

Blaufuss Multimedia Heart Sounds and Cardiac Arrhythmia
    www.blaufuss.org

Frontiers in Bioscience
    www.bioscience.org/atlases/heart

HeartLab
    www.familypractice.com/heartlab/heartlab.htm

Other

Cardiomyopathy Association
    www.cardiomyopathy.org/html/which_card_hcm.htm

Hypertrophic Cardiomyopathy Association
    www.4hcm.org/WCMS/index.php

National Marfan Foundation
    www.marfan.org

Lab Exercise 6-1
Assessment of Vital Signs

Objectives

After completing this lab activity, students will be able to:

1. Measure and record resting and post-exercise blood pressure.
2. Measure and record resting and post-exercise heart rate.
3. Measure and record resting and post-exercise respiration rate.

Competencies Addressed

This lab exercise addresses the following psychomotor competencies from the NATA's *Athletic Training Educational Competencies, 4th ed*:

- Medical Conditions and Disabilities: 4a and 4b

Equipment Needed

- Stethoscope
- Watch displaying seconds
- Blood pressure cuff
- Treadmill or stationary bicycle

Instructions

Part 1: Assess resting blood pressure, heart rate, and respirations in at least five different individuals. Record your results below.

Subject #1:____________________ BP:________ HR:________ Resp:________

Subject #2:____________________ BP:________ HR:________ Resp:________

Subject #3:____________________ BP:________ HR:________ Resp:________

Subject #4:____________________ BP:________ HR:________ Resp:________

Subject #5:____________________ BP:________ HR:________ Resp:________

Part 2: Your partner (one of the subjects from Part 1 above) will perform 15 minutes of moderate exercise (75% of max heart rate) on a stationary bicycle or treadmill. As soon as your partner completes the exercise, assess his or her post-exercise blood pressure, heart rate, and respiration rate. Repeat the measurements 5 minutes and 10 minutes post-exercise. Record your results (p. 134). Answer the analysis questions (p. 134) based on your results.

Lab Exercise 6-1 (continued)
Assessment of Vital Signs

Immediately Post-Exercise
Subject:________________________ BP:_________ HR:_________ Resp:_________

5 Minutes Post-Exercise
Subject:________________________ BP:_________ HR:_________ Resp:_________

10 Minutes Post-Exercise
Subject:________________________ BP:_________ HR:_________ Resp:_________

Part 3: Analysis:

1. Prepare a line graph illustrating the change in systolic BP, diastolic BP, HR, and respirations from pre- and post-exercise intervals. Use your lab partner's vital sign values for the pre-exercise data points.

2. How would these lab findings affect your clinical evaluation of an athlete complaining of chest pain or shortness of breath during practice?

Lab Exercise 6-2
Cardiac Auscultation

Objectives

After completing this lab activity, students should be able to:

1. Locate the four "listening zones" for performing cardiac auscultation.
2. Correctly perform cardiac auscultation in the positions of supine, side-lying, and sitting.

Competencies

This lab exercise addresses the following psychomotor competencies from the NATA's *Athletic Training Educational Competencies, 4th ed*:

- Medical Conditions and Disabilities: 4b

Equipment Needed

- Stethoscope
- Exam table
- Female students will need to wear a tank top or sports bra

Instructions

1. Review the step-by-step instructions for cardiac auscultation provided in Table 6-7.
2. Locate the four listening zones (Figure 6-11) on yourself.
    a. Aortic (right second intercostal space)
    b. Pulmonary (left second intercostal space)
    c. Tricuspid (left, fourth or fifth intercostal space)
    d. Mitral (left fifth intercostal space in midclavicular line)
3. Place the diaphragm of the stethoscope over each of your four listening zones while simultaneously palpating your carotid pulse. This will enhance your ability to hear the heart sounds. The diaphragm should rest directly on the skin rather than on top of clothing. Listen to the heart sounds at each zone for several cardiac cycles.
4. With your lab partner lying supine, locate the four listening zones and listen to the heart sounds through several cardiac cycles.
5. Repeat Step 4 with your lab partner in left side-lying and seated leaning forward.
6. Perform cardiac auscultation on nine additional individuals with at least one of these being evaluated by your lab instructor or ACI.
7. If a teaching stethoscope is available, have each individual listen to and confirm the heart sounds at each zone. Record your completion of these auscultations on the form provided.

Lab Exercise 6-2 (continued)
Cardiac Auscultation

Student: ______________________________ Date:__________________________

Subject	Supine	Left Side-Lying	Seated
1. ____________ Date: __________	__M __T __P __A__	M __T __P __A	__M __T __P __A
2. ____________ Date: __________	__M __T __P __A__	M __T __P __A	__M __T __P __A
3. ____________ Date: __________	__M __T __P __A__	M __T __P __A	__M __T __P __A
4. ____________ Date: __________	__M __T __P __A__	M __T __P __A	__M __T __P __A
5. ____________ Date: __________	__M __T __P __A__	M __T __P __A	__M __T __P __A
6. ____________ Date: __________	__M __T __P __A__	M __T __P __A	__M __T __P __A
7. ____________ Date: __________	__M __T __P __A__	M __T __P __A	__M __T __P __A
8. ____________ Date: __________	__M __T __P __A__	M __T __P __A	__M __T __P __A
9. ____________ Date: __________	__M __T __P __A__	M __T __P __A	__M __T __P __A
10. ____________ Date: ___________	__M __T __P __A__	M __T __P __A	__M __T __P __A

Chapter Seven

Pulmonary System

Chapter Outline and Objectives

Introduction

Review of Anatomy, Physiology, and Pathogenesis

- ❖ Describe basic pulmonary anatomy and function.
- ❖ Review pathophysiological mechanisms of the pulmonary system.
- ❖ Describe the response of the pulmonary system to exercise.

Signs and Symptoms

- ❖ Identify the general signs and symptoms of pulmonary pathology.

Pain Patterns

- ❖ Identify the referred pain patterns associated with pulmonary pathology.

Medical History and Physical Examination

- ❖ Discuss medical history results that are relevant to pulmonary pathology.
- ❖ Perform physical examination tasks relevant to the pulmonary system.
    - Palpation
    - Percussion
    - Auscultation
    - Respiration Rate and Depth
    - Heart Rate
    - Blood Pressure
    - Peak-Flow Meter (Hand-Held Spirometer)

Pathology and Pathogenesis

Disorders of the Lung and Thorax

- ❖ Discuss the signs, symptoms, management, and medical referral guidelines for pulmonary pathology associated with trauma.

- Atelectasis
- Drowning and Near Drowning
- Flail Chest Injury
- Pneumothorax, Tension Pneumothorax, and Hemothorax
- Pneumomediastinum

Pulmonary Obstructive Disorders

❖ Discuss the signs, symptoms, management, and medical referral guidelines for pathology associated with pulmonary obstruction.

- Asthma
- Exercise-Induced Bronchospasm
- Exercise-Induced Anaphylaxis
- Chronic Obstructive Pulmonary Disease

Lung Cancer

❖ Discuss the risk factors, signs, symptoms, treatment, and prognosis associated with lung cancer.

Restrictive Lung Disorders

❖ Discuss the etiology of restrictive lung disorders.

Upper Respiratory Infections

❖ Discuss the signs, symptoms, treatment, and return-to-play guidelines associated with upper respiratory infections.

❖ Differentiate upper respiratory infections from other similar illnesses.

Influenza ("Flu")

❖ Discuss the signs, symptoms, treatment, and return-to-play guidelines associated with influenza.

Pediatric Concerns

❖ Discuss the common pulmonary disorders that affect children.

- Asthma in Children
- Cystic Fibrosis
- Neuromuscular Diseases
- Scoliosis
- Pertussis (Whooping Cough)

This chapter addresses the following competencies from the *Athletic Training Educational Competencies, Fourth Edition*[1]:

Domain	Cognitive	Psychomotor
Acute Care of Injuries and Illnesses	4, 8, 12, 16, 30	4e, 4g
Medical Conditions and Disabilities	1–3, 7–9	4
Pathology of Injuries and Illnesses	4–6	
Pharmacology	3	

Introduction

The pulmonary system extracts oxygen from the air and exchanges it with carbon dioxide in the blood, thus performing a critical life-sustaining function.[2] Pulmonary disorders are the second most frequent cause of disability and the fifth leading cause of death among adults. In addition, an estimated 14 to 15 million people have asthma, many of whom regularly participate in physical activity.[3] Chronic pulmonary diseases can be classified as either obstructive or restrictive.[3] Obstructive diseases (eg, asthma) limit air flow; restrictive conditions (eg, from scoliosis) limit physical lung expansion.[3]

Review of Anatomy, Physiology, and Pathogenesis

The lungs, consisting of the bronchi, alveoli, and a rich blood supply, are the primary organs of the pulmonary system (Figure 7-1). Air enters the nasopharynx, passes down the trachea, through the bronchi and bronchioles, and arrives in the alveoli. The capillary-rich alveoli, the terminal units of the respiratory pathway, exchange gases between the air and the blood. The other airway structures are physiological "dead space" since they do not participate in *respiration* (gas exchange). In some pulmonary disorders, the amount of this physiological "dead space" in the lung increases and creates a functional (ie, non-anatomic) obstruction to respiration.[2]

The upper airway, primarily the nasopharynx, adds warmth and moisture as it filters the incoming air.[2,4] Mucous and tiny hair-like projections (*cilia*) that cover the upper airway and bronchi serve to filter the incoming air. Particles in the air are trapped by the mucous, moved upward by the cilia, and expelled by coughing.

During the process called *ventilation,* air moves into and out of the lungs as an effect of pressure changing within the thorax in accordance with a principal of physics called Boyle's law. Boyle's law states that the relation between the volume and the pressure of a gas is constant; as volume increases, pressure decreases, and vice versa. During inspiration, as the diaphragm and external intercostal muscles contract, the thorax's circumference expands. The visceral and parietal pleura that lines the lungs and thorax maintain a negative pressure in the interpleural space—the space between the two pleura. Thus, when the thorax expands, this negative pressure in the interpleural space expands the lungs by keeping the lungs close to the wall of the thorax. As the pressure inside the thorax falls below atmospheric pressure, the lungs draw in air. Boyle's law demonstrates the effect: for a given volume of air at atmospheric pressure will flow toward lower pressure, which occurs when the lungs expand to increase their volume. Expiration of air occurs as elastic recoil of the ribcage compresses the lungs and alveolar pressure exceeds atmospheric pressure.[4]

Therefore, inspiration requires active muscle contraction, whereas expiration occurs passively, although some muscles can cause forceful expiration if needed.[4] Accessory inspiratory muscles include the abdominals, sternocleidomastoid, and scalenes, and can include the serratus anterior, pectoralis muscles, and upper trapezius as the task of inhalation becomes more difficult. The levator scapulae and trapezius also participate in cases of severe respiratory distress. Accessory muscles of ventilation are not normally active during quiet breathing, but do become active as oxygen demand or the work of breathing increases, as occurs during exercise.[4]

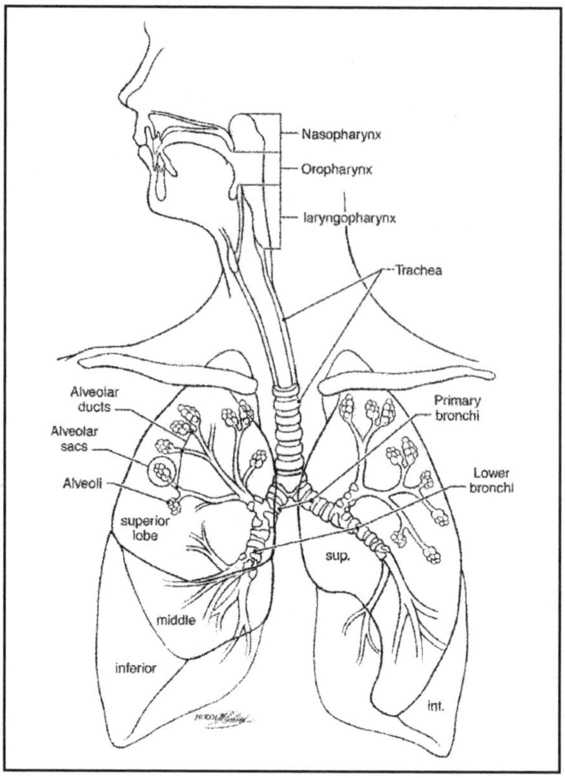

Figure 7-1. Schematic representation of the anatomy of the lungs.

Oxygen and carbon dioxide are exchanged in the alveoli by diffusion in a process called *respiration* (Figure 7-2). The rate of diffusion varies depending on the difference in the partial pressures of the gases at the alveolar wall. The diffusing capacity can be calculated as the volume of the gas entering the blood divided by the difference between the partial pressure of the gas in the aveoli and the partial pressure of the gas in the blood. Oxygen's partial pressure in the atmosphere (and therefore in the aveoli) is greater than its pressure in the alveolar capillaries, so oxygen moves into the blood across the single-celled walls of the alveoli.[2] Likewise, carbon dioxide moves into the alveoli since the partial pressure of carbon dioxide in the capillaries is greater than the pressure in the atmosphere (and the aveoli).[2]

Many complex mechanisms affect pulmonary gas exchange. When either ventilation or blood flow to the lungs is disrupted, the process of binding oxygen to hemoglobin is impaired. The amount of oxygen in the blood falls rapidly when this occurs, leading to hypoxemia, tissue hypoxia, and other severe physiological and metabolic consequences.

Ventilation is regulated by several mechanisms. The first mechanism involves regions of the medulla oblongata that are sensitive to carbon dioxide and pH levels in the blood.[4] Low pH indicates chemical acidity and high pH indicates alkalinity. Carbon dioxide, and most metabolic byproducts in the blood, are acidic and thereby decrease blood pH. The low pH stimulates the breathing center in the medulla oblongata, which increases ventilation rate and depth to expel the acidic waste products and rebalance pH.[2,4]

The second mechanism involves receptors that are sensitive to pressure, called baroreceptors, in the aorta and carotid arteries; these receptors detect changes in

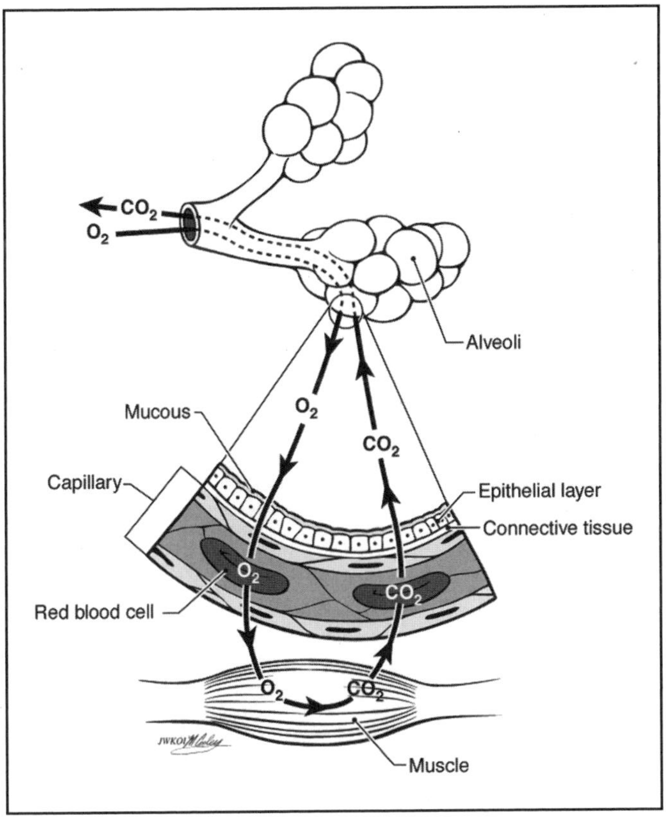

Figure 7-2. Diffusion of gases across the alveolar wall.

blood pressure. Chemoreceptors in the same areas detect decreases in blood oxygen levels. These two types of receptors act in concert to increase ventilation to maintain blood oxygen concentration.[2,4]

The third mechanism involves several processes in the nervous system. Stretch receptors in the intercostal muscles cause inspiration to stop and expiration to begin.[4] Neurons controlling the ventilation muscles (diaphragm, intercostals, and accessory muscles) travel through the phrenic nerve (from nerve roots C3-5), cranial nerve XI (sternocleidomastoid), and through the segmental thoracic nerves that supply the intercostal muscles.[4] Regions of the pons in the brainstem also contribute to the rate and depth of respiration. Damage to the spinal cord above vertebral level C3 or C4 usually necessitates the use of a ventilator. The neurological signal for voluntary control of breathing is passed from the brain through the corticospinal tracts to the diaphragm and intercostal neurons.[2]

Both ventilation and respiration are affected by exercise. First, the lungs receive more blood as heart rate and stroke volume (ie, cardiac output) increases. Next, during exercise the muscles use more oxygen, and the partial pressure of oxygen in the pulmonary vessels decreases. As a consequence, more of the oxygen in the inhaled air diffuses into the alveolar capillaries and is made available to the body. Third, the acid and buffering carbon dioxide produced by vigorously exercising muscles causes a reflexive increase in ventilation when the chemoreceptors of the carotid bodies are stimulated. Last, to meet the growing oxygen demand, the rate of ventilation increases; this increase occurs nearly immediately at the onset of exercise.[2]

Signs and Symptoms

Dyspnea

Dyspnea is a breathlessness or shortness of breath that occurs as blood oxygen level decreases. Airway obstruction, metabolic imbalances, psychological stress such as anxiety, mechanical restriction of the lungs, cardiac pathology, or pulmonary disease can cause dyspnea.[5]

Dyspnea produced by the supine position is called *orthopnea.* Orthopnea is a sign of fluid shift into the lungs, enlarged abdominal organs pushing on the diaphragm, or left-sided heart failure.[5]

Cough

A *cough* is a reflex contraction of the diaphragm that forces a blast of air from the lungs in an attempt to eliminate an irritation in the airway.[6] A dry, nonproductive cough is most often caused by allergic reactions to environmental irritants. A cough producing clear sputum, consisting primarily of watery mucus, suggests an upper airway irritation. *Purulent* sputum, containing pus, or opaque sputum are signs of lower respiratory infection.[5,7] *Hemoptysis,* a productive cough with blood in the sputum, is a sign of damaged lung tissue that requires prompt medical attention.[5-7]

Cyanosis

Cyanosis is a bluish tint in the fingernails, lips, face, and mucus membranes that occurs when oxygen saturation in arterial blood decreases below 85%.[4,5] Sudden onset of cyanosis indicates hypoxemia and is a medical emergency.

Pain Patterns

Pain from pathology in the pulmonary system rarely occurs without accompanying signs and symptoms, including coughing, wheezing, sore throat, and dyspnea. Pulmonary structures can refer pain to the chest, neck, and shoulders, as seen in Figure 7-3.

Lung

Tumors in the apex of the lung (Pancoast tumor) may compress the brachial plexus and vascular structures, causing pain and vascular symptoms (numbness, pallor, cramping) in the upper extremity. Tumors can also compress the bronchi, causing cough, dyspnea, or chest pain. Lung tissue usually does not produce pain until inflammation affects the parietal pleura (see below).[8]

Tracheobronchial

The trachea and proximal bronchial tree will refer pain to the overlying cutaneous areas.

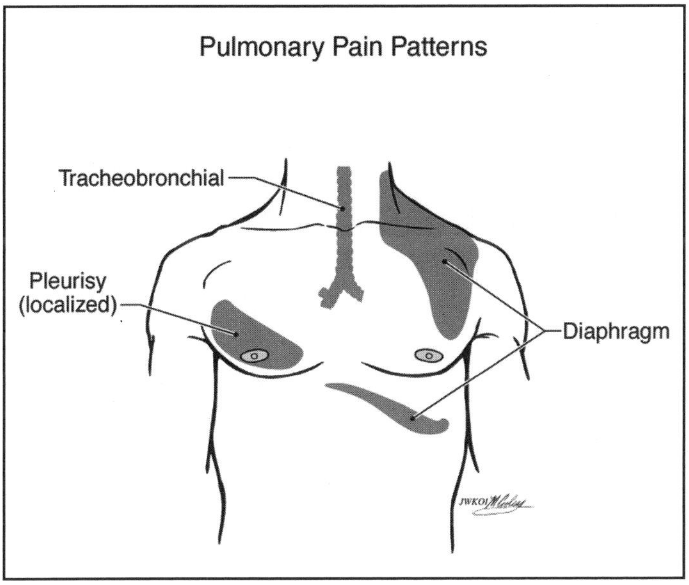

Figure 7-3. Pain patterns of pulmonary structures.

Diaphragm

Diaphragmatic pain usually refers to the ipsilateral shoulder, but may also occur in the neck, the ribs, or spine.[6] Abdominal hemorrhage is characterized by a similar pain referral pattern, resulting from irritation of the central diaphragm (see Chapter Eight).

Pleurisy

Pleural pain, or *pleurisy,* results from inflammation of the parietal pleura. Inflamed pleura creates sharp, stabbing pain over the affected area that worsens with coughing or deep inspiration.[5,6,8] Pleurisy can occur with trauma, infection, tumors, or pulmonary disease.

Medical History and Physical Examination

Family and Personal History

Cigarette smoking is a strong risk factor for virtually all acquired pulmonary disorders. A careful history can reveal a previously undetected chronic pulmonary disorder (intermittent symptoms with respiration, coughing, or sneezing) or infection (fever, recent infection, fatigue). Injury history that includes blunt trauma to the chest or sudden deceleration suggests pneumothorax or other lung injury.[9]

Symptoms

Dyspnea, cough, chest tightness, and decreased capacity for exercise (because of impairment of gas exchange) are common pulmonary symptoms. These symptoms may change with physical activity, deep breaths, speaking, or laughing.[3,10,11]

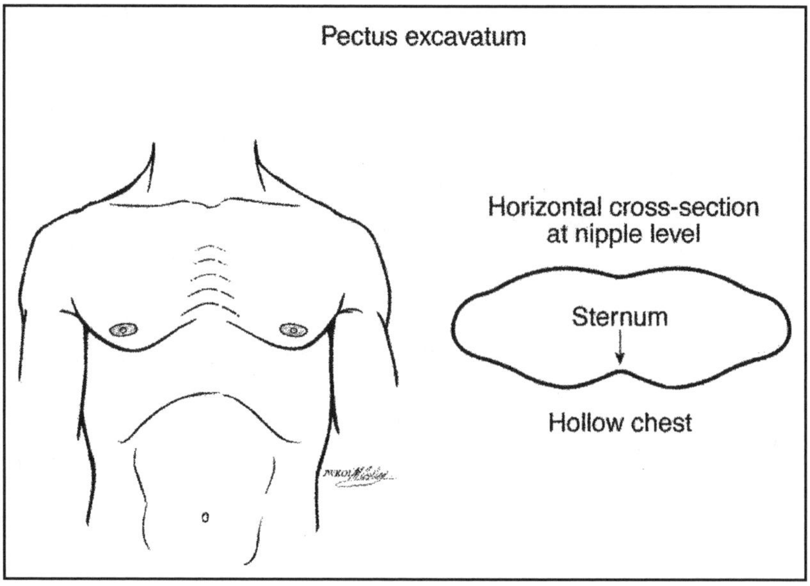

Figure 7-4a. Pectus excavatum.

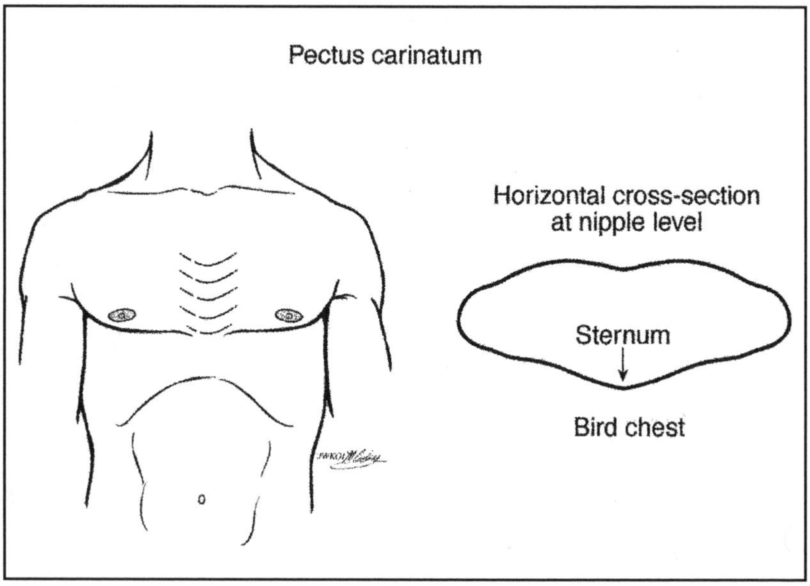

Figure 7-4b. Pectus carinatum.

Inspection

The ribcage and spinal column should be examined for obvious deformities or asymmetry that affects inspiration, such as pectus excavatum (Figure 7-4a), pectus carinatum (Figure 7-4b), scoliosis, or displaced rib fractures. Obesity can restrict ribcage expansion and diaphragm contraction, thus hindering breathing.[7]

Palpation

In sitting or supine, the mechanics of breathing can be evaluated by palpating and observing the motion of the ribcage. Bilateral palpation should be done at the superior, anterior, inferior, and posterior aspects of the ribcage. With normal inspiration, the ribcage moves symmetrically and the ribs and abdomen rise together.

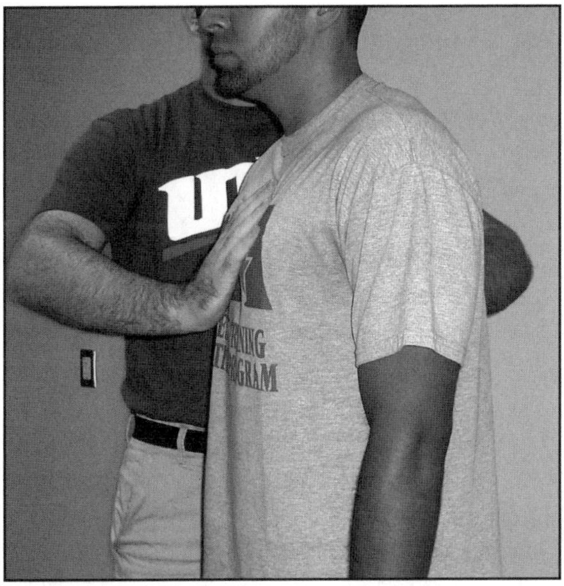

Figure 7-5a. Anterior compression test for a lateral rib fracture.

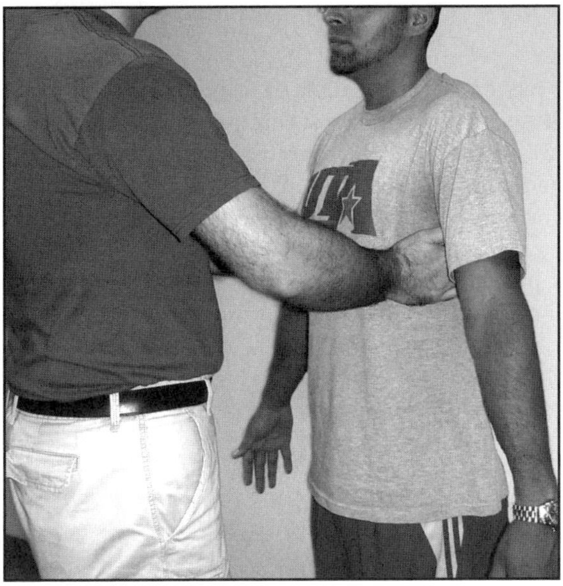

Figure 7-5b. Lateral compression test for an anterior or posterior rib fracture.

Examples of abnormal patterns are: the abdomen rising first; no movement of the ribcage; excessive use of accessory breathing muscles (sternocleidomastoid, abdominals, levator scapula, trapezius, pectoralis major and minor, serratus anterior); or asymmetrical expansion or contraction of the ribcage.[6] Palpation can also reveal *crepitus*, a subcutaneous grinding sensation, which indicates air leaking into the subcutaneous tissues, or *fremitus*, a subtle vibration with breathing, suggesting pulmonary or pleural edema.[9]

If a fracture is suspected, the ribs should be palpated for point tenderness, deformity, or crepitus. The rib compression test can be used to assess for possible rib fracture. If pain is produced with anteroposterior compression of the thorax, a lateral rib fracture should be suspected (Figure 7-5a). Conversely, pain produced by lateral compression of the thorax suggests an anterior or posterior rib fracture (Figure 7-5b)

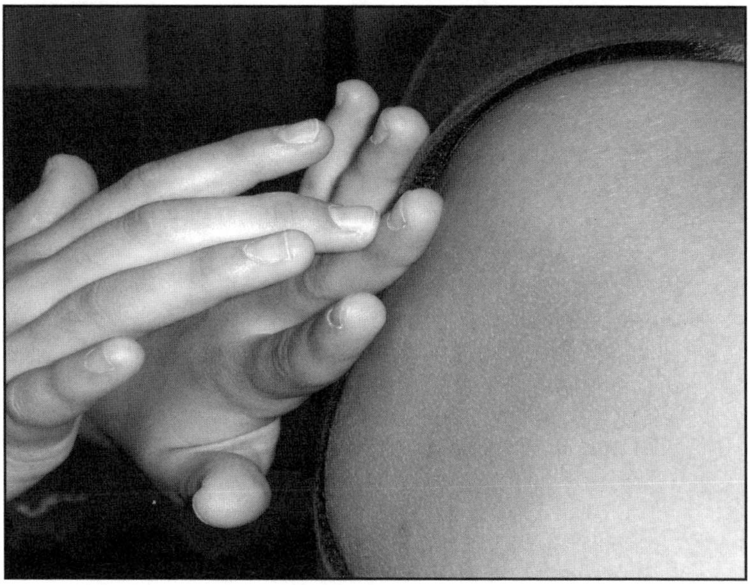

Figure 7-6. Hand posture for pulmonary percussion.

Percussion

Percussion plays an important part in the evaluation of pulmonary pathology, particularly those conditions caused by physical trauma. Percussion can help identify tissues as fluid-filled, air-filled, or solid. The skill of percussion requires practice, not just with the technique, but in listening for and identifying the different types of normal and abnormal sounds. The steps outlined below are for a right-handed examiner.

When performing pulmonary percussion, the examiner should hyperextend the third finger of the left hand. The volar surface of the DIP joint is then placed on the surface to be percussed. The rest of the third finger, as well as all of the remaining fingers should not touch the patient (Figure 7-6). The third finger of the examiner's right hand is used to apply the percussing blows. Position the right wrist in slight hyperextension, with the third finger flexed at the MCP and PIP joints. The tip of the third finger should be used to strike the DIP joint of the left hand. Striking with the pad of the finger is incorrect and will dampen the sound. The percussing blow should be performed with a quick tapping motion. The technique can be practiced on a variety of surfaces that can provide examples of normal and abnormal sounds. Percussing the anterior thigh will produce a flat or dull sound which might equate to the sounds produced by pleural effusion. Percussing your own puffed out cheek will produce a hollow, tympanic sound which might equate to the sounds heard when percussing over a pneumothorax (collapsed lung). If you feel as though you can not hear the percussion sounds well and need to "turn up the volume," press more firmly with the DIP surface of the left hand rather than striking harder with the right hand.

When percussing the thorax and lungs, the examiner should follow the numbered percussion sites illustrated in Figures 7-7a and 7-7b, tapping at least twice at each site. It is important to alternate between contralaterally matched sites to compare percussion sounds.[7] (Lab Exercise 7-1 provides an opportunity to practice pulmonary percussion.)

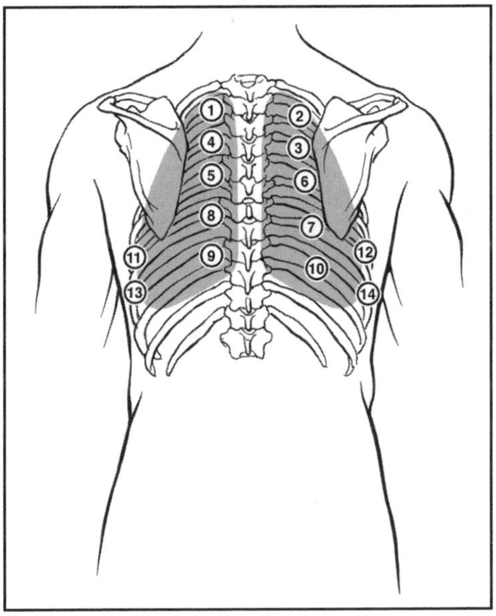

Figure 7-7a. Pattern of pulmonary percussion and auscultation: posterior.

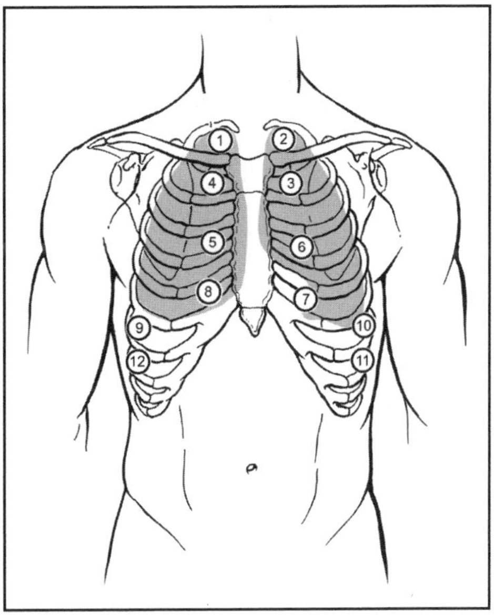

Figure 7-7b. Pattern of pulmonary percussion and auscultation: anterior.

Hyperresonance, percussion creating a sound like a tympanic drum, indicates an abnormal air space in the thorax, as occurs with pneumothorax.[9] Pulmonary edema, pleural edema, and hemothorax produces a dull thud rather than the normal hollow sound over the lungs.[7] Areas of the thorax that do not sound normal to percussion should be auscultated.[7]

Auscultation

When auscultating the lungs, the examiner should follow the same pattern as that used for percussion (see Figures 7-7a and 7-7b). Also as with percussion, auscultation should be performed alternating between contralaterally matched sites.[7,12] The diaphragm of the stethoscope should be placed firmly against the skin, with the examiner listening to at least one full breath at each site. Instruct the patient to take deep breaths with the mouth open. An alternate patient position can be used if examiners have difficulty hearing the lung sounds. This position maximizes the exposure of the thorax and involves having the patient seated, chin to chest, with the arms folded across the chest. (Lab Exercise 7-2 provides practice in auscultation of the lungs.)

Air passing through the stiff upper airway of the trachea and bronchi normally creates some turbulence, which can be auscultated. The softer alveoli tend to dampen transmission of sound, so auscultated sounds over the lung lobes are dull.

Normal breath sounds, when heard outside their normal anatomical regions are considered abnormal.[7] Normal tracheal and bronchial sounds are like wind rushing through a metallic tube, with the bronchial sounds slightly more muffled. The expiratory phase is usually louder than the inspiratory phase for both of these sounds. In contrast, vesicular breath sounds, described as "rustling leaves" and of a lower pitch than bronchial sounds, are heard over most of the thorax, with the inspiratory phase more prominent. Bronchovesicular sounds are similar to vesicular sounds upon inspiration and bronchial sounds upon expiration.[7]

Clearly heard spoken sounds (*bronchophony*), whispered sounds (*whispered pectoriloquy*), or high-pitched but intelligible spoken sounds (*egophony*) with auscultation are all abnormal.[7] These conditions occur when the lung and pleura are so inflamed and filled with exudate that they become "consolidated"—dense and solid rather than spongy and aerated—and can no longer exchange gases.

Inflammation of the pleura, obstruction of a bronchus, or atelectasis all cause "decreased breath sounds," in which the normal breath sounds are less audible or absent.[6,7] A complete absence of the normal breath sounds is, of course, also abnormal and warrants immediate referral.

The *adventitious* sounds, which are heard in addition to the normal breath sounds, include rales, rhonchi, stridor, and pulmonary friction rub.[7] *Rales* (pronounced *rahlz*) are a series of distinct pops or cracks during inspiration that occur when blocked bronchi cause a collapse of distal bronchioles and alveoli (ie, atelectasis).[6,7] *Rhonchi* are continuous rumbling sounds auscultated during both inspiration and expiration, indicating an incomplete obstruction of bronchi or lower trachea producing turbulent air.[6,7] *Stridor* is a harsh, raspy sound that is audible upon inspiration, often even without a stethoscope. Stridor is caused by a sudden and nearly complete obstruction of the airway by a foreign object or inflammation.[7] Stridor is a medical emergency. Stridor that occurs with coughing is called *croup.*[5] A pleural "friction rub" can be auscultated when the visceral and parietal pleura become inflamed. A friction rub sounds like a creaking or a clicking at the end of inspiration and is most commonly auscultated over the posterior and lateral thorax.[7] In addition, pain from the inflamed pleura may cause the person to pause during inspiration and expiration.

Respiration Rate and Depth

Breathing patterns are described by rate, depth, effort, and pattern. Normal breathing in adults is 10 to 15 breaths per minute, shallow (about 500 mL), relatively effortless, and regular. Children's breathing is more rapid (up to 20 breaths per minute). Changes in any of these parameters may suggest pulmonary impairment.

The relative length of inspiration and expiration is one-to-one; both phases last about the same amount of time.[2] In persons with obstructive pulmonary disorders the expiration phase is significantly longer than inspiration.[7]

An increased rate (over 20 breaths per minute) or depth (over 750 mL) of ventilation is called *hyperpnea.* An increase in breathing rate without an increase in depth, known as *hyperventilation,* rapidly decreases the partial pressure of carbon dioxide in the blood and increases pH, producing a state called respiratory alkalosis. Hyperventilation can be triggered by acidosis, in which the blood pH has increased due to a metabolic disorder such as diabetes mellitus (see Chapter Nine), or various psychological states such as anxiety or panic.

Hyperpnea is a medical emergency; psychogenic hyperventilation is not. Having a person hold their breath can discern metabolic hyperpnea from hyperventilation. Persons with hyperpnea have difficulty holding their breath because that will worsen their hypoxemia. In addition, other pulmonary signs, such as cyanosis and chest pain, are usually present. Psychogenic hyperventilation improves when the breath is held because it allows the carbon dioxide concentration and pH to return to normal.

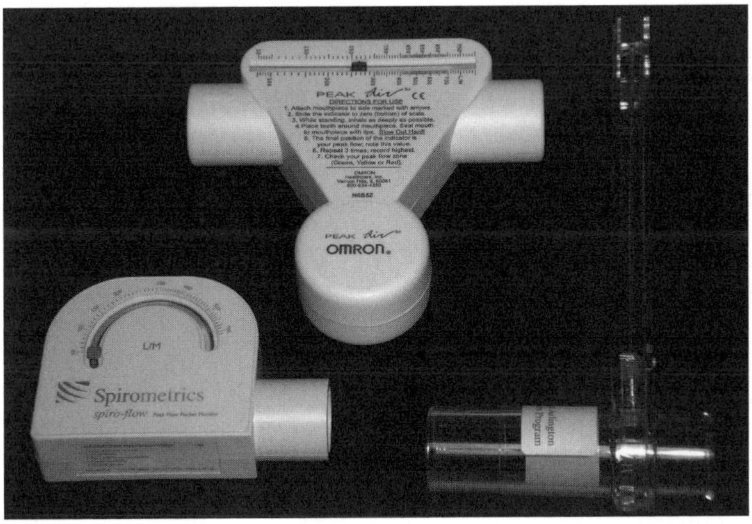

Figure 7-8. Peak flow meters.

Heart Rate

See Chapter Six. In general, the heart rate and respiration rate both increase and decrease together. Thus, a pulmonary condition that increases respiration rate will usually also increase the heart rate.

Blood Pressure

See Chapter Six. As the amount of oxygen in the blood decreases, the blood pressure rises to maintain the delivery of oxygen to the tissues.

Peak-Flow Meter (Hand-Held Spirometer)

A *spirometer* is an instrument used to measure lung volumes during ventilation. Spirometers typically found in athletic training environments are hand-held devices called peak-flow meters, which are portable and more practical than laboratory spirometers for clinical use (Figure 7-8). As the subject blows into a small tube after taking a full inspiration, an analog scale or dial indicates the volume of peak expiratory flow (PEF), which is the highest volume of air they can exhale. Usually measured in liters per minute (L/min), PEF is an indication of airway function and is often used to monitor the effectiveness of medications in managing asthma.[13] (Lab Exercise 7-3 provides practice in using a peak-flow meter.)

First, a "personal best" PEF is established over several days as a baseline measure. Then peak-flow meter measures are taken and compared to baseline each day immediately before physical activity. For persons with moderate to severe asthma, a PEF less than 80% of personal best indicates an impending acute bronchospasm, known as an asthma attack.[13-15] Prescribed medication (bronchodilators) may be used to restore PEF to near baseline value. If the medication does not restore PEF, as indicated by repeating the test, the person is held out of vigorous physical activity for that day.[16] If PEF falls below 50% despite taking medication, the person should be transported for emergency medical care.

Pathology and Pathogenesis

Pathology of the pulmonary system can affect the interstitial lung tissue, the wall of the thorax, or the bronchi. Pulmonary pathology may be caused by environmental influences, trauma, genetic factors, or immune responses. Table 7-1 outlines the mechanisms and signs and symptoms of the major pulmonary disorders.

Disorders of the Lung and Thorax

Atelectasis

Atelectasis (pronounced *at-uh-LECK-ta-sis*) is the collapse of a lung segment's alveoli; it is not itself a disease, but a consequence of disease or injury. Atelectasis is usually a result of a complete obstruction by an object or mucous lodged in the bronchi (Figure 7-9).[2] Atelectasis leads to pulmonary hypertension and cor pulmonale and increases risk for development of pneumonia. Patients who are bedridden are most at risk, but lung injury such as a severe blow to the thorax can also cause atelectasis. The signs of atelectasis are dyspnea, cough, and hemoptysis. Auscultation may detect diminished breath sounds or rales in the affected area. Depending on the amount of tissue damage, full recovery or return to sports can take a long time.[17]

Drowning and Near Drowning

Drowning causes many deaths each year among children, adolescents, and young adults. Water aspiration, when water is inhaled into the lungs, physically damages lung tissue, leading to atelectasis and infection. In addition, a drowning victim may asphyxiate—die from respiratory and ventilatory failure—as a result of a reflex spasm of the larynx.[18] Among near-drowning survivors, neurological and renal complications are the most obvious and disabling consequences. Time of immersion and temperature of the water determines the extent of tissue damage in these systems.

The inability to breathe underwater causes *anoxia,* a lack of oxygen, which produces severe, irreversible neurological and renal damage within minutes. Cold water temperatures, however, allow for longer immersion due to the mammalian diving reflex, which reduces metabolic demand.[18] A drowning rescue should continue resuscitation efforts until advanced medical care is obtained. While 90% of those rescued while drowning survive, 20% have permanent complications. Rapid, progressive respiratory failure can occur 12 to 24 hours after a near-drowning incident, so all such victims should be transported to a hospital for evaluation and observation.

Flail Chest Injury

A "flail chest" results from multiple anterior or posterior rib fractures creating a free-floating segment of ribcage (Figure 7-10). The affected region collapses upon inspiration and bulges upon expiration, referred to as "paradoxical excursion" of the chest. Flail chest injury is a medical emergency and is often accompanied by pneumothorax (collapsed lung).

Pneumothorax, Tension Pneumothorax, and Hemothorax

Pneumothorax, or a "collapsed lung," is the medical term for the presence of air in the pleural space, resulting either from a sudden increase in lung pressure or

Table 7-1
Types of Major Pulmonary Pathology

Pathology	Mechanism	Signs and Symptoms
Atelectasis	Bronchial obstruction	Dyspnea, cough, hemoptysis, diminished breath sounds or rales
Pneumothorax	Puncture of the pleura, leading to collapse of the pleural space	Acute chest pain, hyperpnea, decreased or absent breath sounds, hyperresonance upon percussion, subcutaneous crepitus, contralateral tracheal shift
Asthma	Intermittent bronchospasm, causing bronchial obstruction	Anxiety, dyspnea, coughing, wheezing, panting speech, cyanosis
Exercise-induced bronchospasm	Bronchospasm caused by environmental irritants (eg, cold, allergens) and exercise	Dyspnea, fatigue, abdominal discomfort, peripheral edema
Exercise-induced anaphylaxis	Anaphylactic shock precipitated by exercise	Cough, stridor, urticaria (hives), shock
Chronic obstructive pulmonary disease	Lower airway obstruction caused by mechanical insufficiency, bronchospasm, or inflammation	Cough, dyspnea, barrel chest, signs of chronic illness
Lung cancer	Chronic chemical or mechanical irritation of lung tissue	Cough, weight loss, fatigue, various pulmonary symptoms
Cystic fibrosis	Genetic abnormality of exocrine glands, causing blockage of the airway and intestines	Cough, wasting, signs of pulmonary infection

trauma causing pleural injury, such as a rib fracture.[2,9,17,19] The negative pressure in the pleural space that holds the lungs inflated is lost, and the lung retracts toward the bronchial tree (Figure 7-11). Without the negative pleural pressure, the lung cannot reinflate when the thorax expands.

Symptoms of pneumothorax include acute pleuritic chest pain and dyspnea. Signs including hyperpnea, decreased or absent breath sounds upon auscultation, crepitus (palpable subcutaneous air in the thorax), and hyperresonance upon percussion may be noted over the affected lung.[9,17,19] If the pleural space continues to collect air, a *tension pneumothorax* results, in which the intrathoracic pressure rises rapidly with respect to the environment (Figure 7-12). The trachea and mediastinum,

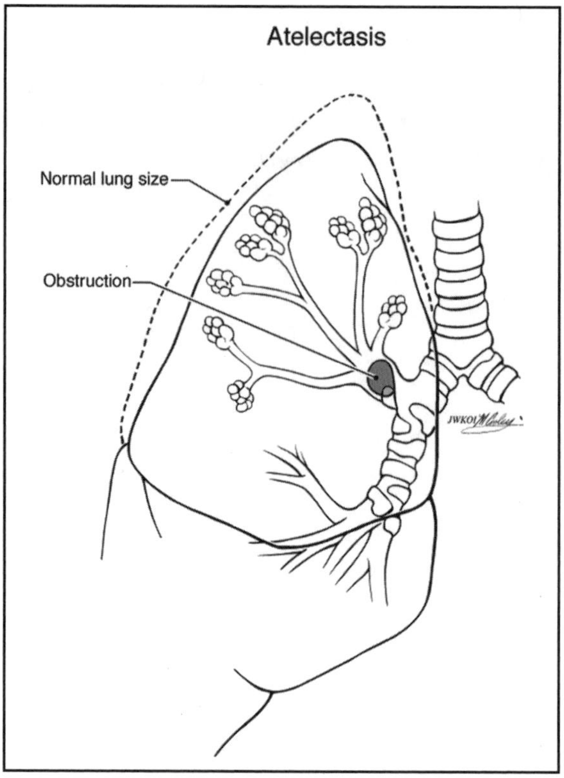

Figure 7-9. Atelectasis.

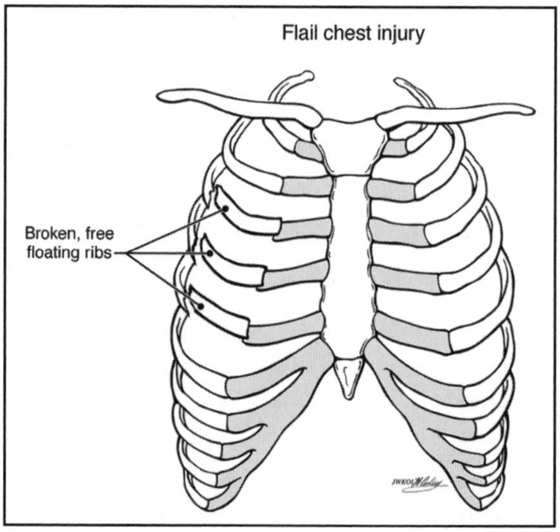

Figure 7-10. Flail chest injury.

the chest compartment that contains the heart and other structures, may deviate to the side opposite the collapsed lung and the thorax may twist asymmetrically.[17] If uncorrected, the pressure from the tension pneumothorax occludes the major vessels and compresses the heart, resulting in death. Treatment requires decompression with a chest tube, inserted surgically through the thorax wall. The tube provides an outlet to relieve the pressure of the air in the thorax.

Suspected pneumothorax is treated by splinting the thorax by hugging a pillow, calming the patient to control coughing or gasping for air, monitoring vital signs,

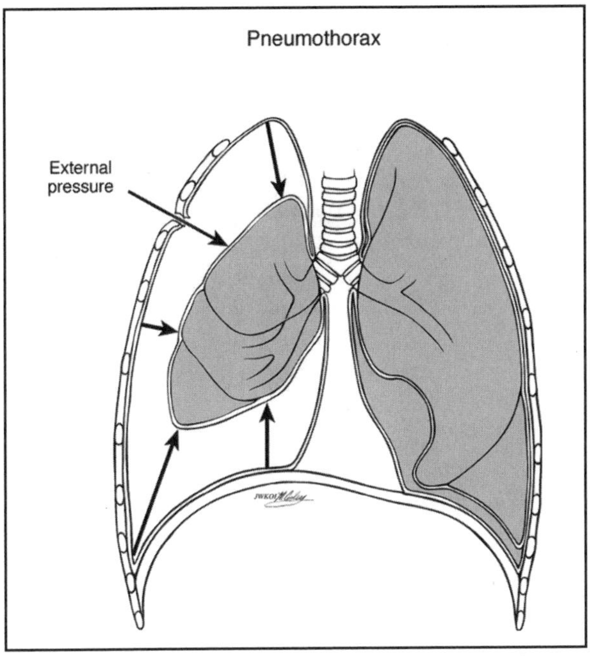

Figure 7-11. Pneumothorax.

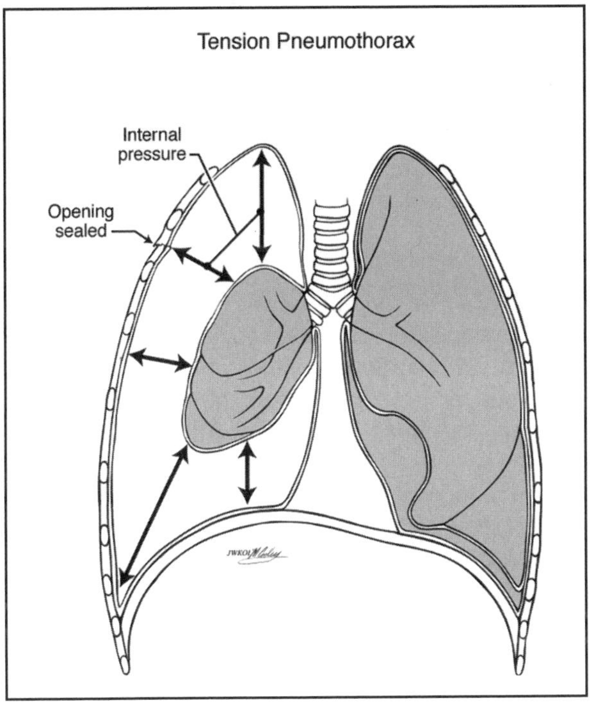

Figure 7-12. Tension pneumothorax.

sealing any open wounds with an occlusive dressing, and immediate emergency transport.[19] Returning to sports after pneumothorax (not tension pneumothorax or hemothorax) can occur within days of discharge from the hospital, if other injuries (eg, rib fractures) permit.[17] 911

Figure 7-13. Hemopneumothorax.

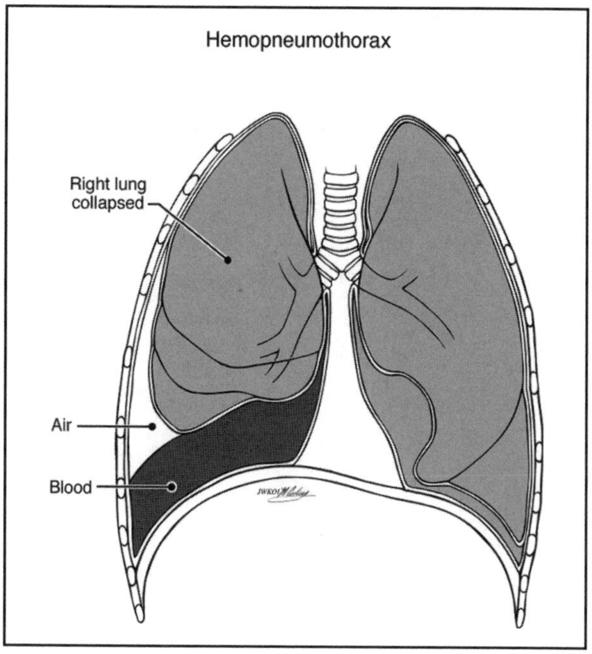

If blood enters the pleural cavity, the condition is called *hemothorax*. The presence of both blood and air in the thorax is a *hemopneumothorax* (Figure 7-13).[2] The signs and symptoms of hemothorax are similar to pneumothorax, but splashing can sometimes be auscultated in the lower lung lobes with changes in posture. Tension pneumothorax, hemopneumothorax, and pneumothorax with concomitant traumatic injuries require extensive medical care and a longer course of recovery.

Pneumomediastinum

Air can also spontaneously leak into the mediastinum, the anatomic space between pulmonary compartments, in a condition referred to as pneumomediastinum. Spontaneous pneumomediastinum occurs after a forceful effort that increases pressure in the thorax (eg, Valsalva maneuver, cough, or sneeze).[20,21] Asthma, diabetes, illicit drug use, anorexia nervosa, and pulmonary disorders are significant risk factors for this condition.[20]

Chest pain similar to pneumothorax appears, but is localized to the sternum rather than the lateral thorax.[21] Neck pain or difficulty swallowing (*dysphagia*) may also be reported.[6,20] Pneumomediastinum is usually not an emergency, usually resolving within 10 days unless a more serious condition (eg, pulmonary embolism, pneumothorax) is also present. Physical activity can be gradually resumed once there are no symptoms and the condition does not recur.[20]

Pulmonary Obstructive Disorders

The bronchi contain smooth muscle that widen or narrow the bronchial lumen. When these muscles contract abnormally, the bronchi may narrow to the extent that passage of air is impaired, creating, in effect, an obstruction. Bronchitis, rhinitis, and sinusitis, inflammation of the bronchi, nostrils, and sinuses, respectively, occur in the upper airway and can also cause obstruction in the airway. Typically, mild allergic reactions (*atopy*) cause rhinitis, infection or allergy cause sinusitis, and infection or environmental irritants cause bronchitis.

Asthma and exercise-induced bronchospasm are the most common obstructive disorders in physically active people. Other types of chronic obstructive pulmonary disorders (COPDs), such as emphysema and chronic bronchitis, are common in the general population.

Asthma

Asthma is a chronic abnormal autonomic response of the bronchial muscles that produces intermittent acute bronchospasm, partial airway obstruction, and chronic bronchial inflammation and edema.[10,22,23] Airway obstruction results from the combined effects of inflammation and bronchospasm.[16,23,24] The NATA has issued a detailed position statement regarding the recognition, evaluation, and management of asthma in athletes, including exercise-induced asthma.[15] Table 7-2 summarizes the recommendations of the NATA position statement.

Asthma affects between 5% and 10% of the population and is caused by various genetic and immune system factors.[23,24] Asthma causes epithelial cell damage and fibrous changes in the bronchioles, which can lead to a chronic reduction in air flow.

Symptoms of acute bronchospasm include a sensation of chest constriction, sudden fatigue, and anxiety.[3,13] Clinical signs are dyspnea, coughing, wheezing, prolonged expiration, panting speech, which may also be accompanied by leaning forward to assist breathing, cyanosis, and, in severe cases, seizure.[16] Hyperpnea and tachycardia occur when there is significant obstruction, as breathing becomes increasingly more difficult and hypoxemia increases.[16] Auscultation reveals decreased breath sounds and inspiratory rhonchi.[16]

Asthmatic bronchospasm may be precipitated by allergens (see Chapter Four), infection, cold or dry air, drugs, and certain emotional states.[10,13,14,24] Goals of asthma treatment include limiting bronchial inflammation, controlling symptoms, preventing exacerbation, maintaining normal pulmonary function, and limiting the side effects of medication.[14,23]

Asthma medications are administered through either inhaled or oral routes.[13,23] As discussed in Chapter Three, inhalation allows the medication to be delivered directly to the lungs, allowing it to have a quicker onset with fewer systemic side effects. There are three main types of inhalers commonly used by people who have asthma: metered dose inhalers (MDI), dry-powder inhalers (DPI), and breath actuated MDIs (Figure 7-14). The standard MDI is the most common type of inhaler used and delivers a metered dose of medication in the form of an aerosol mist. This type of delivery, however, requires good technique in timing the inhalation to coincide with the propelled mist. Poor technique results in a decreased amount of medication actually reaching the lungs. Plastic spacers can be used to extend the distance between the inhaler and the mouth and help reduce the effects of poor technique on medication delivery (Figure 7-15). For optimum dosing, patients should be instructed in the proper techniques for using their inhalers. Table 7-3 provides step-by-step instructions for using a standard MDI.[25]

Asthma is managed using anti-inflammatory medications (corticosteroids, mast cell stabilizers, and antileukotrienes) to control the underlying chronic inflammation and provide long-term control and bronchodilators (β_2–agonists) to provide

Table 7-2

Recommendations from the NATA's Position Statement Regarding the Management of Asthma in Athletes

- During the preparticipation examination, athletes should be screened for asthma.
- The athletic trainer should be aware of the signs and symptoms that are suggestive of asthma, including chest tightness, coughing, shortness of breath, wheezing, and limitation of physical activity due to breathing difficulty.
- Pulmonary testing may be indicated for athletes with a history of asthma or athletes in whom the diagnosis of asthma cannot be excluded by medical history alone.
- An asthma action plan should be incorporated into the overall emergency plan of a sports medicine service.
- Athletes who have asthma should have a rescue inhaler available at all times, and the athletic trainer should have access to a nebulizer for emergencies.
- Alternate workout sites should be considered when possible to avoid allergens that may trigger an asthma attack.
- Patients with asthma should have regular follow-up visits with their physician to monitor and modify the individualized treatment regimen.
- Athletic trainers should be familiar with the pharmacological interventions used in the treatment of asthma.
- Proper warm-up may provide a refractory period lasting up to 2 hours.
- Athletes should be educated about asthma, including signs and symptoms, potential triggers, proper use of spirometry, pharmacological and nonpharmacological supportive treatments, use of metered dose inhalers and nebulizers, and that asthma need not limit participation in sports and other physical activities.
- Athletic trainers should be aware of other medical conditions that may mimic the signs of asthma, including vocal cord dysfunction and other upper respiratory diseases.
- Patients with asthma should be encouraged to exercise.
- Athletic trainers should be able to differentiate between restricted, banned, and permitted asthma medications relative to participation in organized competitive sports.
- Web sites are available for more information, including the American Academy of Allergy, Asthma & Immunology (www.aaaai.org); the American Thoracic Society (www.thoracic.org); the Asthma and Allergy Foundation of America (www.aafa.org); and the American College of Allergy, Asthma & Immunology (www.acaai.org).

quick relief from acute bronchospasm.[13] It is important that asthmatics understand the difference between these two types of medication. While anti-inflammatories should be taken on a daily basis, bronchodilators should be used on an as needed basis. Noncompliance with the anti-inflammatory medications can lead to more frequent acute attacks and more scarring within the lungs. Likewise, inappropriate use of an anti-inflammatory to treat an acute asthma attack can lead to serious consequences. Confusion between these two types of drugs is compounded when both medications are delivered by inhaler. Athletic trainers should be familiar with

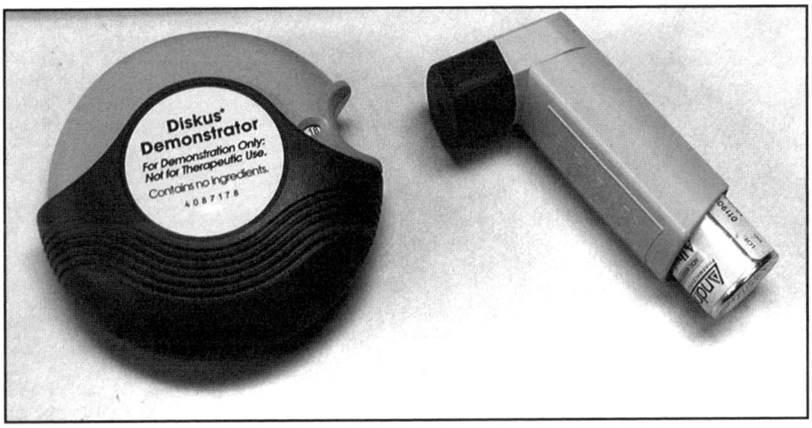

Figure 7-14. Types of inhalers used by people who have asthma.

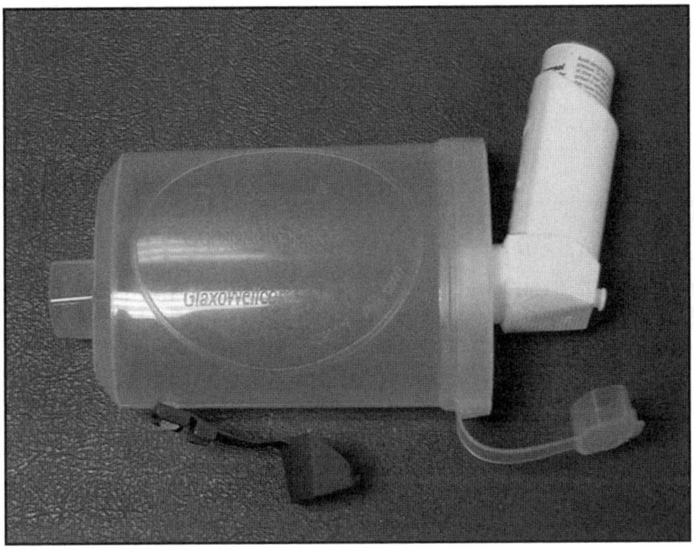

Figure 7-15. Plastic spacer used to improve medication delivery from an inhaler.

the asthma drugs used by their patients and play an active role in ensuring their proper use. Table 7-4 provides a listing of the common drugs used to treat asthma and their routes of delivery.

A severe asthma attack can produce a pneumothorax, acute right heart failure, hypoxemia, and metabolic collapse.[16] To manage an acute asthma attack, the person should sit, take deep breaths and exhale through pursed lips, which increases pressure throughout the airway. An attempt should be made to calm the person emotionally. Administration of a bronchodilator, if prescribed, is indicated; the typical dose is one puff followed by a second dose five minutes later. Recovery should occur gradually and in less than 1 hour. Severe attacks that do not respond to these measures should be treated as an emergency.

Exercise-Induced Bronchospasm

Exercise-induced bronchospasm (EIB), also known as exercise-induced asthma, is more common than asthma, affecting approximately 15% of the population; 90% of people with asthma and 35% to 40% of people with allergies experience

Table 7-3

Procedures for Using a Typical Metered Dose Inhaler

Step 1.	Prepare the MDI according to the directions on the container (eg, shake canister).
Step 2.	Hold the inhaler upright and tip the head back slightly.
Step 3.	Exhale slowly.
Step 4.	Place the inhaler (or spacer with inhaler attached) in the mouth and seal the lips securely around the mouthpiece of the inhaler (or spacer).
Step 5.	Press down on the inhaler to release the medication and at the same time take a slow, deep inhalation.
Step 6.	Hold the breath for about 10 seconds before exhaling.
Step 7.	If another puff is needed of a quick-relief inhaler, wait about 1 minute before taking the second puff. This will give time for the first puff to begin working and may improve the effectiveness of the second puff.
Step 8.	When using a corticosteroid, rinse mouth out with water.

Table 7-4

Medications Commonly Used to Treat Asthma

Generic Name	Trade Name	Type	Action	Route of Delivery
albuterol	Proventil	Bronchodilator	Quick relief	Inhalation
cromolyn	Intal	Mast cell stabilizer	Long term	Inhalation
fluticasone	Flovent	Corticosteroid	Long term	Inhalation
ipratropium	Atrovent	Anticholinergic	Quick relief	Inhalation
montelukast	Singulair	Antileukotriene	Long term	Oral
pirbuterol	Maxair	Bronchodilator	Quick relief	Inhalation
prednisolone	Prednisolone	Corticosteroid	Quick relief	Oral
salmeterol	Serevent	Bronchodilator	Long term	Inhalation
zafirlukast	Accolate	Antileukotriene	Long term	Oral

EIB.[10,26-28] EIB occurs 5 or 10 minutes into an exercise session and becomes progressively worse as activity continues. Spontaneous recovery occurs 30 to 60 minutes after stopping exercise.[3,10,11,26,29] In contrast to asthma, EIB that is not associated with asthma does not produce chronic inflammation in the bronchioles.

Cool or dry air and breathing through the mouth during vigorous exercise have been identified as factors that may exacerbate EIB. Allergens, infection, or pollution have also been identified as potential triggers.[11,26-28] Symptoms include unusual dyspnea and central chest pain during exercise.[3,10,11,26] Coughing after strenuous exercise is another common sign of EIB, which may also be accompanied by an ache in the gut. Syncope and cyanosis may appear if air flow into the lungs is significantly obstructed, producing hypoxemia.[3,10,11,26]

Diagnosis is made by measuring the amount of air that can be moved from the lungs in one second before and after exercise on a treadmill or cycle ergometer. EIB is identified if the post-exercise value is more than 15% below the pre-exercise value.[27] Preventative treatment involves control of underlying asthma (if present), preventative medication, and environmental precautions, mainly avoiding cold, dry air during exercise.[3] In addition, a prolonged warm-up (60 minutes before competition, exercise for 10 to 15 minutes at 50% maximal heart rate, rest 15 minutes before beginning full exercise session) induces mild EIB followed by a refractory period during which EIB will not recur.[11,26,29] If control of onset of bronchospasm cannot be obtained, switching sports or exercise in humid, warm environments may be indicated.[3] Bronchodilators, either oral or inhaled, effectively control EIB, but have undesired side effects for physical activity, such as anxiety, tremor, and tachycardia. In addition, many of these medications are banned by competitive athletic associations.[11,26]

Acute EIB is managed much like an acute asthma attack. The person is removed from exercise, reassured emotionally, evaluated to rule out exercise-induced anaphylaxis (see below), and monitored until symptoms resolve. EIB that persists for more than 60 minutes, or produces syncope or cyanosis at any time, is an emergency.

Exercise-Induced Anaphylaxis

A history of breathing problems during exercise combined with chronic use of nonsteroidal anti-inflammatories (NSAIDs) increase the risk of exercise-induced anaphylaxis (EIA), an abnormal immune response to vigorous physical activity.[26] The anaphylactic reaction causes a widespread release of histamine, an inflammatory chemical that causes vasodilatation throughout the body. This reaction also causes acute bronchospasm. Recognition of EIA is important; in contrast to asthma and EIB, which are not typically emergencies, EIA is always life-threatening.

EIA causes a "flush" sensation in the head and neck during exercise that is rapidly followed by coughing, stridor, and shock.[10] Multiple skin lesions (*urticaria* or hives) one-half inch to one inch in size may appear.[26] Wheezing and other signs of bronchospasm are usually not present, but a resonant or barking-type cough (*croup*) may appear and the person may report a choking sensation as the condition progresses and the airway becomes progressively more obstructed.[26,30] Hypotension and tachycardia herald the onset of shock.

Administration of epinephrine (via EpiPen [Meridian Medical Technology, Bristol, Tenn]; see Chapter Three), maintaining an airway, administering supplemental oxygen, and emergency transport to a hospital are indicated. Intravenous medications, such as adrenaline, are required to reverse the vasodilation and open the airway.[26] Modifying behavior, such as avoiding known irritants or exercising several hours after exposure to an irritant, and use of antihistamines may be preventative.[30]

Chronic Obstructive Pulmonary Disease

Chronic obstructive pulmonary disease (COPD) is a classification for diseases involving partially blocked airways. Examples of COPD include bronchitis, emphysema, and cystic fibrosis.[7,22] Obstruction caused by mechanical insufficiency, bronchospasm, or inflammation traps air in the lower airway increasing residual volume, the air remaining in the lungs, and decreasing the volume of air exchanged during ventilation, called vital capacity. These effects mean that less fresh air is available for gas exchange. In addition, carbon dioxide concentration increases and oxygen concentration decreases in the lungs, thus decreasing the diffusion gradient for these gases between the alveoli and capillaries and impairing gas exchange.[22]

Acute bronchitis is most frequently a result of an infection or chemical irritant that produces an inflammatory response; viral infection is the most common cause.[28] Early signs and symptoms include fever, nonproductive cough, sore throat, and musculoskeletal chest pain from violent and persistent coughing. Acute bronchitis progresses to a productive cough, wheezing, and systemic signs of infection, such as fever. Cough suppressants, rest, and hydration are the usual course of treatment; antibiotics should only be prescribed if a bacterial organism is identified.[28] If neglected, the edema and irritation produced by acute bronchitis provide an ideal environment to produce a severe bronchial infection.

Chronic bronchitis is caused by prolonged or repeated exposure to irritants that inflame the bronchial mucous membranes. The chronic inflammation decreases the functional diameter of the bronchi and impairs airflow. As the distal bronchioles become completely obstructed, air is trapped in the alveoli. This causes hypoxemia and cyanosis because the trapped air is quickly depleted of oxygen, and causes pulmonary hypertension because the hypoxemia causes vasoconstriction of the pulmonary vasculature. Right ventricular hypertrophy develops in response to the pulmonary hypertension (cor pulmonale), which in turn leads to the development of peripheral edema as blood return to the heart is impaired.

Wheezing and dyspnea appear, and fever may develop. The cough associated with chronic bronchitis is more productive in the mornings and evenings; the cough is an attempt to clear the airway of mucous and other fluids produced by the inflammation. A cough that is present 3 months a year for 2 consecutive years and accompanied by reduced expiratory capacity with no other medical explanation suggests chronic bronchitis.[22]

Emphysema, a complication of chronic pulmonary disease and prolonged smoking, is not likely to be encountered in physically active persons.[22] Emphysema is a chronic inflammatory reaction to chemicals in smoke that destroys the alveolar walls, capillaries, and lung elasticity, and decreases the lung area that is available for gas exchange. The signs and symptoms are dyspnea, increased breathing effort, a barrel-chested (hyperinflated) appearance, and signs of infection and cor pulmonale. The lung damage in emphysema is irreversible and prognosis for recovery is poor.

Lung Cancer

Lung cancer causes more cancer-related deaths in America among both genders than any other type of cancer. There are approximately 170,000 cases diagnosed each year, and more than 160,000 deaths annually are attributed to lung cancer. Lung cancer is associated with smoking; people who smoke are at a much larger risk for lung cancer. Up to 90% of lung cancer occurs in persons who smoke. Smoking is thus the major risk factor for development of lung cancer.[31] Smoking and use of other tobacco products also greatly increases the risk of oral and throat cancers. Chronic exposure to other chemicals (asbestos, hydrocarbons, polyethylenes, etc) and radiation also increases the risk of lung cancer.[31]

Lung cancer is rarely diagnosed before age 35, most frequently occurring among people over age 45. In early stages, pulmonary symptoms may be mild, such as a persistent productive cough, which is so common among people who smoke that it may be ignored.[31] As the lung cancer advances, loss of appetite, weight loss, and fatigue from impaired pulmonary function may occur.[31] Depending on the location of the tumor within the lung, dyspnea, stridor, pneumonia, pleurisy, and hemoptysis may appear. A tumor in the superior lung may grow large enough to impinge on the brachial plexus, causing shoulder and arm pain. Diagnosis is made with chest x-rays and laboratory tests.

Treatment is surgical resection of the affected portion of the lung, radiation therapy, chemotherapy, or a combination of these techniques. Treatment depends on the stage and extent of the tumor. Due to difficult early detection, prognosis is generally poor.[31] Less than 15% of patients survive 5 years after diagnosis. Bony metastases are very common and may cause chest (ribs), neck, or back (vertebrae) pain. The lungs also very commonly develop metastatic tumors from cancer of other organs.[31] Survival for lung cancer is poor. Five-year survival for early stage lung cancer is less than 50%; for advanced lung cancer, 5-year survival is less than 2%. Certain types of lung cancer (small cell carcinoma) have 5-year survival rates less than 10% even when detected in the earliest stage.

Restrictive Lung Disorders

Scarring of the lung from trauma, surgery, chemotherapy, or radiation can physically limit lung volume and, consequently, limit pulmonary function.[3] Decreased air flow decreases the amount of oxygen being delivered to the lungs and, consequently, the body. Physical activity is limited by the decreased respiratory function and capacity.[3]

Upper Respiratory Infections

Several types of viruses produce upper respiratory infections (URIs).[6,10-13] For example, most common colds (*coryza*) are the result of infection by a rhinovirus.[10,13] URIs produce a common set of signs and symptoms, including rhinitis, rhinorrhea, sore throat, nonproductive cough, sneeze, headache, malaise, chills, low-grade fever, laryngitis, and arthralgia.[4,10,12] The number of coughs, sneezes, and need to blow the nose per day can be used to track progression of an URI since their frequency decreases as recovery occurs.[12] Most cases of URIs last approximately 7 to 10 days.

Ear infections and sinus infections are two complications that may arise from URIs. Acute sinusitis will present with a similar clinical picture to the common cold, often making it difficult to differentiate the two infections. Differentiating symptoms of sinusitis can include tooth pain, facial or sinus pressure and pain, nasal congestion or discharge, and foul breath.[14]

URIs are contagious, spreading from person to person through contact with an infected person's respiratory secretions.[10] Hand-to-hand contact after touching the mouth, nose, or eyes appears to be the most efficient mode of transmission.[12] The virus is active for at least 8 days following the initial infection, during which the person may transmit the virus; communicability is highest in the first 72 hours.[12,13] Frequent hand washing and avoidance of persons known to have an URI can prevent its spread. For most effective hand washing, you should continuously scrub your hands for approximately 20 seconds or the time it takes to sing one verse of the happy birthday song.

Recognition of URI and support of the immune system with rest, fluids, and nutrition can limit the duration of the infection. Antibiotics, which are effective against bacterial infections, usually have no role in the treatment of a viral URI. Over-the-counter medications can be used to treat the symptoms and therefore reduce the individuals discomfort during the course of the infection. Analgesics such as acetaminophen and ibuprofen are effective in treating the headache and fever associated with URIs. Aspirin should not be used by children and adolescents under the age of 12 due to the risk of developing Reye's syndrome. Although rare, Reye's syndrome has been reported in children who had viral infections and ingested aspirin. This potentially life-threatening illness is signaled by altered mental status and severe vomiting. Antihistamines are effective in treating the runny nose and sneezing. Daytime dosing or dosing in individuals who need to remain alert should include loratadine (Claritin [Schering-Plough, Kenilworth, NJ]), fexofenadine (Allegra [Sanofi Aventis, Bridgewater, NJ]), or other second-generation antihistamines (see Chapter Three). Since diphenhydramine (Benadryl [McNeil Consumer Healthcare, Fort Washington, Pa]) is known to produce drowsiness, it is a better choice for bedtime dosing. An antitussive, like dextromethorphan, can be used to suppress a dry hacking cough. Sucking on cough drops containing dextromethorphan or menthol can also suppress the cough and provide some anesthetic relief to a sore throat. Codeine and hydrocodone are generally more effective in cough suppression; however they have a higher potential for dependency and are only available by prescription. Decongestants are effective in reducing nasal congestion and are available in oral form as well as in sprays, inhalers, and drops. Pseudoephedrine is a common oral nasal decongestant and can provide relief within 30 minutes of dosing. Nasal decongestant sprays should only be used for a short period of time (3 to 5 days) since they can result in rebound congestion. Also, some nasal decongestants are banned by certain drug-testing authorities.

Due to the multitude of symptoms associated with URIs, many individuals choose a multisymptom reliever product such as Tylenol Cold and Sinus (McNeil Consumer Healthcare) or NyQuil (Procter & Gamble, Cincinnati, Ohio), which may contain a pain reliever, antihistamine, decongestant, and cough suppressant. The specific antihistamine included in the product determines whether it is better suited for day time or night time dosing (as discussed in Chapter Three). Although these medications are more convenient than taking several different medications, they can be associated with adverse reactions when taken with other medications. For example, taking a NSAID along with a multisymptom cold product containing ibuprofen can lead to gastric discomfort due to the additive effect of taking two NSAIDs. Athletes should be aware that some multisymptom cold relievers containing decongestants may cause them to fail a drug test. Also of note when treating athletes, athletic trainers should be aware that taking systemic antihistamines and decongestants can contribute to heat-related illnesses.

Athletes who are experiencing symptoms of URI should limit their activities until the fever resolves to avoid fatigue and dehydration and to prevent infecting their teammates.[10,12] Some physicians use the "neck rule" in determining return-to-play in individuals with a URI. Individuals with symptoms above the neck only (runny nose, sore throat, etc) and no fever may return to activity. Persons with below the neck symptoms (cough, body aches, etc) or fever should not exercise until 24 hours after the symptoms are gone.[4,14] If no evidence of cardiac, pulmonary, gastrointestinal, or other systemic involvement appears, full activity can resume within a few days.[6,7,10,13]

Influenza ("Flu")

"Flu" is often incorrectly used as a general term for a URI, but more correctly describes a disease caused by the influenza virus. Influenza infections occur annually, usually beginning in the fall, peaking in winter, and lasting into early spring. Influenza virus occurs in three recognized strains, called A, B, and C; the A strain is the one most commonly associated with large seasonal outbreaks of flu. The A strain of the influenza virus mutates slightly each year, appearing as variants or strains, rendering vaccination only partially effective. Vaccination is the injection of deactivated virus antigens, which stimulates antibody formation. The antibodies then recognize the virus upon infection and can mount a more effective immune response.

Influenza virus travels from person to person in respiratory secretions, which are either inhaled as airborne droplets or picked up by touching contaminated objects. After *incubation* (time between infection and appearance of symptoms) of two days, fever, myalgia, headache, and upper respiratory symptoms (rhinitis, rhinorrhea, sore throat, sneezing) appear. As infection progresses, a productive cough (ie, with sputum, signifying a lower respiratory infection) develops, as well as pharyngitis, conjunctivitis, and nausea.

The active stage lasts 2 to 3 days, followed by a reduction in fever, diaphoresis, and fatigue (ie, "breaking" fever) that may last several additional days. Secondary infections of the respiratory tract with additional bacteria or viruses may coexist, producing hemoptysis, recurrent fever, purulent sputum, or progressive dyspnea. As mentioned above, aspirin is not recommended for use among children with viral infections due to the risk of developing Reye's syndrome.

Treatment for influenza is generally supportive to address the symptoms. The use of an expectorant, such as guaifenesin, can help thin mucus secretions allowing them to be removed from the respiratory tract by coughing. Nausea is a common side effect reported by some individuals when taking guaifenesin. The body's immune response is the primary mechanism by which the infection is addressed. People with weaker immune responses, including young children and older people, cannot fight the viral infection as effectively. As a result, influenza can be fatal in these groups; hospitalization is often required to maintain hydration.

Occasionally antiviral medications are used prophylactically to prevent the spread of the virus throughout an athletic team or to reduce the duration of the virus when administered at the first sign of symptoms. Amantadine (Symmetrel [Endo Pharmaceuticals, Chadds Ford, Pa]) and rimantadine (Flumadine [Forest Laboratories, New York, NY]) are both effective in preventing and reducing the duration of influenza A. Zanamivir (Relenza [GlaxoSmithKline, Brentford, Middlesex, UK]) is effective in treating both influenza A and B. Possible side effects associated with these medications include nausea, nervousness, anxiety, lightheadedness, and insomnia.

Pediatric Concerns

Asthma in Children

Asthma causes a large number of missed school days and is one of the most common chronic illnesses in children. Exposure to respiratory viruses in infancy or childhood has been suggested as a precipitating factor; the first asthma attack may at first appear to be a simple case of coryza (the common cold) before progressing to bronchospasm. Childhood attacks vary in severity, but are similar in clinical presentation to adolescent or adult asthma attacks: wheezing, dyspnea, nonproductive cough, and use of accessory breathing muscles. If the attack progresses in severity, cyanosis and tachycardia appear; in extreme cases, wheezing is not heard because the airway is collapsing. A rapid progression may require emergency care.

Asthma in children is treated by avoidance of known allergens and medication, similar to patients of other ages.

Cystic Fibrosis

Cystic fibrosis (CF) is the most commonly inherited disorder among Caucasian Americans.[3,32] The genetic abnormality affects the exocrine glands, primarily those of the respiratory system, pancreas, and intestines.[32] Thick secretions from these glands block the airway, which tends to become infected.[3,22] Pneumonia, a bacterial pulmonary infection, is recurrent, progressively disabling, and eventually fatal. Blockage of glands also occur in the pancreas and instestines, producing the respective effects of malnutrition from a lack of pancreatic enzymes to aid digestion and peritonitis from intestinal obstruction followed by rupture. Either effect may also cause death. Only half of people with CF will live to 30 years of age.[3,22,32]

Treatment for cystic fibrosis includes nutritional support, regular pulmonary hygiene to clear secretions, and antibiotic medications.[3,22,32] Mild to moderate intensity exercise is recommended to improve aerobic fitness, survival time, and overall function.[3]

Neuromuscular Diseases

Respiratory disability accompanies chronic neuromuscular diseases (see Chapter Thirteen) that affect the respiratory muscles or neural control of breathing.[3] In addition, chest wall deformities, either congenital or acquired, can restrict lung volumes and impair pulmonary function.[3] Deformities of the thorax such as pectus excavatum, pectus carinatum, and scoliosis, should be referred for medical examination to rule out underlying cardiac or congenital disorders.[3]

Scoliosis

Severe scoliosis, an abnormal curvature in the spinal column, can impair the inflation of one or both lungs, thus decreasing vital capacity and overall pulmonary function. Persons with scoliosis are not restricted from sports participation unless the curve is progressing rapidly, prohibits trunk movement, or inhibits ventilation to a substantial degree.[3] Sports participation for persons who have had surgical spinal fixation to correct scoliosis depends on residual pulmonary impairment and the limitations of the surgical hardware or trunk strength and motion.[3] The treating surgeon should provide a release specifying in which sports the person may participate.

Pertussis (Whooping Cough)

Infection with the bacteria *Bordetella pertussis* causes the respiratory infection known as pertussis, or whooping cough. The bacteria release a toxin which impairs the function of the cilia in the respiratory tree. The result is that secretions are not removed from the airway and the patient begins to cough violently in an effort to expel thickened mucus from the bronchial tree. The cough has a long inspiratory phase followed by a sudden violent cough; during inspiration, the narrowed airways produce the characteristic "whooping" sound. Pertussis is highly contagious, with 80% of persons in contact with the infected patient themselves becoming infected. *B. pertussis* is not carried by a vector, but is strictly transmitted from person to person.

Following a relatively asymptomatic incubation phase of 7 to 21 days, the disease has three clinical stages. First, the catarrhal stage lasts 1 to 2 weeks and resembles a simple URI, with low-grade fever, sneezing, and coughing. It is during this first stage that the bacteria is most communicable to other persons through aerosalization of respiratory secretions. Second, the paroxysmal stage is characterized by the whooping cough, gradually increasing in frequency and severity over a week and persisting for 6 to 10 weeks. Third, the convalescent stage heralds recovery, with gradual cessation of the cough over 2 to 3 weeks. For several months after pertussis infection, patients are susceptible to recurrence of the whooping-type cough with other respiratory infections. Fever remains low-grade during the three clinical stages. Treatment is supportive to maintain hydration and facilitate mucus secretions, and usually involves antibiotics. Other children in the patient's family should be isolated from the child who is ill, as should all persons who have not completed the pertussis vaccination series.

Vaccination programs had decreased the prevalence of pertussis in the 1970s and 1980s in the United States, but since about 2000 the disease has again been on the rise. The reasons for this increase are unclear, but may be related to inappropriate timing of vaccination. Approximately 12,000 cases per year are currently reported, most among children less than 4 years of age, although older children and adolescents may also be affected. Older children typically have a less severe clinical presentation, but pose a risk to younger siblings and other children.

Summary

The pulmonary system exchanges oxygen and carbon dioxide between the body and the environment, a process called respiration, by inspiring and expiring air, a process called ventilation. Dyspnea, cough, cyanosis, thoracic chest pain, and abnormal breathing patterns are the most common signs and symptoms of pulmonary pathology. Percussion and auscultation are used to evaluate potential pulmonary disorders. Pulmonary pathology can occur in the lung tissue, by collapse of the interpleural space, as obstructive conditions, or as restrictive disorders.

Case Study

Sarah, a 20-year-old basketball player who transferred to your school this year, is having difficulty with her in-season conditioning program. During the 3-mile outdoor runs that were added a few weeks ago, she reports that a few minutes into the runs she gets a tightness in her chest that takes her breath away, makes her cough, and keeps her from continuing. About a half an hour later, she recovers fully and can complete the weight lifting part of the workout. The conditioning coach thinks she just doesn't want to participate in the runs.

During your medical history, you discover that Sarah's condition is worse in colder weather, she has never been diagnosed with asthma or any other breathing problem, and that the shortness of breath has never caused her to feel like she was going to faint. She does not smoke.

Normal breath sounds are heard upon auscultation of her lungs. Heart rate, respiration rate, and blood pressure are all normal (she came to see you before the workout).

Critical Thinking Questions

1. What conditions would you include in your differential diagnosis? Why?
2. What further tests might be needed to confirm or rule out a diagnosis?
3. How would the most likely diagnoses be managed?

References

1. National Athletic Trainers' Association. *Athletic Training Educational Competencies.* 4th ed. Dallas, TX: National Athletic Trainers' Association; 2005.
2. Ganong WF. *Review of Medical Physiology.* 22nd ed. New York, NY: McGraw-Hill Medical; 2005.
3. Homnick DN, Marks JH. Exercise and sports in the adolescent with chronic pulmonary disease. *Adolesc Med.* 1998;9:467-481.
4. Dantzker DR, Tobin MJ. Anatomical and physiological considerations. In: Andreoli TE, Carpenter CCJ, Plum F, Smith Jr LH, eds. *Cecil Essentials of Medicine.* 2nd ed. Philadelphia, PA: WB Saunders Co; 1990:126-135.
5. Loudon RG. Approach to the pulmonary patient. In: Beers MH, Berkow R, eds. *The Merck Manual of Diagnosis and Therapy.* 17th ed. Whitehouse Station, NJ: Merck Research Laboratories; 1999:511-521.
6. Dantzker DR, Tobin MJ. Approach to the patient with respiratory disease. In: Andreoli TE, Carpenter CCJ, Plum F, Smith Jr LH, eds. *Cecil Essentials of Medicine.* 2nd ed. Philadelphia, PA: WB Saunders Co; 1990:124-126.
7. Arnall D, Ryan M. Screening for pulmonary system disease. In: Boissonnault WG, ed. *Examination in Physical Therapy Practice: Screening for Medical Disease.* 2nd ed. New York, NY: Churchill-Livingstone; 1995:69-100.
8. Stopka CB, Zambito KL. Referred visceral pain: what every sports medicine professional needs to know. *Athl Ther Today.* 1999;4:29-36.
9. Kizer KW, MacQuarrie MB. Pulmonary air leaks resulting from outdoor sports: a clinical series and literature review. *Am J Sports Med.* 1999;27:517-520.
10. Mellman MF, Podesta L. Common medical problems in sports. *Clin Sports Med.* 1997;16:635-662.
11. Virant FS. Exercise-induced brochospasm: epidemilogy, pathophysiology, and therapy. *Med Sc Sports Exerc.* 1992;24:851-855.
12. Bickley LS, Szilagyi PG. *Bates' Guide to Physical Examination and History Taking.* 9th ed. Philadelphia, PA: Lippincott Williams & Wilkins; 2005.
13. Houglum JE. The basics of asthma therapy for athletes. *Athl Ther Today.* 2001;6:16-21.
14. Dishuck J, Harrelson GL, Harrelson L. Educating the asthmatic athlete. *Athl Ther Today.* 2001;6:26-32.

15. Miller MG, Weiler JM, Baker R, Collins J, D'Alonzo G. National Athletic Trainers' Association position statement: management of asthma in athletes. *J Athletic Training.* 2005;40:224-245.
16. Ellis EF. Asthma. In: Beers MH, Berkow R, eds. *The Merck Manual of Diagnosis and Therapy.* 17th ed. Whitehouse Station, NJ: Merck Research Laboratories; 1999:556-568.
17. Amaral JF. Thoracoabdominal injuries in the athlete. *Clin Sports Med.* 1997;16:739-753.
18. Dean NL. Near drowning. In: Beers MH, Berkow R, eds. *The Merck Manual of Diagnosis and Therapy.* 17th ed. Whitehouse Station, NJ: Merck Research Laboratories; 1999:2459-2460.
19. Cvengros RD, Lazor JA. Pnuemothorax: a medical emergency. *J Athl Training.* 1996;31:167-168.
20. Ferro RT, McKeag DB. Neck pain and dyspnea in a swimmer: spontaneous pneumomediastinum presentation and return-to-play considerations. *Physician Sportsmed.* 1999;27(10):67-71.
21. Leiber JD, Phan NT. Pneumomediastinum and subcutaneous emphysema in a synchronized swimmer. *Physician Sportsmed.* 2005;33(8):40-43.
22. Dantzker DR, Tobin MJ. Obstructive lung disease. In: Andreoli TE, Carpenter CCJ, Plum F, Smith Jr. LH, eds. *Cecil Essentials of Medicine.* 2nd ed. Philadelphia, PA: WB Saunders Co; 1990:140-147.
23. Jain P, Golish JA. Clinical management of asthma in the 1990s: current therapy and new directions. *Drugs.* 1996;52(Suppl 6):1-11.
24. Spahn JD, Szefler SJ. The etiology and control of bronchial hyperresponsiveness in children. *Curr Opin Pediatr.* 1996;8:591-596.
25. Houglum JE, Harrelson GL, Leaver-Dunn D. *Principles of Pharmacology for Athletic Trainers.* Thorofare, NJ: SLACK Incorporated; 2005.
26. Kyle JM. Exercise-induced pulmonary syndromes. *Sports Med.* 1994;78:413-421.
27. Kovan JR, Mackowiak TJ. Exercise-induced asthma. *Athl Ther Today.* 2001;6:22-25.
28. Pope JS, Koenig SM. Pulmonary disorders in the training room. *Clin Sports Med.* 2005;24:541-564.
29. Nichols AW. Nonorthopedic problems in the aquatic athlete. *Clin Sports Med.* 1999;18:395-411.
30. Truwit J. Pulmonary disorders and exercise. *Clin Sports Med.* 2003;22:161-180.
31. Gould BE. Respiratory disorders. *Pathophysiology for the Health-Related Professions.* Philadelphia, PA: WB Saunders Co; 1997:213-252.
32. Rosenstein BJ. Cystic fibrosis. In: Beers MH, Berkow R, eds. *The Merck Manual of Diagnosis and Therapy.* 17th ed. Whitehouse Station, NJ: Merck Research Laboratories; 1999:2366-2371.

Online Resources

Auscultation

Auscultation Assistant
www.med.ucla.edu/wilkes/intro.html

RALE Repository
www.rale.ca

Virtual Stethoscope
http://sprojects.mmi.mcgill.ca/mvs/mvsteth.htm

Pathology

American Academy of Asthma, Allergy, and Immunology
www.aaaai.org

American Lung Association
www.lungusa.org

National Heart, Lung, and Blood Institute
www.nhlbi.nih.gov

Lab Exercise 7-1
Pulmonary Percussion

Objectives

After completing this lab activity, students should be able to:

1. Locate the "percussion sites" for performing pulmonary percussion on the posterior thorax.
2. Correctly perform pulmonary percussion following the listening zone pattern for the posterior thorax.
3. Locate the "percussion sites" for performing pulmonary percussion on the anterior thorax.
4. Correctly perform pulmonary percussion following the listening zone pattern for the anterior thorax.

Competencies

This lab exercise addresses the following psychomotor competencies from the NATA's *Athletic Training Educational Competencies, 4th ed*:

- Medical Conditions and Disabilities: 4b

Equipment Needed

- Female students will need to wear a tank top or sports bra

Introduction

Pulmonary percussion can be used to identify the areas within the thorax that are air-filled, fluid-filled, or solid. These different tissue densities can be heard as hollow or dull sounds with percussion. Being familiar with the normal sounds with percussion can assist you in identifying abnormal sounds. For example, bleeding within a lung (hemothorax) will cause a change in the sound produced with percussion from hollow to dull. For optimum results, the hand placement and technique of percussion must be practiced.

Instructions

1. Place the DIP joint of your left middle finger on the surface to be percussed. Using the middle finger of your right hand, quickly strike the tip of your finger on the DIP joint of the left hand. The motion involves a quick wrist motion.
2. Practice the hand placement and percussing technique on a table top, your own thigh, and your puffed out cheek. Each of these surfaces will produce a different type of sound.
3. Working with your lab partner, identify the 14 percussion sites located on the posterior chest (see Figure 7-7a). Percuss over each site and then move to the contralateral site for comparison.
4. Working with your lab partner, identify the 12 percussion sites located on the anterior chest (see Figure 7-7b). Again, percuss over each site and then move to the contralateral site for comparison.
5. Perform pulmonary percussion on four additional individuals, **with at least one of these being evaluated by your lab instructor or ACI**.

Lab Exercise 7-1 (continued)
Pulmonary Percussion

Student:______________________________ Date:__________

Subject	Anterior Chest	Posterior Chest	Date
1. ____________	____________	____________	________
2. ____________	____________	____________	________
3. ____________	____________	____________	________
4. ____________	____________	____________	________

Lab Exercise 7-2
Pulmonary Auscultation

Objectives

After completing this lab activity, students should be able to:

1. Locate the "listening zones" for performing pulmonary auscultation on the posterior thorax.
2. Correctly perform pulmonary auscultation following the listening zone pattern for the posterior thorax.
3. Locate the "listening zones" for performing pulmonary auscultation on the anterior thorax.
4. Correctly perform pulmonary auscultation following the listening zone pattern for the anterior thorax.

Competencies

This lab exercise addresses the following psychomotor competencies from the NATA's *Athletic Training Educational Competencies, 4th ed*:

- Medical Conditions and Disabilities: 4b

Equipment Needed

- Stethoscope
- Female students will need to wear a tank top or sports bra

Introduction

Pulmonary auscultation is performed similarly to cardiac auscultation; however, the "listening zones" differ in their number and location (see Figures 7-7a and 7-7b). Patients should be instructed to breath with their mouth open. The diaphragm of the stethoscope should be placed directly on the skin rather than over clothing.

1. Working with your lab partner, identify the 14 listening zones located on the posterior chest (see Figure 7-7a). Auscultate over each listening zone, listening to several breath cycles at each site. If you have difficulty hearing the lung sounds, you can try an alternate patient position that maximizes the thorax exposure. Instruct your lab partner to place his or her arms across the chest and put his or her chin to his or her chest.
2. Working with your lab partner, identify the 12 listening zones located on the anterior chest (see Figure 7-7b). Again, auscultate each listening zone, listening to several breath cycles at each site.
3. Perform pulmonary auscultation on four additional individuals **with at least one of these being evaluated by your lab instructor or ACI**.
4. If a teaching stethoscope is available, have each individual listen to and confirm the lung sounds at each zone. Record your completion of these auscultations on the form provided.

Lab Exercise 7-2 (continued)
Pulmonary Auscultation

Student:______________________________ Date:__________

Subject	Anterior Chest	Posterior Chest	Date
1. ________	________	________	________
2. ________	________	________	________
3. ________	________	________	________
4. ________	________	________	________

Lab Exercise 7-3
Assessment of Peak Flow Expiratory Rate

Objectives

After completing this lab activity, students will be able to:

1. Instruct a patient how to properly use a handheld spirometer to assess PEFR.
2. Determine a patient's baseline PEFR.
3. Interpret daily PEFR values to determine a patient's ability to participate in their sport.

Competencies

This lab exercise addresses the following psychomotor competencies from the NATA's *Athletic Training Educational Competencies, 4th ed*:

- Medical Conditions and Disabilities: 4

Equipment Needed

- Two different models of hand-held spirometers
- Calculator
- Pencil or pen

Instructions

Part 1: Assessment of baseline PEFR

1. Using the assessment instructions outlined in the chapter, instruct your lab partner how to properly use the hand-held spirometer.
2. Instruct your lab partner to perform three trials and record the highest value, which becomes his or her baseline or "personal best."

Lab Partner	1st Trial	2nd Trial	3rd Trial	Baseline	Spirometer Model
1.______________	________	________	________	________	______________
	________	________	________	________	______________
2.______________	________	________	________	________	______________
	________	________	________	________	______________
3.______________	________	________	________	________	______________
	________	________	________	________	______________

Lab Exercise 7-3 (continued)
Assessment of Peak Flow Expiratory Rate

Part 2: Determination of zones for management of asthma.

1. Using the baseline measurements obtained in Part 1 for each of your lab partners, calculate the green, yellow, and red zones for managing your partners' asthma (use the readings obtained from one of the spirometer models).

Lab Partner #1:________________ Spirometer Model:__________________

Baseline:__________________________

Green Zone:________________________

Yellow Zone:_______________________

Red Zone:__________________________

Lab Partner #2:________________ Spirometer Model:__________________

Baseline:__________________________

Green Zone:________________________

Yellow Zone:_______________________

Red Zone:__________________________

Lab Partner #3:________________ Spirometer Model:__________________

Baseline:__________________________

Green Zone:________________________

Yellow Zone:_______________________

Red Zone:__________________________

Chapter Eight

Gastrointestinal and Hepatic-Biliary Systems

Chapter Outline and Objectives

Introduction

Review of Anatomy, Physiology, and Pathogenesis

- Describe basic gastrointestinal and hepatic-biliary anatomy and function.
- Review pathophysiological mechanisms of the gastrointestinal and hepatic-biliary systems.
- Describe the response of the gastrointestinal and hepatic-biliary systems to exercise.

Signs and Symptoms

- Discuss the general signs and symptoms of gastrointestinal and hepatic-biliary pathology.

Pain Patterns

- Describe the referred pain patterns associated with gastrointestinal and hepatic-biliary pathology.

Medical History and Physical Examination

- Discuss medical history findings relevant to gastrointestinal and hepatic-biliary pathology.
- Perform physical examination tasks relevant to the gastrointestinal and hepatic-biliary systems.
    - Auscultation
    - Percussion
    - Palpation

Pathology and Pathogenesis

Gastrointestinal Infections

❖ Describe signs, symptoms, treatment, and return-to-play criteria for gastrointestinal infections.
- Viral Gastroenteritis
- Food Poisoning
- Traveler's Diarrhea

Upper Gastrointestinal Disorders

❖ Describe signs, symptoms, treatment, and return-to-play criteria for upper gastrointestinal disorders.
- Dyspepsia
- Gastroesophageal Reflux
- Hiatal Hernia
- Peptic Ulcer
- Gastritis

Lower Gastrointestinal Disorders

❖ Describe signs, symptoms, treatment, and return-to-play criteria for lower gastrointestinal disorders.
- Inflammatory Bowel Diseases
- Irritable Bowel Syndrome
- Appendicitis
- Diverticulosis and Diverticulitis
- Hernia
- Hemorrhoids
- Colorectal Cancer

Abdominal Trauma

- Spleen Trauma and Splenomegaly
- Liver Trauma

Hepatic-Biliary Diseases

- Hepatitis
- Cirrhosis
- Gallstones and Gallbladder Disease
- Pancreatitis

This chapter addresses the following competencies from the *Athletic Training Educational Competencies, Fourth Edition*[1]:

Domain	**Cognitive**	**Psychomotor**
Acute Care of Injuries and Illnesses	4, 14, 16, 30	4
Medical Conditions and Disabilities	1–3, 12, 16	3, 4
Pathology of Injuries and Illnesses	4–6	
Pharmacology	3, 14, 16	

INTRODUCTION

Intensity and duration of exercise can alter the functions and digestive processes of the gastrointestinal (GI) system. Consequently, GI symptoms, including nausea, vomiting, abdominal pain, diarrhea, and constipation, are common in athletes and the general population.[2,3] For instance, over 10% of people are affected by irritable bowel syndrome and experience GI symptoms almost daily.[3]

Trauma, infection, and disease can affect the organs of the GI system, producing very similar signs and symptoms regardless of etiology. Pathological conditions of the liver and gallbladder (hepatic-biliary system), both intimately related to the GI system, are included in this chapter. Trauma to GI organs and the abdomen are relatively rare in sports, but are also difficult to recognize and can have grave consequences.[4,5] Any athlete who sustains significant trauma to the abdomen should be examined and monitored closely.[5]

REVIEW OF ANATOMY, PHYSIOLOGY, AND PATHOGENESIS

The structures and organs of the GI system include the mouth, esophagus, stomach, small intestine (duodenum, jujenum, and ileum), large intestine, rectum, and anus (Figure 8-1). Figure 8-2 shows the relative position of the abdominal organs by quadrant. The functions of the upper GI system, from the mouth to the duodenum, are to take in and digest food. The lower GI system, from the jujenum to the rectum, absorbs nutrients and water, and eventually expels the waste products of digestion.[6]

Gastric (stomach) emptying accelerates with the onset of exercise.[3,7] Once exercise intensity reaches about 75% of aerobic capacity, however, gastric emptying slows.[3,7] Overall, lower GI (bowels) motility increases with regular exercise.[3] Since gravity assists the GI system, upright activity increases bowel motility in persons who have been immobile. During exercise, small intestine motility slows as a result of decreased blood flow and exercise-induced hormone release.[7] Jostling or other movement of the large bowel in the gut during exercise may cause diarrhea or mild abdominal cramping.[5,7] Proper hydration can prevent many of these exercise-induced GI symptoms.[3]

The liver, gallbladder, and exocrine pancreas each secrete digestive enzymes into the duodenum through the same opening, called the ampulla of Vater. In addition, the liver filters the blood from the intestines, colon, spleen, and pancreas before it returns to the heart, allowing the liver to absorb nutrients and catabolize toxins. In addition, the liver regulates metabolism of fats and cholesterol and stores large amounts of carbohydrate. It also forms bile, which contains pigments and salts that emulsify fat during digestion. Most of the bile salts are recycled through the GI-hepatic circulation, whereas the pigments are excreted.

Bile flows directly into the duodenum when food is present. Otherwise, it is stored in the gallbladder and becomes more concentrated. Disorders of the biliary (liver and gallbladder) system produce high levels of bilirubin, a yellow pigment, in the blood which leads to *jaundice*, a yellow discoloration of the skin, eyes, and mucosa. In addition, digestion and absorption of fats are impaired from a lack of bile salts in the small intestine.

Figure 8-1. Organs of the upper and lower gastrointestinal system.

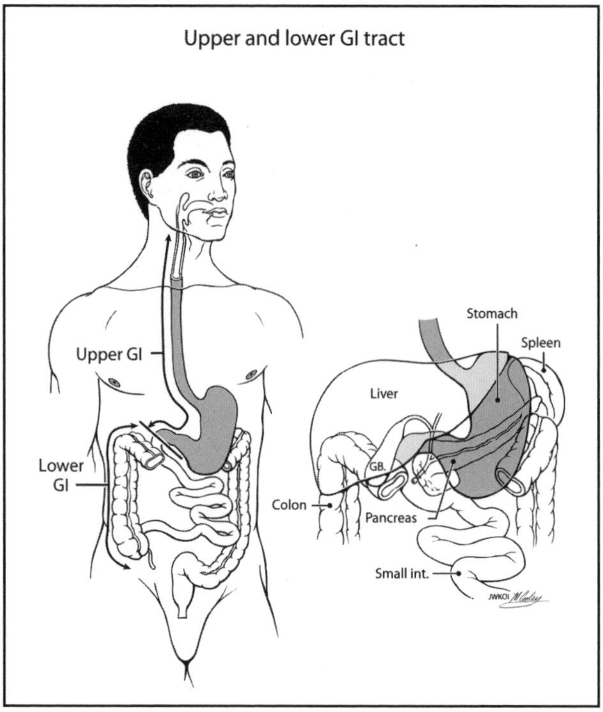

Figure 8-2. Abdominal quadrants and their contents.

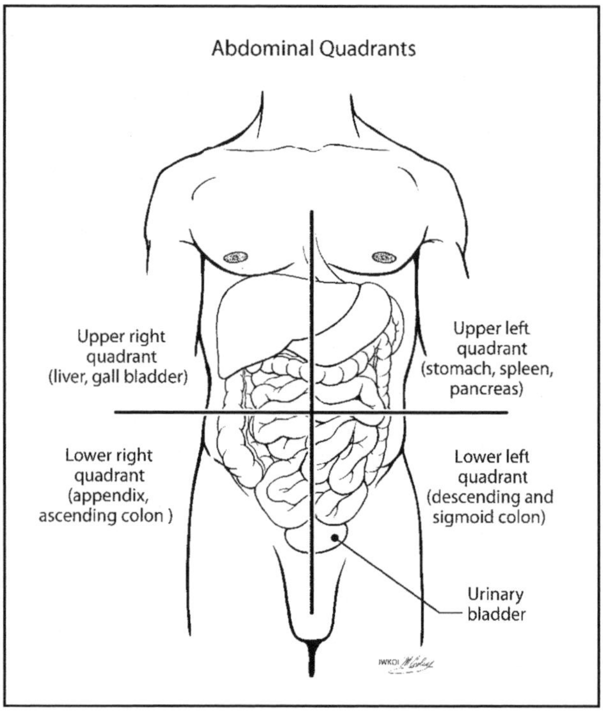

The pancreas consists of two functional segments. The endocrine pancreas, discussed in Chapter Ten, secretes hormones (insulin, glucagons, and somatostatin) that regulate blood carbohydrate levels. The exocrine pancreas secretes several enzymes important to digestion of carbohydrates, proteins, and fats. Diseases affecting the exocrine pancreas thus affect digestion.

Signs and Symptoms

Nausea and Vomiting

Nausea and vomiting (*emesis*) are hallmarks of upper GI disorders. Nausea and vomiting occur when nerve endings in the upper GI are irritated by chemical, mechanical, or autonomic (vagus nerve) stimuli.[3] This stimulation of the upper GI nerve endings reverses peristalsis, pushing its contents back into the stomach. Contraction of the abdominal muscles increase intraabdominal pressure and force the stomach contents up the esophagus and out of the mouth.

When blood appears in vomitus, the condition is called *hematemesis*. A person with nose or mouth trauma may accidentally swallow and then vomit bright red blood. If blood collects in the stomach, as occurs with pathological upper GI bleeding, the vomitus appears like coffee grounds. Gastric ulcers, excessive use of nonsteroidal anti-inflammatory drugs ([NSAIDs] or other drugs), alcohol abuse, or major systemic illness can produce upper GI bleeding. Rarely, extremely intense exercise can cause acute gastric hemorrhage and hematemesis.[7]

Abdominal Pain

Location (ie, abdominal quadrant), severity, and quality of abdominal pain should be noted. Description of the pain may aid in discerning the affected structure or likely pathology. Severe, progressive cycles of intense cramping-type pain (called *colic*) is produced by acute inflammation or obstruction in an abdominal organ or duct; the cramping sensation results from the rhythmic contractions of these organs.[8] Acute, localized constant pain indicates inflammation of the parietal peritoneum (*peritonitis*).[8] Nontraumatic, mild abdominal cramps usually indicate lower GI disorders.[3] NSAIDs may temporarily eliminate pain of GI origin.

Abdominal Rigidity

Protective spasm of the muscles of the abdominal wall caused by pain from injury, internal bleeding, or disease in the abdominal organs is called *rigidity*. Rigidity is detected during palpation in contrast to the normal suppleness of the abdomen. Rigidity usually occurs in a specific quadrant or region rather than the whole abdomen. Significant abdominal pain and difficulty flexing the trunk accompanies rigidity. Abdominal rigidity indicates a significant injury or disease process and requires immediate medical attention.

Loss of Appetite and Significant Loss in Body Weight

Loss of appetite may indicate an upper GI problem.[3] A recent loss of significant body weight suggests poor nutritional absorption, dehydration from recurrent vomiting or diarrhea, or increased metabolic demand from a chronic disease. Infection and cancer also induce both loss of appetite by affecting the satiety center in the medulla oblongata and weight loss by increasing metabolism while decreasing food intake.[3]

Night Pain

Abdominal pain that wakes a person at night is nearly always a symptom of serious pathology. Night pain is a result of the parasympathetic nervous system, which is more active at night, stimulating the GI organs and producing symptoms as function of the affected organ increases.

Prandial or Postprandial Symptoms

Prandial (while eating) and *postprandial* (after eating) symptoms suggest GI or biliary pathology. Stomach pain begins about an hour after eating, as the food passes into the duodenum. Similarly, duodenal pain occurs 2 hours or more after a meal as food passes into the jejunum. Food usually irritates a gastric ulcer but may relieve a duodenal ulcer. In addition, caffeine, alcohol, and spicy foods may irritate gastroesophageal reflux or peptic ulcer. Fatty foods may exacerbate gallbladder or pancreas pathology.[6]

Change in Bowel Habits or Stool Quality

Changes in the frequency, regularity, or ease of defecation indicate lower GI pathology.[6] Changes in consistency, odor, or color of the stool (feces) are suggestive of disease in the lower GI or biliary systems.[6] Two types of disturbed bowel habits are diarrhea and constipation.

Diarrhea describes frequent or loose bowel movements caused by increased bowel motility, malabsorption syndromes, infection, or a combination of these factors.[9] In general, an infectious agent stimulates the cells in the small intestine and colon to release sodium, potassium, and water into the bowel. The result is a watery stool that moves quickly through the large intestine. Diarrhea leads to dehydration, electrolyte imbalance, and, in severe cases, shock. Effective treatment involves hydration, electrolyte replacement (usually through sodium-glucose preparations), and medications (bismuth subsalicylate [Pepto-Bismol, Procter & Gamble, Cincinnati, Ohio] or loperamide [Imodium, McNeil Consumer Healthcare, Fort Washington, Pa]) to reduce bowel output. The "BRAT" diet (bananas, rice, applesauce, and toast) is also effective in managing diarrhea.

Increased urgency or diarrhea also occasionally occurs with vigorous exercise.[2,3] Some medications and drugs cause temporary diarrhea. For instance, antibiotics allow overproduction of intestinal bacteria (causing colitis), which increases intestinal motility.

Constipation is abnormal retention of feces as a result of hardened (dehydrated) stool or decreased bowel motility. Poor diet (high-sugar, low-fiber), dehydration, medications (eg, analgesics that decrease bowel motility), stress, inactivity, or GI disease can contribute to constipation. Chronically retained stool becomes impacted and cannot progress through the bowel, causing a bowel obstruction that requires surgery. Appropriate lifestyle changes relieve constipation due to a poor diet or inactivity, although laxatives may be needed in more severe cases.

Rectal Blood

Bleeding from the rectum, either bright red or detected occultly in the feces (*hematochezia*), is a sign of lower GI pathology.[2] Simple causes include hemorrhoids or anal fissures, but requires a physician to rule out irritable bowel syndrome, cancer, or parasitic GI infection.[2,7] Black stools with a tar-like consistency, called *melena*, suggests upper GI bleeding; the blood coagulates as it passes through the lower GI to produce this effect. Some medications can also cause melena, which may be ascertained during the medical history.

Jaundice

Jaundice, or *icterus*, is yellow discoloration of skin, eyes, and mucous membranes that occurs with high bilirubin levels in the blood. Pathology of the liver, gallbladder, exocrine pancreas, or the common bile duct for these organs causes jaundice.[10] The urine progressively darkens and the stool progressively lightens in color as bilirubin increases in the blood and the kidneys filter it out into the urine while concentration decreases in the bowel.

PAIN PATTERNS

Upper Gastrointestinal

Referred pain from the upper GI (Figure 8-3a) can be similar to that of the heart (see Chapter Six), but history and accompanying signs and symptoms usually clarify the system of origin.[3,7] The esophagus causes substernal pain, although occasionally pain is also noted in the epigastric area or radiating to the back.[7] The stomach also produces epigastric pain, but may refer to the back or the shoulder if the diaphragmatic pleura also becomes irritated.[11]

Lower Gastrointestinal

Pain from the small and large intestines present diffuse middle to lower abdominal pain (Figure 8-3b).[11] The visceral pain is accompanied by localized peritoneal pain and abdominal rigidity as the condition worsens.

The appendix classically produces initially midabdominal pain that gradually migrates to the right lower quadrant, one-third to one-half the distance from the anterior superior iliac spine toward the umbilicus (*McBurney's point*).[11] Pain from acute appendicitis may also refer to the central abdomen, hip, thigh, or lower back.

Liver

The liver refers pain to the epigastric region and right upper quadrant (RUQ), and can refer pain to the right shoulder, thoracic, or cervical spine if the diaphragm becomes irritated.[11]

Gallbladder

The gallbladder produces a characteristic pattern along the right T8 dermatome, radiating to the right scapula as a sharp, stabbing sensation.[11] Gallbladder pain may begin as a sensation of heartburn.

Pancreas

The pancreas produces epigastric pain referring to the middle or lower back. If the diaphragm becomes irritated, pain occurs in the left shoulder.

Figure 8-3a. Referred pain patterns for the upper gastrointestinal system.

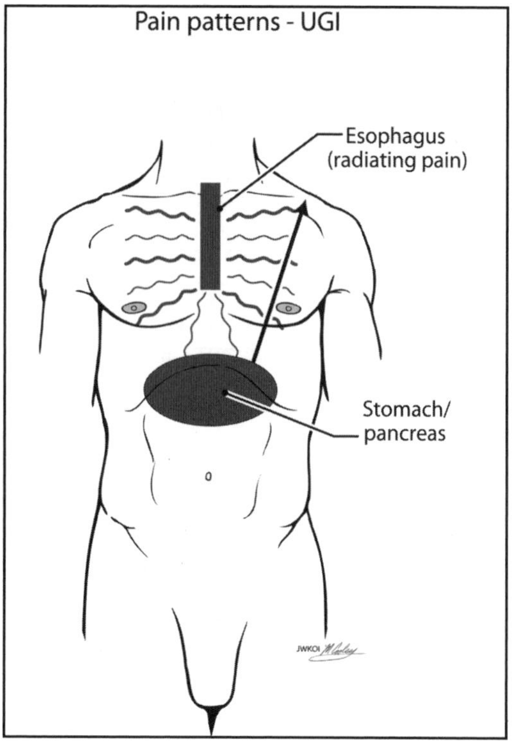

Figure 8-3b. Referred pain patterns for the lower gastrointestinal system.

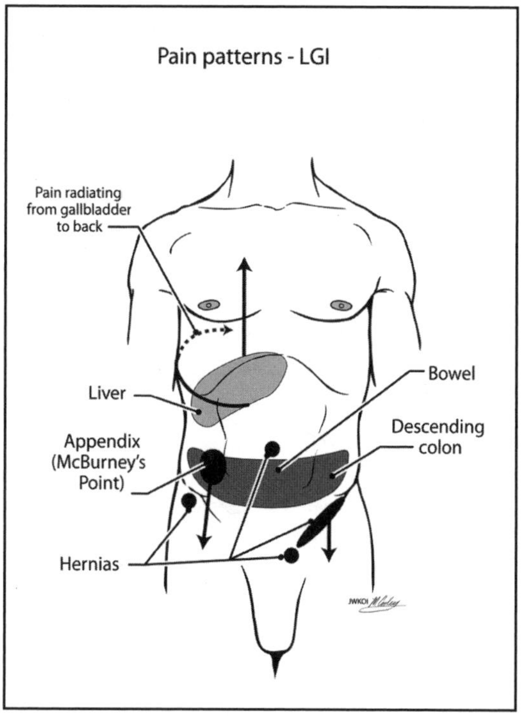

Spleen

The spleen, an abdominal organ that filters abnormal red blood cells and functions as part of the immune system, refers pain to the left upper quadrant (LUQ) and left shoulder. Referred pain from the spleen to the left shoulder is known as *Kehr's sign*.

Medical History and Physical Examination

Family and Personal History

A complete GI history should be conducted for any person reporting nausea, vomiting, or abdominal pain as a primary complaint.[3] Recent GI illness, change in diet, current training regimen, and recent travel can be related to the etiology of GI pathology.[2] Childhood diseases, recent surgery, current medications, and history of a similar condition should be ascertained.[8] Symptoms produced at night or while eating are usually more serious than postprandial heartburn or exercise-induced indigestion.[3] Regular use of caffeine, alcohol, nicotine, drugs, or medications should be noted.[6]

Direct trauma can damage the organs of the GI and hepatic-biliary systems.[5] Significant injuries to the liver, jujenum, or colon are rare in sports. Trauma from the end of a blunt instrument (bicycle handlebars, baseball bat) or that produces bruising or rib fractures should raise suspicion of internal organ damage. A sudden deceleration of the thorax can cause the contents of the abdomen to collide with the ribcage, thus causing injury.[4]

Very recent trauma to the abdomen or thorax may not present signs or symptoms for hours despite significant injury.[4] Symptoms should be reevaluated at regular intervals for several hours following abdominal trauma.[5] Progressive deterioration of vital signs (shock) and persistent abdominal pain indicate serious injury.

Inspection

An abnormally protruding abdomen indicates *ascites* (excess peritoneal fluid), distended bowels from an obstruction, or excessive gas in the bowels.[8] An asymmetric abdomen is a sign of ascites shifting with gravity, hepatomegaly (right enlargement), or splenomegaly (left enlargement).[6]

Other signs may be observable by close inspection. Small, bulging masses in the lower abdomen may be herniated bowel, particularly if tender or manually reducible. Pulsing may be observed with an aortic or iliac artery aneurysm (see Chapter Six).[8] Jaundice may be noted in the skin or sclera of the eyes. Severe abdominal muscle spasms cause a characteristic flexed or sidelying "fetal" posture, with both arms crossed across the belly.

Examination of the Abdomen

Physical examination of the abdomen should include auscultation, percussion, and palpation (see Lab Exercise 8-1).[5,6,8,12] When examining the abdomen, the patient should be placed in a hook-lying position (supine with knees bent and feet flat on the table; Figure 8-4). This position relieves some of the stress on the abdomen while lying supine. Instructing the patient to raise his or her arms above his or her head

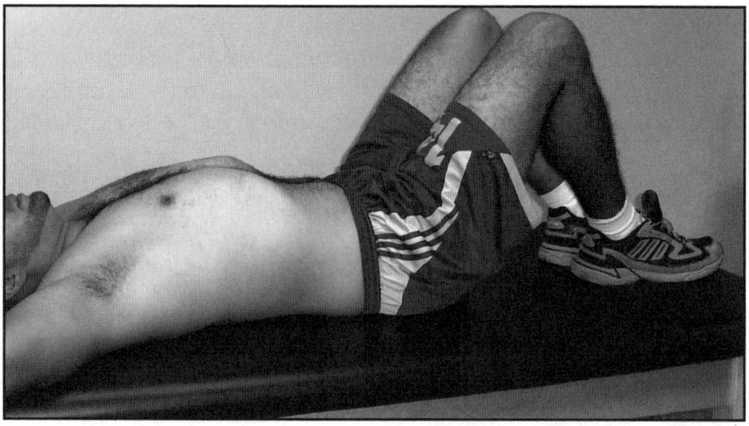

Figure 8-4. Hook-lying position for abdominal examination.

Table 8-1	
Signs and Symptoms of Bowel Obstruction	
• Vomiting	• Inability to pass gas
• Progressive cramping pain	• Diminished bowel sounds
• Distended abdomen	• Tympanites
• Foul breath odor	• Systemic signs

will also improve examination as it causes the liver and spleen to extend slightly below the ribcage. Auscultation and percussion should be performed before palpation, as palpation may disturb the contents of the GI leading to false findings.

Auscultation should be performed for approximately 1 to 3 minutes within each quadrant to listen for bowel sounds. Bowel sounds will be heard as tinkling, clicking or gurgling sounds, with a normal rate of 5 to 35 sounds per minute.[13] It may take up to a minute or so to begin hearing bowel sounds. Decreased or absent bowel sounds may indicate a bowel obstruction. Other signs and symptoms of bowel obstruction are given in Table 8-1.

Percussion of the abdomen can be performed to identify the approximate location of the liver and spleen as they extend beyond the ribcage. Also, percussion can be used to detect changes in resonance. Internal bleeding within the abdomen can produce a dull thud on percussion in place of the normal hollow sound. The technique for abdominal percussion is similar to that used for pulmonary percussion (see Chapter Seven).

Superficial palpation should be performed using the palmer aspect of the fingers rather than poking with a single finger (Figure 8-5a). Deep palpation is performed similarly; however, the other hand is placed on top of the palpating hand (Figure 8-5b). When palpating the abdomen, the examiner should feel for tenderness, rigidity, and abnormal masses. The liver and spleen should be palpated below the ribcage in the RUQ and LUQ, respectively. Palpation of these structures can often times be enhanced by placing one hand under the appropriate quadrant and the other hand on top of the quadrant palpating the organ (Figure 8-6).

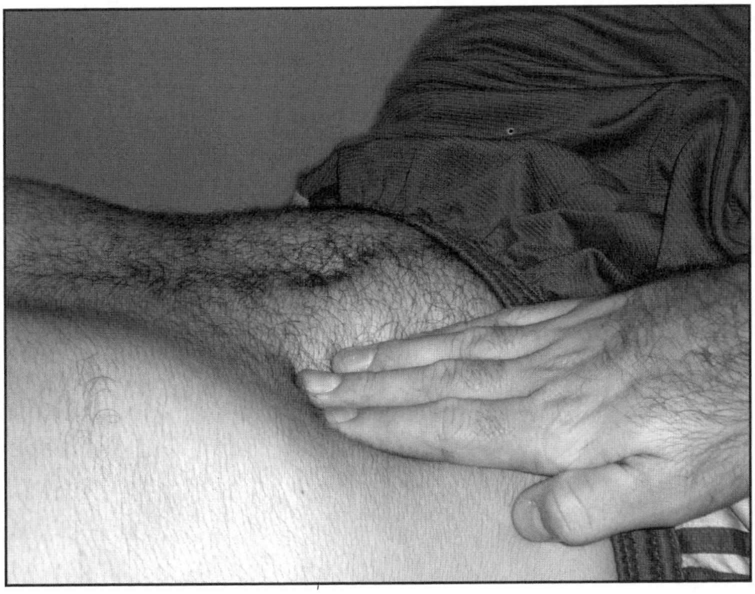

Figure 8-5a. Palpation of abdomen.

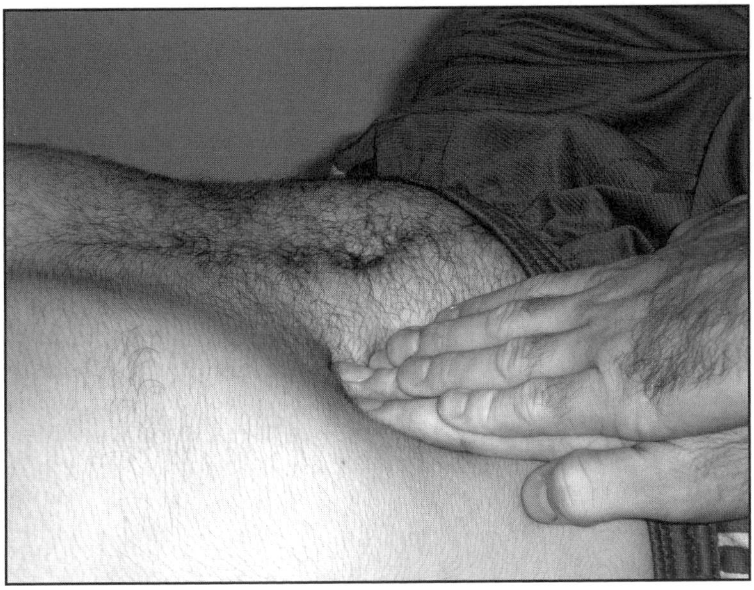

Figure 8-5b. Deep palpation of abdomen.

Differentiating musculoskeletal trauma, such as fractured ribs or strained abdominal muscles, from abdominal organ trauma or pathology can be difficult. If palpation of the abdomen is painful, but pain during palpation is decreased significantly if the patient contracts their abdominal muscles (by raising the head in supine), injury to the internal organs is likely.[6] In addition, placing the palm of the left hand flat on the quadrants or over specific abdominal organs and striking briskly with the ulnar edge of the right fist, an exam technique called *hammering*, increases the pain caused by injured organs.[12]

The test for rebound tenderness involves manually depressing the abdomen, on either the same or opposite side as the symptoms, and then quickly releasing the

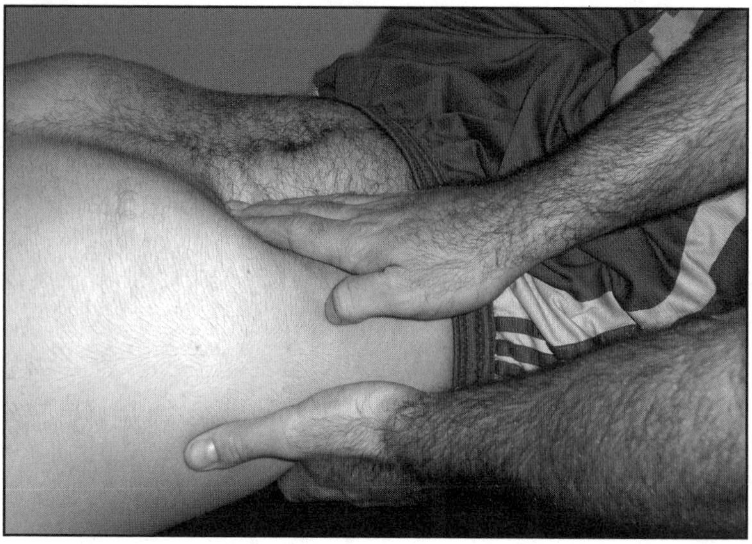

Figure 8-6. Enhancement of abdominal palpation.

pressure. Pain produced by this manuever suggests peritonitis.[5,6,14] Another test for peritonitis is the *"jar" test*, also known as *Markle's sign*.[15] The person stands on his or her toes then suddenly drops flatly onto their heels; a sharp increase in abdominal pain is positive for peritonitis.[14]

Initial physical examination may not suggest intra-abdominal injury, thus requiring repeated examinations.[5] Almost half of emergency room patients who have abdominal pain initially have a negative physical examination, but actually end up having significant abdominal injuries.[3,5] Hence, emergency transportation should occur upon the first sign that the condition is worsening after an abdominal injury.

Many GI disorders are associated with severe vomiting and diarrhea which can lead to dehydration. The clinical detection of dehydration can be made by measuring the blood pressure and heart rate in both supine and standing (orthostatic vital signs).[13] When moving from a supine to a standing position, it is normal for the blood pressure to decrease by 20 points and the pulse to increase by 20 points. If the blood pressure decreases by more than 20 points or the pulse increases by more than 20 points, dehydration should be suspected.

Pathology and Pathogenesis

Gastrointestinal Infections

GI infections include viral gastroenteritis, food poisoning, and so-called "traveler's diarrhea."[16] *Viral gastroenteritis* ("stomach flu") causes severe vomiting, diarrhea, and abdominal spasms, and is accompanied by fever and myalgia.[16,17] The virus is contracted by ingesting food that has been contaminated with virus, most commonly a result of infected food preparers improperly washing their hands after using the restroom; it is also contracted by ingesting raw seafood or water that has been contaminated by sewage. This is known as the "fecal-oral" route of transmission. The illness, which lasts a few days, is usually self-limiting and rarely life-threatening in healthy young people.[16] Primary treatment includes rest and hydration.[16,17] Occasionally, hydration by intravenous fluids is required if the person cannot hold down water or other fluids. Antidiarrheal and antiemetic (inhibits vomiting) medications are not recommended since they delay elimination of the virus from the body.[16] Return to participation usually occurs within a week, depending on resolution of symptoms and restoration of hydration.

Food poisoning occurs with ingestion of food-borne bacteria, most commonly a species of *Staphylococcus*.[16] The bacteria, usually passed into food from the hands or respiratory secretions of a food handler, produces a toxin as it multiplies on poorly refrigerated meat or dairy products.[16] Within an hour or two of ingestion, severe vomiting and diarrhea occur and persist for several hours. Rest and hydration are usually the only treatment needed. Again, antiemetic and antidiarrheal medications are not recommended since they delay elimination of the bacteria.[16]

Another type of food poisoning is caused by a strain of *Escherichia coli* (*E. coli*) that lives in the intestines of cattle. During slaughter or preparation, the E. coli contaminate the meat as it is being prepared for consumption. The bacteria is communicated when meat, particularly ground meat, is not properly cooked, food preparers do not wash their hands after working with raw meat, or raw meat comes in contact with other food. The *E. coli* strain produces a toxin in the human GI system, leading to bloody diarrhea and severe abdominal cramping. Once infected, the bacteria can be communicated from person to person through contact with infected feces; most often, this occurs among groups of children or when the hands are not washed after using the restroom. Treatment is generally supportive (hydration); antidiarrheal medications should not be used because they allow the bacteria to remain in the body a longer period of time. There is no evidence that antibiotics lessen the duration or intensity of the infection. Occasionally, the toxins destroy red blood cells, which leads to kidney failure; this is a severe condition that results in a 5% rate of death even when intensive care is provided.

"Traveler's diarrhea" is so named since infectious diarrhea can occur in persons from the United States while traveling to foreign countries, particularly Asia and South America. Bacteria (*Salmonella*, etc) or viruses are transmitted through the fecal-oral route from improper hand washing, poor handling of uncooked food, improperly cooked food, and contamination of public water sources. Traveler's diarrhea is similar to other GI infections, producing diarrhea, abdominal spasms, and fatigue from dehydration and decreased caloric intake that may last up to 3 days.[16] Avoidance of potentially contaminated foods and water (ie, consume only bottled fluids and packaged foods) and the use of prophylactic bismuth subalicylate (Pepto-Bismol) every 6 hours throughout travel can prevent infection while traveling. Treatment is similar to viral gastroenteritis and food poisoning, involving primarily rest and hydration. Antidiarrheal medications can be used to control traveler's diarrhea unless fever (indicating gastroenteritis) or bloody stool (hematochezia) occurs.[16]

Upper Gastrointestinal Disorders

Burning pain in the chest, nausea, vomiting, and loss of appetite are the hallmarks of upper GI pathology.[3]

Dyspepsia

The most common upper GI condition is dyspepsia, also known as indigestion or heartburn, which produces an uncomfortable burning sensation under the sternum.[9] Irritation of the mucosum in the upper GI from reflux of gastric acids, medications, drugs, alcohol, and caffeine, or from certain nondisease states such as pregnancy, can cause dyspepsia.[9,18] Dyspepsia can usually be successfully managed with dietary changes or over-the-counter (OTC) antacids designed to reduce gastric acid.

Antacids are fast acting and generally provide relief within 15 minutes of dosing. They should be taken after meals and at bedtime. Their duration of effect can be extended by taking them within 1 hour of meals. Antacids can interfere with the absorption of other medication; therefore, they should not be taken along with other medications. A general rule of thumb is to separate dosing of antacids and other drugs by at least 2 hours.[19] Antacids are not as effective in treating heartburn as proton pump inhibitors (PPIs) or H_2-blockers; therefore, individuals with chronic heartburn should see their physician to discuss alternative medications.

The symptoms of dyspepsia are common to other, more serious GI disorders, including gastroesophageal reflux, peptic ulcer, and liver disease.[9] Other signs, such as weight loss, abnormal masses in the abdomen, hematochezia, or fever, however, do not occur with benign dyspepsia, and therefore warrant referral.

Gastroesophageal Reflux

Gastroesophageal reflux (GERD) occurs when the esophageal sphincter, controlling flow of food from the esophagus into the stomach, malfunctions after ingestion of certain types of foods, medications, or drugs (caffeine, alcohol). Symptoms are produced by acid from the stomach entering the esophagus, which has a thinner mucosal layer than the stomach.[18] Exercise involving repeated vertical impact forces, such as running, can also induce GERD by causing stomach acids to enter the esophagus.[7] Psychoemotional stress stimulates the vagus nerve, causing secretion of excess stomach acid and abnormal stomach contractions that may push acid into the esophagus.

GERD causes symptoms similar to those of dyspepsia, but are usually more frequent, more intense, and of longer duration. Most often, GERD can be controlled with dietary and lifestyle changes (avoidance of irritating foods or activities, stress management) and use of prescription medications. If the condition prevents participation in physical activity, persists for several weeks, or becomes significantly worse, the patient should be referred to a physician. Occasionally prescribed medication is required and, in rare instances, surgery.[7]

PPIs and H_2-blockers inhibit acid production in the stomach, are both more effective in treating GERD than antacids. Common PPIs include esomeprazole (Nexium [AstraZeneca, Wilmington, Del]), lansoprazole (Prevacid [Tap Pharmaceuticals, Lake Forest, Ill]), omeprazole (Prilosec [AstraZeneca]), and pantoprazole (Protonix [Wyeth Pharmaceuticals, Madison, NJ]). H_2-blockers include cimetidine (Tagamet [GlaxoSmithKline, Brentford, Middlesex, UK]), famotidine (Pepcid [Merck, Whitehouse Station, NJ]), and ranitidine (Zantac [GlaxoSmithKline]). The PPIs will often have an enteric coating, and therefore, should not be crushed, chewed, or split. For optimum use, they should be taken approximately 30 minutes before a meal. PPIs are generally more effective in treating GERD and are associated with a 30% greater rate of healing with the esophagus.[19]

Hiatal Hernia

A herniation is the abnormal protrusion of an organ through its surrounding tissue. A hiatal hernia is the protrusion of part of the proximal stomach through the diaphragm and into the thorax. This displacement impairs the function of the lower esophageal sphincter, which regulates the flow of food from the esophagus into the stomach. The effect is an increased risk of gastroesophageal reflux, although many people who have small hiatal hernias have no symptoms and apparently no effects. Symptoms are worse when lying down because the stomach acids flow more easily into the esophagus and are relieved by sitting as gravity pulls the acid back into the stomach. Diagnosis is made using barium fluoroscopy to image the upper GI system. Treatment involves medication to reduce stomach acid and surgery in recalcitrant cases.

Peptic Ulcer

A peptic ulcer occurs when the gastric juices digest the submucosal layers of the stomach or duodenum.[6] The mucosal layer of the stomach is normally protected from stomach acid by the mucosal barrier, which consists of secreted mucus and bicarbonate. Anything that disrupts this protective barrier increases the risk of peptic ulcer. Chronic infection by *Helicobacteri pylori* has been strongly associated with development of peptic ulcers; this bacteria interferes with the protective mucosal barrier of mucus and bicarbonate.[20] Chronic use of NSAIDs, such as aspirin and ibuprofen, also increase risk of peptic ulcers because they inhibit prostaglandins, which are necessary for the secretion of mucus and bicarbonate in the stomach. Some diseases that increase acid secretion in the stomach can also lead to ulcers by overwhelming the mechanisms in the protective barrier. Ulceration into the muscular layer produces scarring, and erosion beyond the muscular layer can perforate blood vessels, causing severe gastric hemorrhage and shock.[20]

Risk of peptic ulcer increases with advancing age, chronic use of NSAIDs (eg, for arthritis), and regular heavy use of nicotine and alcohol. Ulcers can occur in physically active persons who are under psychological and physiological stress.[6]

A peptic ulcer produces intermittent pain in the upper or middle abdomen that radiates to the thoracic spine, chest, and neck.[6] The symptoms may improve or worsen after eating and may disappear and recur over several weeks or months. Abdominal pain at night is very common. If the condition persists, recurrent vomiting and loss of appetite may cause weight loss.[6] A perforated ulcer may produce bloody vomitus (hematemesis), "coffee-grounds" vomitus, or melena.[6]

Avoidance of foods known to irritate the condition and use of antacids usually provide symptomatic relief.[20] Prescription antibiotics for *H. pylori* and acid-reducing medications such as PPIs (with the exception of Nexium) and H_2-blockers often succeed in healing peptic ulcers, with a 5% to 10% recurrence rate. Relatively few patients with ulcers require surgery, which is performed to stop excessive gastric bleeding or to biopsy for a suspected malignancy.[20]

Gastritis

Gastritis describes stomach inflammation resulting from a disease causing erosion of the entire mucosa, chronic use of NSAIDs, *Helicobacter pylori* infection, or autoimmune diseases.[6] Gastritis can be acute or chronic, erosive or nonerosive.

Acute erosive gastritis occurs in patients with severe chronic illnesses, such as severe burns, head or spinal trauma, shock, mechanical ventilation, and hepatic or renal failure. These conditions cause severe gastric stress by impairing the mucosal barrier mechanism, leading to the erosion of the mucosa. Treatment of the causative medical condition takes precedence.

Chronic erosive gastritis is most commonly attributed to long-term use of NSAIDs, alcohol abuse, irritable bowel disease, or viral infection.[20] Nausea, vomiting, and vague upper abdominal pain may be present in such cases. Dietary restrictions and symptomatic treatment with antacids are used as treatment, although recurrences are frequent.

Acute and chronic nonerosive gastritis is frequently a result of *H. pylori* infection, potentially causing gastric irritation, mucosa breakdown, peptic ulcers, and stomach cancer.[20] Symptoms, when present, are similar to erosive gastritis and peptic ulcer. A course of antibiotics eliminates the bacteria and the gastritis.

Lower Gastrointestinal Disorders

The signs of lower GI (jujenum, colon, and rectum) pathology are persistent diarrhea or hematochezia. Diarrhea is a symptom, not a disease. Most commonly, infection causes diarrhea that resolves with simple supportive interventions, such as hydration and electrolyte replacement, within 5 days.[9] A pattern of similar GI signs and symptoms among family or teammates suggests an infectious origin. In such cases, the affected individuals should be temporarily isolated from others to prevent cross-contamination.

Bismuth subsalicylate (Pepto-Bismol) and loperamide (Imodium) are both OTC medications that are effective in treating diarrhea. As mentioned previously, bismuth subsalicylate is especially effective in treating traveler's diarrhea. Person's with a known allergy to aspirin should not take bismuth subsalicylate.[19]

Radical changes in diet, excessive alcohol consumption, mechanical vibration of the bowels from running long distances, and psychoemotional stress can also cause a bout of diarrhea. An athlete with diarrhea should be withdrawn from participation until the syndrome resolves to prevent dehydration. Return-to-play is allowed once normal, fully hydrated body weight is restored.

Occasionally, diarrhea is the chief compliant in a person with more serious pathology, particularly if it is notably unusual in color or odor, or accompanied by fever, vomiting, or severe abdominal cramps. Recurrent or persistent diarrhea, particularly leading to weight loss or accompanied by other systemic signs and symptoms (fever, fatigue, etc) requires urgent referral to a physician.[2]

Inflammatory Bowel Diseases

The inflammatory bowel diseases, Crohn's disease and ulcerative colitis, are genetic autoimmune disorders in which the small intestine and colon initiate an immune reaction against their own cells. This reaction causes widespread ulceration, fibrosis, and necrosis in the small and large intestines.[21] Onset of the disease is usually in adolescence or early adulthood and the condition often coexists with other immune disorders.

Inflammatory bowel diseases can cause a variety of signs and symptoms, including abdominal pain, chronic diarrhea, hematochezia, weight loss, a palpable abdominal mass (particularly in the right lower quadrant), loss of appetite, skin rash, and intermittent joint pain.[21] A key to recognition is the chronic recurrence of whichever signs and symptoms are present. Inflammatory bowel diseases are not curable, but they are usually not disabling and can be medically managed with diet, lifestyle changes, medication, and surgery as needed. Treatment with medication often involves a combination of drugs depending on the symptoms. Combination therapies include the use of corticosteroids, NSAIDs, antibiotics, and immunosuppressants.[19] Approximately 30% of patients with ulcerative colitis and 70% of patients with Crohn's disease will require surgery.[21]

Persons with inflammatory bowel disease should be monitored during physical activity to ensure adequate hydration. Exacerbation of symptoms are common with heavy exercise or physical activity, but inflammatory bowel disease is not necessarily a contraindication to sports; the treating physician should make this determination.

Irritable Bowel Syndrome

A similar, but less severe and far more common condition is irritable bowel syndrome (IBS), thought to be a reaction to psychophysical stress and poor diet.[22] IBS produces intermittent abdominal pain and cramping, and is most prevalent among young women.[18,22] This disorder affects the motility of the intestines, causing either diarrhea or constipation, or alternating episodes of both. Bloating or abdominal distention may also appear as gas builds up in the colon. Relief of abdominal pain usually occurs after defecation.[22]

IBS does not cause inflammation in the bowels, which distinguishes it from other disorders. In addition, IBS rarely interrupts sleep.[22] Stress reduction, dietary changes, and reasonable physical activity are the usual course of treatment.[18] Alcohol, nicotine, and caffeine use should be curtailed, and a physician should review any medication use. Medication may be prescribed to assist with decreasing stress or relieving symptoms.[22] OTC antidiarrheals and laxatives are the primary medications used to treat IBS. Bulk-forming laxatives (psyllium [Metamucil, Procter & Gamble] or methylcellulose [Citrucel, GlaxoSmithKline]) are usually preferred over stool softeners (docusate [Colace, Roberts Pharmaceutical Corp, Eatontown, NJ]) or osmotic laxatives (magnesium hydroxide [Milk of Magnesia, Bayer Healthcare Pharmaceuticals, Montville, NJ]).[19] With appropriate treatment, most affected people are not substantially limited by IBS.

Appendicitis

The appendix lies in the lower right quadrant of the abdomen, where the terminal ileum becomes the cecum and then the ascending colon. When the appendix becomes acutely inflamed by physical irritants or infection, a general, progressively increasing epigastric abdominal pain appears. The abdominal pain eventually migrates to the lower right quadrant (the right iliac region). McBurney's point, about one-third of the distance from the anterior superior iliac spine to the umbilicus, becomes exquisitely sensitive to palpation, and rebound tenderness or a positive "jar sign" is present (see Lab Exercise 8-1). Passive extension or active flexion of the right hip may be painful because the inflammation sometimes affects the psoas muscle.[12] Loss of appetite and nausea are usually present, although vomiting is rare.[4] Other signs of infection may be present, such as fever and malaise.

The usual treatment is surgical removal of the appendix, although nonsurgical medical treatment is sometimes successful. Return to activity after surgery occurs in 1 to 2 weeks in children and 3 to 4 weeks in adults.[4] If the condition goes untreated, the appendix may inflame to the point that it ruptures, spilling its infected contents into the peritoneal cavity. A ruptured appendix is a medical emergency and requires prompt surgical treatment. Early recognition and proper management of appendicitis are key to preventing rupture.

911

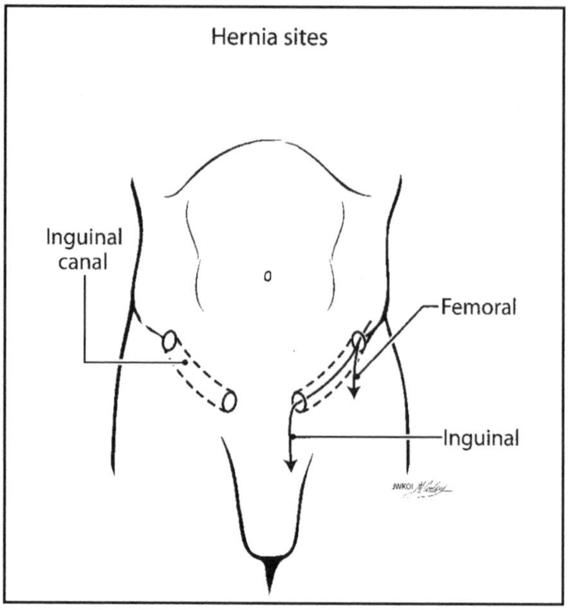

Figure 8-7. Location of indirect, direct, and femoral hernias.

Diverticulosis and Diverticulitis

Multiple herniations of the mucosa and submucosa of the intestine through the muscular layer of the intestinal wall is a condition called diverticulosis. Ten percent of Americans, and as many as half of the elderly population, have this anatomical disorder. In most cases diverticulosis is asymptomatic.

If feces becomes trapped in a herniated section or such a section becomes obstructed, an inflammation of the herniated section, called *diverticulitis*, results. Symptoms include severe abdominal cramping and constant pain in the lower left quadrant; this pain may radiate to the back.[6] Additional signs include alternating constipation and diarrhea, fever, and rectal bleeding. The pain and cramping usually worsen a few hours after eating and may briefly resolve after defecation.

Treatment with a high-fiber diet and light exercise to encourage bowel motility is common. In more severe cases involving infection or a complete bowel obstruction (causing an ischemic bowel segment), antibiotics and emergency surgery may be required.

Hernia

Herniation occurs when an organ or part of an organ protrudes through a defect in the tissue surrounding that organ.[6,12] A segment of small intestine can herniate into the inguinal canal, under the inguinal ligament and into the femoral canal (which contains the neurovascular bundle) (Figure 8-7), or through the linea alba near the umbilicus. Inguinal, femoral, and umbilical hernias often cause a palpable bulge at the herniation.[4,6] With an indirect inguinal hernia, the herniated segment travels down the inguinal canal and into the scrotum, where the bowel loop may be palpated by the athlete during showering or self-examination. History may include a sudden tearing sensation that occurred during a specific physical exertion, although many persons do not remember a particular episode. Many hernias are detectable only by medical imaging and may be completely asymptomatic.[4,6]

The primary symptom of hernia is a burning pain in the groin. This pain worsens with activity, an increase in abdominal pressure (Valsalva maneuver), or body position.[6] Pain from an inguinal or femoral hernia may radiate into the anterior thigh if it irritates the femoral nerve. An umbilical hernia produces pain in the abdominal wall near the point of herniation. The intestinal segment may herniate only intermittently, and thus cause only intermittent symptoms. Herniation of a large bowel segment that does not retract, a condition called strangulation of the bowel, requires surgical repair to prevent bowel ishcemia or obstruction.[6] Modern surgical techniques allow laproscopic hernia repair. Gradual return to physical activity can be expected in about 1 week after laproscopic surgery; open surgical repair requires an additional week or two of recovery.[4]

Hemorrhoids

Hemorrhoids, also called "piles," are veins in the rectum or anus that become dilated. The reason for the dilation is poorly understood, but is thought to be related to genetic predisposition, frequent constipation, and liver disease (both of which increase pressure in the anorectal veins). Internal hemorrhoids occur inside the rectum; external hemorrhoids protrude through the anal border. In either case, bright red blood may appear with defecation, although no pain occurs unless the rectum or anus is fissured (split in tissue) or the veins become strangulated (ischemic). Pain and itching accompany external hemorrhoids, particularly during sitting.

Very common, very bothersome, but usually not medically serious, hemorrhoids are treated with changes in diet, to soften the stool and reduce constipation, and topical medications to relieve symptoms. Topical medications are available in a variety of dosage forms including creams, suppositories, ointments, and pads. Although minimal, some systemic absorption may occur with medications, depending on the dosage form. Occasionally surgery is needed to provide relief.

Colorectal Cancer

Cancer of the colon and rectum causes the second most cancer deaths in the United States annually. Age over 50 years, a family history of colorectal cancer, history of other colon disorders, presence of polyps in the colon, and a high-fat, high-sugar, low-fiber diet are risk factors for colorectal cancer. Colorectal cancer can exist for a long time before symptoms are noticed. Bleeding from the rectum or bloody stools is usually the first sign. Change in bowel habits, including intermittent diarrhea and constipation, and a continuing sense of bowel fullness even after a bowel movement are other potential symptoms of colorectal cancer. Depending on the stage of the cancer, treatment will usually involve surgery, chemotherapy, radiation, or a combination of these. Prognosis depends on the stage of the disease when diagnosed. Early detection is associated with a 5-year survival rate of nearly 100%; the survival rate in advanced disease is very low.

Abdominal Trauma

Persistent abdominal pain, localized tenderness, abdominal rigidity, or upper GI signs (nausea, vomiting, etc) after a blow to the ribs or abdomen requires emergency referral. If an athlete sustains a blow that fractures ribs, causes bruising in the abdomen, causes abdominal cramping, or produces rigidity, a physician should examine him or her as soon as possible.[4] In sports, the spleen and liver are the abdominal organs most susceptible to injury.

Spleen Trauma and Splenomegaly

The spleen stores platelets and other types of blood cells and filters the blood to remove small particles and deformed or old red blood cells. The spleen lies on the left side of the abdomen under the region from the ninth to the eleventh ribs. A direct blow to the LUQ is thus the most common mechanism of injury.[4] Signs and symptoms of splenic injury include shock, nausea, vomiting, rigidity in the LUQ, abdominal pain, and pain referred to the left shoulder (known as Kehr's sign).[3,4] The pain in the left shoulder is a result of diaphragmmatic irritation caused by inflammation and bleeding of the spleen. Occasionally, signs of serious injury to the spleen appear gradually and are difficult to recognize. The spleen's ability to "splint" itself through clotting may cause a delay in the presentation of symptoms. Later disruption of the clot or "splint" will cause symptoms to develop hours or days after the original injury, leading to severe shock and death. Any suspicion of splenic injury, by history, symptoms, or signs, requires immediate withdrawal from participation and urgent medical referral.

People with *splenomegaly*, a pathological enlargement of the spleen, often from medical conditions such as mononucleosis (see Chapter Four), require at least 3 weeks of rest before resuming physical activity, and 1 month or more before returning to strenuous athletic activity.[3,9] Splenomegaly greatly increases the risk of splenic rupture, so physician clearance is required before return to contact or collision sports.[3,4]

Liver Trauma

Trauma to the liver is more subtle in its clinical presentation than trauma to the spleen.[3,4,23] The mechansim of liver injury is a direct blow to the RUQ; liver injury is less common than splenic injury. Persistent abdominal pain, RUQ tenderness, and upper GI signs (nausea, vomiting, etc.) are signs of liver injury and warrant an emergency medical examination.[4,23] Many liver injuries recover naturally and do not require surgery, but all such injuries should be monitored overnight in a hospital and followed by a physician upon discharge.[4,5,23] Recovery, from either surgical or nonsurgical treatment, can take weeks or months.[23] A liver injury severe enough to require surgery often results in a permanent exclusion from sports.[4]

Hepatic-Biliary Diseases

Hepatitis

Hepatitis, meaning literally "inflammation of the liver," occurs primarily with viral infection or liver toxicity; the inflammation response affects liver function, which causes the signs and symptoms. Viral infection is the leading cause of hepatitis in the United States.

Hepatitis types (A, B, C, and D) refer to the different viruses that infect the liver.[24] Hepatitis A virus is transmitted through close personal contact (oral-oral route) or by contamination when food preparers do not wash their hands appropriately (oral-fecal route). Hepatitis B, C, and D require direct exposure to body fluids, including blood, urine, feces, saliva, mucous, tears, vomit, semen, or vaginal secretions.[24,25] Children and adolescents usually acquire hepatitis A, whereas young adults are more likely to contract hepatitis B or hepatitis C. Hepatitis D occurs primarily as a complication of type B. Hepatitis B and hepatitis C are more damaging to the liver than hepatitis A or hepatitis D.

Health care workers are at increased risk for contracting viral hepatitis since they are exposed to many people who have chronic illnesses.[6] Vaccines are available for hepatitis viruses A and B, and vaccination is recommended for all health care workers. Frequent handwashing and strict adherence to standard precautions (ie, gloves; mask and gown as needed) also offer protection against exposure and spread of hepatitis.[24,25]

Three stages of hepatitis infection are described: initial, icteric, and recovery. The initial stage may be asymptomatic, although the hepatitis virus is highly communicable during this time.[24] During this stage, general systemic signs and symptoms may appear, including fatigue, loss of appetite, nausea, diarrhea, weight loss, and joint pain.[6] As hepatitis progresses, urine darkens and stool lightens in color as a result of the pigment bilirubin increasing in concentration in the blood.[6,24] During this stage, the liver swells and becomes tender to palpation.

The icteric stage begins three or four weeks later, producing jaundice that lasts 6 to 8 weeks as the systemic signs slowly resolve. Near the end of this stage, the liver begins to return to normal size, but the spleen enlarges and cervical lymph nodes may swell. The virus is no longer communicable at this point.

The recovery stage, when it occurs, can last 4 months or longer. Fatigue is the most prominent symptom as liver function normalizes.[24]

Specific medical treatments do not exist for hepatitis, although antiviral agents and supportive measures are usually administered. Practicing infection control measures, such as rigorous handwashing when working with food or between patient contacts, and inoculating health care workers are prudent preventative measures. Most people infected with hepatitis A recover fully. Recovery from the other types of hepatitis depend on the aggressiveness of infection and timing of medical intervention. Hepatitis B can be fatal.

Toxic hepatitis is an inflammation of the liver that occurs after exposure to certain chemicals or drugs, including antibiotics, oral contraceptives, psychotropics, and cytotoxic drugs used to treat cancer. The chemicals damage liver cells, which become necrotic and cause an inflammatory response. The symptoms and signs depend on the extent of the necrosis. Clinical presentation resembles viral hepatitis, including jaundice, fatigue, loss of appetite, dark urine and light stools, fever, joint pain, and RUQ pain. Treatment is removal of the offending agent and strict avoidance of the toxin.

Chronic hepatitis can develop from viral infection, chronic exposure to toxins, or idiopathic (unknown) etiology.[24] Chronic hepatitis produces liver necrosis and irreparable scarring, called cirrhosis. Many secondary syndromes develop, such as arthritis, kidney disorders, and anemia, as waste products unprocessed by the diseased liver flood the bloodstream. Chronic hepatitis is treated with steroids to reduce the inflammation; unfortunately, the steroids themselves cause many complications and side effects. The prognosis for chronic hepatitis is poor.

Cirrhosis

Cirrhosis is the result of the combined effects of chronic liver disease and malnutrition that irreversibly damages liver cells. Cirrhosis produces cellular damage and necrosis, which lead to fibrotic changes in the liver. The fibrous tissue eventually interferes with the liver's vascular supply and function, leading to ascites, splenomegaly, central and peripheral neurological effects, and various GI system signs and symptoms. Cirrhosis is incurable; the fibrous scarring does not heal. Medical treatment includes addressing the underlying cause (eg, alcohol abuse or hepatitis) to prevent further necrosis and supportive measures. Cirrohsis caused by chronic hepatitis often requires a liver transplant. Overdose of acetaminophen can also cause liver necrosis, requiring a liver transplant.

Alcohol abuse is the leading cause of liver disease in America.[6] Prolonged consumption of large amounts of alcohol leads to hepatitis, cirrhosis, hepatic failure, and death. To quit drinking in such cases is critical, but is difficult both physically and psychologically. Chapter Fourteen discusses alcohol abuse in more detail.

Gallstones and Gallbladder Disease

Gallstones (cholelithiasis) and gallbladder disease (cholecystitis) both produce intermittent RUQ pain that worsens after meals that include fatty foods. Secretion of bile increases when fatty foods are eaten; the increased activity of the gallbladder produces the pain when disease or gallstones are present.

Gallstones account for nearly 20% of all hospital admissions among adults. An increased risk of gallstones is associated with age over 40 years, obesity, a high cholesterol diet, and diabetes. Females are at higher risk, most likely because of elevated estrogen levels, oral contraceptive use, or multiple births; increased estrogen levels inhibit production of bile acid, which leads to collection of cholesterol and bilirubin in the gallbladder. Gallstones are comprised primarily of cholesterol and bilirubin.

Cholecystitis results when gallstones block the cystic duct, the gallbladder's attachment to the common bile duct. Fever, jaundice, vomiting, RUQ tenderness, and referred right shoulder or right scapular pain suggest an acute gallbladder attack.[6] Right shoulder pain is the result of irritation of the diaphragm by the inflammed gallbladder. Chronic cholecystitis may present severe RUQ pain, accompanied by intolerance for spicy or fatty foods, heartburn, belching, constipation, or diarrhea. Laproscopic surgery can remove the gallstones or gallbladder to relieve symptoms. Recovery depends on the size and extent of the gallstones.

Pancreatitis

Acute pancreatitis occurs when the pancreatic enzymes become active within the pancreas rather than the duodenum. The activated enzymes self-digest the pancreatic cells, causing an inflammatory response.[26] The inflammation cascades into severe peritonitis, sudden and excruciating epigastric and LUQ pain, left shoulder pain, LUQ rigidity, and possibly shock. Infection can lead quickly to septicemia (bacteria in the bloodstream) and death. Acute pancreatitis is a medical emergency that has a dramatic clinical presentation of severe illness.[26]

Summary

Many GI disorders can be attributed to lifestyle, including diet, nicotine and alcohol use, and physical inactivity. Other serious disorders are caused by infection, chronic disease processes, or obstruction of the GI tract or its organs' ducts. Common signs and symptoms of GI disorders include nausea, vomiting, diarrhea, constipation, and abdominal pain. The liver, gallbladder, spleen, and exocrine pancreas produce upper abdominal pain that may refer to the shoulders as inflammation of those organs irritate the diaphragm. Pathology in these organs usually disturb digestion. Medical emergencies of the abdomen, containing the GI system, hepatic-biliary system, and spleen, often produce peritonitis, recognizable by abdominal pain, tenderness, localized rigidity, and positive rebound or jar signs. Peritonitis causes fever or shock as it progresses, thereby demanding immediate medical care.

Case Study

One of the football coaches runs into your office and states that he thinks Bill, the offensive line coach, is having a heart attack. Bill is a 45-year-old male who is obese and has high cholesterol.

On your way to Bill's office, the assistant coach tells you that he and Bill had gone for chili cheeseburgers and french fries a couple of hours ago for lunch. Immediately after lunch Bill had complained of an upset stomach, but he usually gets an upset stomach after a big meal. It usually goes away in a couple of hours.

When you get to Bill's office, you find him bent over in obvious pain. His skin appears to be a very pale green, and he's bent over vomiting into his wastebasket. He is fully alert and oriented. He describes his pain as a severe ache in the right shoulder and shoulder blade. He denies having any chest pain.

Bill's heart rate is strong and regular at 90 beats per minute. His respirations also appear strong and regular, and he denies having any problems breathing. You notice while taking his pulse that he feels warm to the touch, and he is sweating profusely. You palpate his abdomen and find that he is acutely tender in the RUQ.

Critical Thinking Questions

1. Based on Bill's clinical presentation, do you think he is having a heart attack? What other conditions might be causing his signs and symptoms?
2. What tests might you do to determine if Bill is having a heart attack or suffering from a different condition?
3. What other steps might you take to manage Bill's condition?

References

1. National Athletic Trainers' Association. *Athletic Training Educational Competencies.* 4th ed. Dallas, TX: National Athletic Trainers' Association; 2005.
2. Butcher JD. Runners' diarrhea and other intestinal problems of athletes. *Am Fam Physician.* 1993;48(4):623-627.
3. Green GA. Gastrointestinal disorders in the athlete. *Clin Sports Med.* 1992;11(2):453-470.
4. Amaral JF. Thoracoabdominal injuries in the athlete. *Clin Sports Med.* 1997;16(4):739-753.
5. Ryan JM. Abdominal injuries and sport. *Br J Sports Med.* 1999;33(3):155-160.
6. Koopmeiners MB. Screening for gastrointestinal system disease. In: Boissonnault WG, ed. *Examination in Physical Therapy Practice: Screening for Medical Disease.* 2nd ed. New York, NY: Churchill-Livingstone Inc; 1995:101-116.
7. Moses FM. The effect of exercise on the gastrointestinal tract. *Sports Med.* 1990;9(3):159-172.
8. Stone R. Primary care diagnosis of acute abdominal pain. *Nurse Practitioner.* 1996;21(12):19-20, 23-26, 28-30, 35-41.
9. Mellman MF, Podesta L. Common medical problems in sports. *Clin Sports Med.* 1997;16(4):635-662.
10. Ganong WF. *Review of Medical Physiology.* 22nd ed. New York, NY: McGraw-Hill Medical; 2005.
11. Stopka CB, Zambito KL. Referred visceral pain: what every sports medicine professional needs to know. *Athl Ther Today.* 1999;4(1):29-36.
12. Bickley LS, Szilagyi PG. *Bates' Guide to Physical Examination and History Taking.* 9th ed. Philadelphia, PA: Lippincott Williams & Wilkins; 2005.

13. Putukian M. Assessment of abdominal conditions in athletes. *Athl Ther Today.* 2000;5(6):20-29.
14. DeGowin RL, Brown DD. *DeGowin's Diagnostic Examination.* 7th ed. New York, NY: McGraw-Hill; 2000.
15. George B, Markle IV. A simple test for intraperitoneal inflammation. *Am J Surg.* 1973;125:721-722.
16. Sevier TL. Infectious disease in athletes. *Med Clin North Am.* 1994;78(2):389-412.
17. Boyce TG. Gastroenteritis. In: Beers MH, Berkow R, eds. *The Merck Manual of Diagnosis and Therapy.* 17th ed. Whitehouse Station, NJ: Merck Research Laboratories; 1999:283-292.
18. Casey E, Mistry DJ, MacKnight JM. Training room management of medical conditions: sports gastroenterology. *Clin Sports Med.* 2005;24(3):525-540.
19. Houglum JE, Harrelson GL, Leaver-Dunn D. *Principles of Pharmacology for Athletic Trainers.* Thorofare, NJ: SLACK Incorporated; 2005.
20. Finn S, Hirschowitz BI. Gastritis and peptic ulcer disease. In: Beers MH, Berkow R, eds. *The Merck Manual of Diagnosis and Therapy.* 17th ed. Whitehouse Station, NJ: Merck Research Laboratories; 1999:245-255.
21. Sachar DB, Walfish J. Inflammatory bowel diseases. In: Beers MH, Berkow R, eds. *The Merck Manual of Diagnosis and Therapy.* 17th ed. Whitehouse Station, NJ: Merck Research Laboratories; 1999:302-311.
22. Olden K. Functional bowel disorders. In: Beers MH, Berkow R, eds. *The Merck Manual of Diagnosis and Therapy.* 17th ed. Whitehouse Station, NJ: Merck Research Laboratories; 1999:312-317.
23. Ray R, Lernire JE. Liver laceration in an intercollegiate football player. *J Athl Training.* 1995;30(4):324-326.
24. Simon JB. Hepatitis. In: Beers MH, Berkow R, eds. *The Merck Manual of Diagnosis and Therapy.* 17th ed. Whitehouse Station, NJ: Merck Research Laboratories; 1999:377-385.
25. Buxton BP, Daniell JE, Buxton BHJ, Okasaki EM, Ho KW. Prevention of hepatitis B virus in athletic training. *J Athl Training.* 1994;29(2):107-112.
26. Freedman SD. Pancreatitis. In: Beers MH, Berkow R, eds. *The Merck Manual of Diagnosis and Therapy.* 17th ed. Whitehouse Station, NJ: Merck Research Laboratories; 1999:269-274.

Online Resources

Gastrointestinal

American College of Gastroenterology
www.acg.gi.org/patients

Colorectal Cancer Network
http://www.colorectal-cancer.net

Emedicine's online Gastroenterology textbook
www.emedicine.com/med/GASTROENTEROLOGY.htm

National Digestive Diseases Information Clearinghouse
www.digestive.niddk.nih.gov/ddiseases/a-z.asp

Hepatic-Biliary

American Liver Foundation
www.liverfoundation.org

Gallstones (National Institute of Diabetes and Digestive and Kidney Diseases)
www.digestive.niddk.nih.gov/ddiseases/pubs/gallstones

Hepatitis Foundation International
www.hepfi.org

Lab Exercise 8-1
Assessment of the Abdomen

Objectives

After completing this lab activity, students will be able to:

1. Auscultate the abdomen to identify normal bowel sounds.
2. Percuss the abdomen to identify normal tissue density within each abdominal quadrant.
3. Identify and palpate the major structures located within each abdominal quadrant.

Competencies

This lab exercise addresses the following psychomotor competencies from the NATA's *Athletic Training Educational Competencies, 4th ed*:

- Medical Conditions and Disabilities: 3, 4a, 4b

Equipment Needed

- Stethoscope
- Blood pressure cuff
- Watch displaying seconds

Instructions

Part 1: Auscultation of the Abdomen

It is important to listen to the bowel sounds **before** you palpate the abdomen. Palpating the abdomen first may disturb the intestinal contents and produce false bowel sounds. Normal peristalsis produces sounds like gurgles, tinkling, or clicks with a rate of 5 to 34 per minute. **Note:** It may take up to 2 minutes before bowel sounds are heard. Injury or illness may inhibit or shut down the normal peristaltic mechanism, causing a decrease in or complete absence of sounds.

1. Position your subject supine in the hook-lying position with his or her arms by his or her side (see Figure 8-4).
2. With the stethoscope placed directly on the skin, listen for the presence or absence of sounds as well as the pitch or tone of sounds.
3. Listen within each quadrant.
4. On the diagrams provided (p. 200), describe the sounds you heard within each quadrant.

Lab Exercise 8-1 (continued)
Assessment of the Abdomen

Diagrams for Part 1:

Subject #1: ______________________

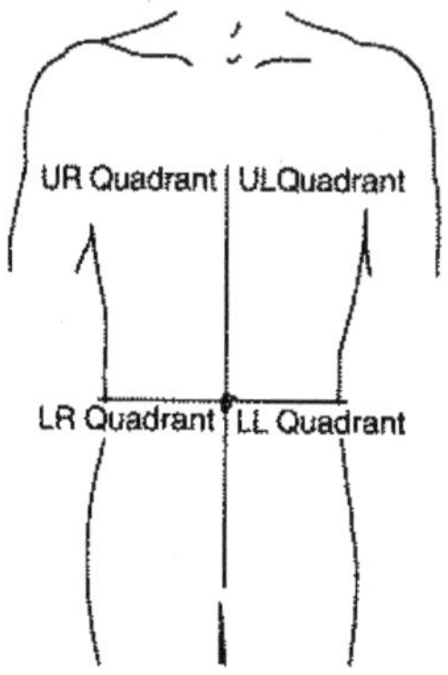

Subject #2: ______________________

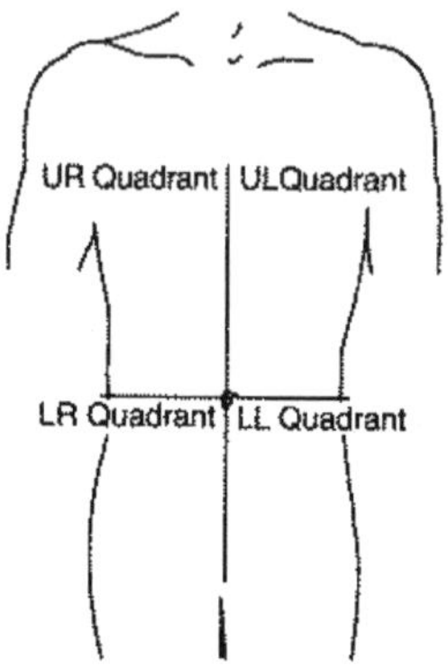

Subject #3: ______________________

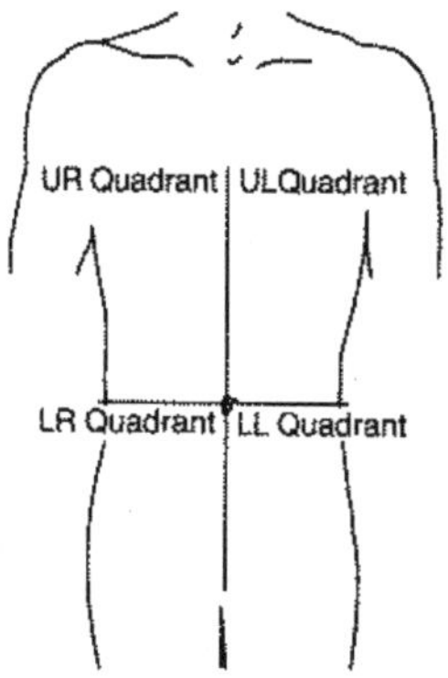

Subject #4: ______________________

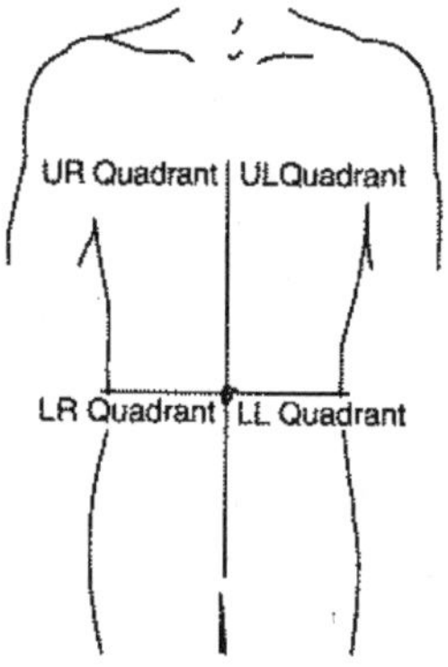

Lab Exercise 8-1 (continued)
Assessment of the Abdomen

Part 2: Percussion

You can assess tissue density by percussing the abdomen. Hollow organs will sound different than solid organs (dull thump). Internal bleeding within the abdominal cavity can change the percussion sound from hollow to more of a solid, dull sound. The percussion technique is the same as that used in pulmonary percussion.

1. Position your subject in the hook-lying position.
2. Place the distal phalanx of the third finger from the left hand flat on the area that you want to percuss.
3. Using the tip of the right third finger, quickly strike the DIP joint of the finger resting on the abdomen.
4. You should hear a hollow echo sound or a dull thump sound.
5. Repeat Steps 1 through 4 throughout each of the four quadrants.
6. In the upper right quadrant, percuss over the ribcage into the abdomen, listening for the dullness associated with the liver. Percussion can be used to identify the size and position of the liver below the ribcage.
7. In the upper left quadrant, percuss over the ribcage into the abdomen, listening for the dullness associated with the spleen. Percussion can be used to identify the size and position of the spleen below the ribcage.
8. Describe and record the sounds that you hear within each quadrant on the diagrams provided (p. 202).

Lab Exercise 8-1 (continued)
Assessment of the Abdomen

Diagrams for Part 2:

Subject #1: ______________________

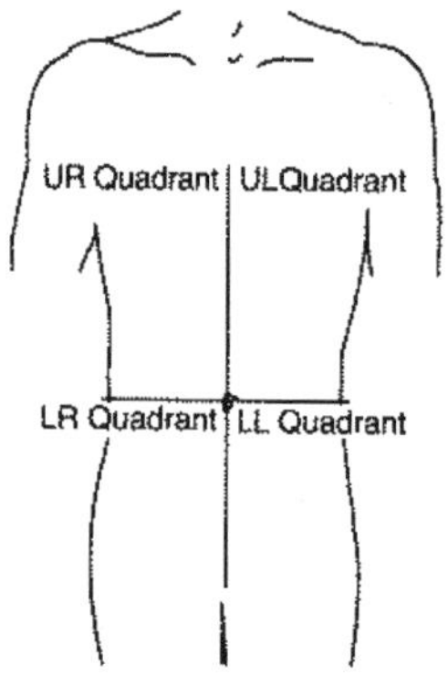

Subject #2: ______________________

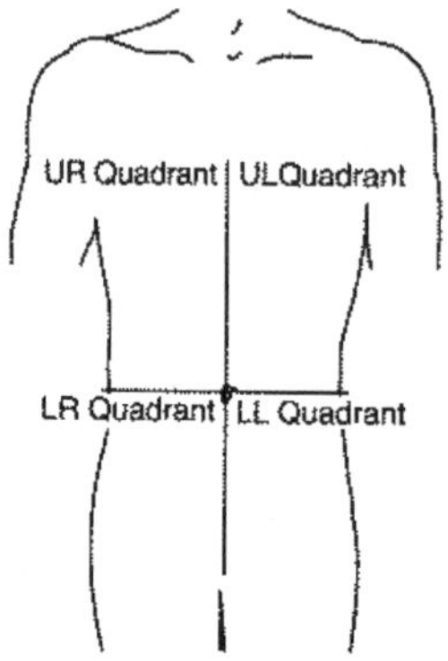

Subject #3: ______________________

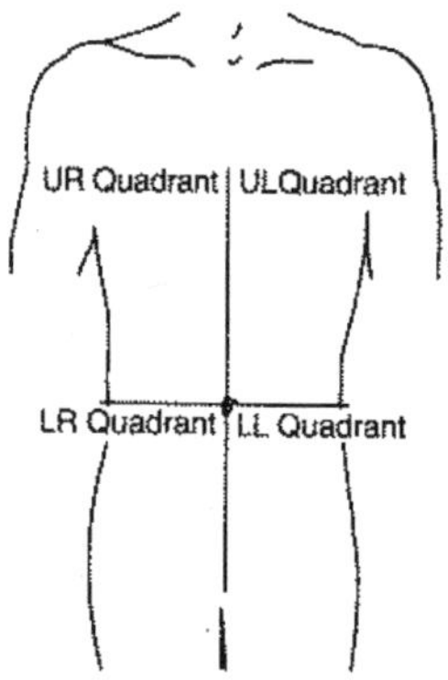

Subject #4: ______________________

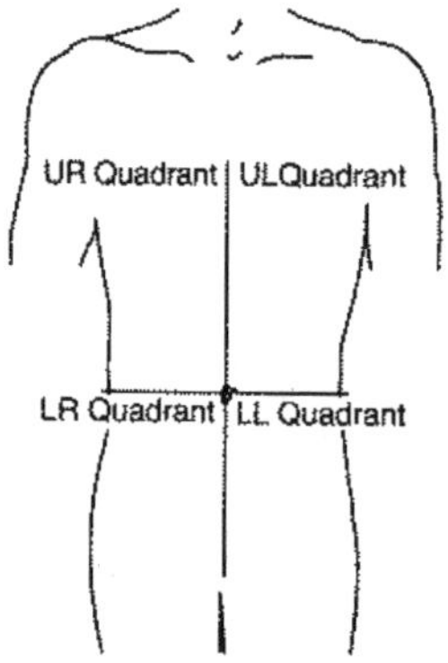

Lab Exercise 8-1 (continued)
Assessment of the Abdomen

Part 3: Palpation

Palpation of the abdomen is performed after auscultation and percussion. Each abdominal quadrant should be palpated for rigidity, pain or point tenderness, and rebound tenderness.

1. Position your subject in the hook-lying position.
2. Palpate each quadrant of the abdomen with the palmer aspect of the phalanges (not a single finger). It is important to become comfortable with how a "normal" abdomen presents.
3. For deeper palpation, one hand should be placed on top of the other (see Figure 8-5b). Again, palpate each quadrant. Palpation can be further enhanced by placing one hand under the abdomen and palpating upward (see Figure 8-6.)
4. The liver, gallbladder, and spleen can be palpated more easily by having the subject raise his or her arms above his or her head.
5. Repeat Steps 1 through 4 with at least **four** different subjects with at least one of these being evaluated by your lab instructor or ACI.

Subject #1____

Subject #2____

Subject #3____

Subject #4 ____

Chapter Nine

Renal and Urogenital Systems

Chapter Outline and Objectives

Introduction

Review of Anatomy and Pathogenesis

- Describe the basic renal and urogenital structures and their functions.
- Describe the pathophysiological mechanisms of the renal and urogenital systems.
- Describe the response of the renal and urogenital systems to exercise.

Signs and Symptoms

- Identify the general signs and symptoms of renal pathology.
- Identify the general signs and symptoms of urogenital pathology.
  - Hematuria
  - Change in Urinary Habit
  - Nipple Discharge
  - Hypertension
  - Anemia
  - Sexual Dysfunction
  - Menstrual Irregularities

Pain Patterns

- Identify the referred pain patterns associated with pathology of the renal and urogenital systems.
  - Kidneys, Ureters, and Bladder
  - Male Urogenital System
  - Female Urogenital System

Medical History and Physical Examination

- Describe medical history findings associated with renal and urogenital pathology.
- Describe the physical examination procedures associated with renal and urogenital pathology.

- Inspection
- Palpation
- Urinalysis

Pathology and Pathogenesis

- ❖ Describe medical history findings associated with renal and urogenital pathology.
- ❖ Discuss the signs, symptoms, management, and medical referral guidelines for pathology involving the renal system.

Renal and Bladder Trauma

- ❖ Discuss the signs, symptoms, management, and medical referral guidelines for pathology involving the urogenital system.

Renal, Bladder, and Genital Infections

- ❖ Urinary Tract Infection
- ❖ Sexually Transmitted Infections
    - Gonorrhea
    - Chlamydia
    - Syphilis
    - Genital Warts
    - Herpes
- ❖ Pelvic Inflammatory Disease

Renal Disorders

- ❖ Urolithiasis
- ❖ Renal Failure

Male Urogenital Disorders

- ❖ Monorchidism
- ❖ Prostate Disorders
- ❖ Prostate Cancer
- ❖ Scrotum and Testicular Trauma
- ❖ Testicular Torsion
- ❖ Varicoceles
- ❖ Testicular Cancer

Female Urogenital Disorders

- ❖ Endometriosis
- ❖ Pregnancy
- ❖ Ruptured Ectopic Pregnancy
- ❖ Female Athletic Triad
- ❖ Breast Disorders
- ❖ Breast Cancer
- ❖ Ovarian Cysts
- ❖ Cervical, Ovarian, and Uterine Cancers

Pediatric Concerns

- ❖ Primary Amenorrhea
- ❖ Kidney Trauma
- ❖ Cryptorchidism

This chapter addresses the following competencies from the *Athletic Training Educational Competencies, Fourth Edition*[1]:

Domain	Cognitive	Psychomotor
Acute Care of Injuries and Illnesses	4, 16, 30	
Medical Conditions and Disabilities	1–3, 14, 16, 20	4f
Orthopedic Clinical Examination and Diagnosis	1, 6, 16	
Pathology of Injuries and Illnesses	3–6	
Risk Management and Injury Prevention	15	

INTRODUCTION

The renal system is responsible for regulating body fluid levels and removing waste products from the blood. The urinary system functions to excrete these waste products from the body. The genital system contains the organs of reproduction that are specific to each gender. Trauma, infection, tumors, hormonal imbalances, and congenital conditions can cause pathology in the renal and urogenital systems. In addition to disorders of the renal and urogenital systems, this chapter includes discussions of other gender-specific medical conditions that affect physical activity.

REVIEW OF ANATOMY, PHYSIOLOGY, AND PATHOGENESIS

Renal-Urinary System

The renal-urinary system, which consists of the kidneys, ureters, bladder, and urethra (Figure 9-1), filters the blood, regulates body fluids, and eliminates metabolic waste from the blood. The kidneys remove waste products and excess water from the blood and regulate electrolyte levels in the body. These substances are collected and sent through the ureters to the bladder, exiting the body through the urethra as urine. The kidneys contribute to homeostasis by providing hormonal and osmotic (fluid balance) control of blood pressure (BP), regulating red blood cell production, and regulating calcium levels.[2,3]

Urine normally contains water, salt, and the by-products of protein metabolism, namely urea, creatine, and various acids. Urine may also normally contain small amounts of glucose, dead cells, crystallized salts, and mucus. Blood cells and whole proteins should not be present in urine since they are too large to be normally absorbed through the renal system.[3] The detection of protein during urinalysis is thus by definition pathological.

The kidneys have a dual role in the control of BP. First, the kidneys secrete the hormone renin, an enzyme which converts angiotensinogen, a protein that circulates in the blood, to angiotensin I. In the presence of angiotensin-converting enzyme (ACE), angiotensin I becomes angiotensin II. Angiotensin II increases vascular resistance by causing vasoconstriction, which in turn increases BP. Thus, the secretion of renin by the kidneys leads to an increase in BP. Angiotensin II also increases the reabsorption of sodium by the renal tubules. Renin secretion is stimulated by falling BP detected by receptors in the kidneys and by increasing catecholemines and

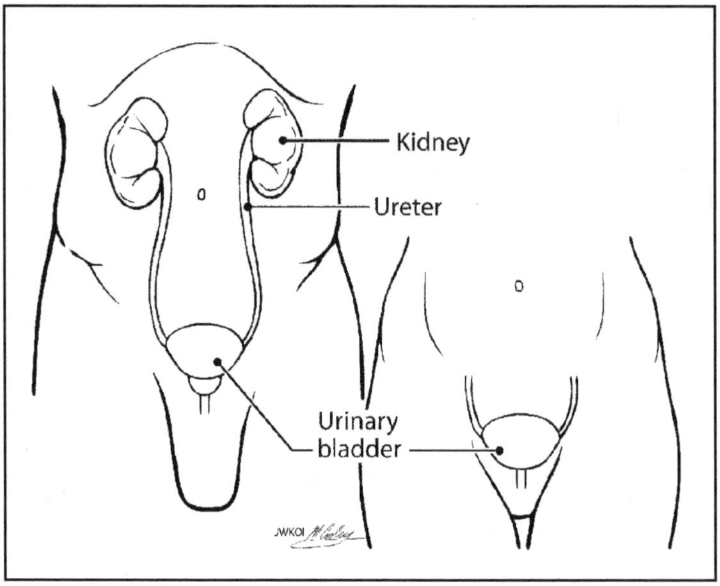

Figure 9-1. Organs of the renal system and urogenital tract.

norepinephrine released by sympathetic nervous system activity. Renin secretion is inhibited by angiotensin II and by increases in electrolyte (sodium, chlorine, and potassium) levels that are detected by receptors in the kidneys. The second function of the kidneys in regulating BP is to eliminate excess fluid, thus maintaining a consistent fluid level in the body and the blood.[2,4] The regulation of fluid level directly affects BP.

If the overall fluid level drops, as occurs with severe bleeding or dehydration, BP decreases. When BP decreases for any reason, the kidneys release renin to restore BP. Conversely, if the kidney is unable to remove excess fluid from the body or if the blood retains excess fluid (*hypervolemia*), BP increases as the increased volume of fluid in the vascular system exerts more pressure on the vascular walls.[2] With chronic secretion of renin or hypervolemia, systemic hypertension results. Chronic hypertension, whether caused by hormonal or fluid imbalances, damages the nephrons of the kidney, which accentuates and perpetuates the problem.

During resistance exercise, systolic and diastolic BP increases in proportion to exercise load. Persons with cardiovascular or kidney problems are thus advised to avoid resistance training. During endurance exercise, systolic BP first increases moderately, then levels off, and gradually decreases back to normal as exercise continues. Diastolic BP changes very little during endurance exercise. Moderate intensity endurance exercise is thus usually recommended for persons with pathology of the cardiovascular or renal systems, or who have hypertension.

The kidneys can be damaged by trauma, toxins, chronic disease, obstruction of urine collection or flow, and chronically high concentrations of glucose (as occurs in diabetes mellitus), urea, or creatine in the blood.[3] Regardless of the etiology, kidney pathology affects the function of the nephrons; nephrons are the basic unit of the kidney and consist of a glomerulus (the vascular component) and the tubular system for collecting and concentrating urine.[3] Simply stated, pathology changes the kidney's filtering process. The kidney either extracts elements from the blood that it should not, fails to extract elements it should, or both. The osmotic pressure in the kidney capillaries (glomeruli) becomes closer to the osmotic pressure in the blood.

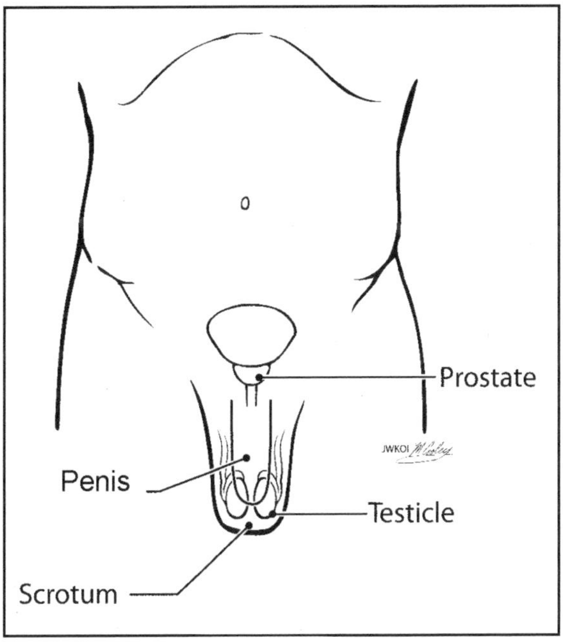

Figure 9-2. Organs of the male genital system.

The nephron then begins to absorb a large amount of fluid in an effort to restore proper osmotic tension. The increased fluid in turn affects the ability of the kidney to draw solutes (waste products) into the urine, so the waste products accumulate in the blood.

Over time, the build up of metabolic by-products in the blood damages other organ-systems. The most notable effects occur in the cardiovascular and neurological systems. Chronic kidney disorders often result in hypertension as they impair the kidneys' role in regulation of BP. Disturbance of acid-base balance produces metabolic imbalances (acidosis or alkalosis) that either depress or excite the central nervous system.

Reproductive System

The male genital system includes the prostate gland, spermatic cord, testes, epididymis, vas deferens, seminal vesicles, urethra, and penis (Figure 9-2). The female genital system includes the ovaries, fallopian tubes, uterus, cervix, and vagina (Figure 9-3). Some organs of the genital system are stimulated by hormones of the hypothalamus (gonadotropin-releasing hormone, prolactin-releasing hormone, and prolactin-inhibiting hormone), and pituitary gland (prolactin, follicle-stimulating hormone, and luteinizing hormone) to release gender specific hormones. The testes produce testosterone and the ovaries produce estrogen, although both sexes have small circulating amounts of the opposite gender's hormones. The "sex hormones" induce puberty, the development of sexual maturation and secondary sex characteristics, and regulate sexual health and function. Testosterone stimulates development of the penis, prostate, and seminal vesicles during puberty, as well as causing enlargement of the larynx and thickening of the vocal cords, producing the characteristic deeper voice of males. Testosterone also influences the growth of face and body (axilla, chest) hair, aggressive behaviors, muscular development, and sebaceous gland activity. Estrogen stimulates uterine and ovarian blood flow and

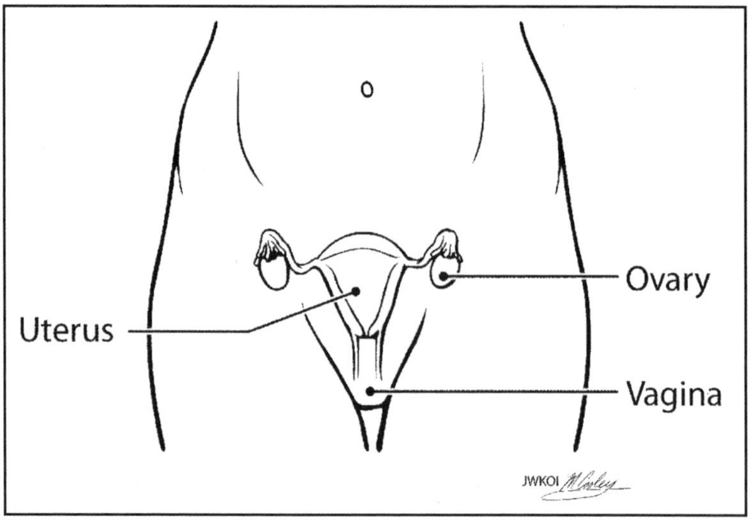

Figure 9-3. Organs of the female genital system.

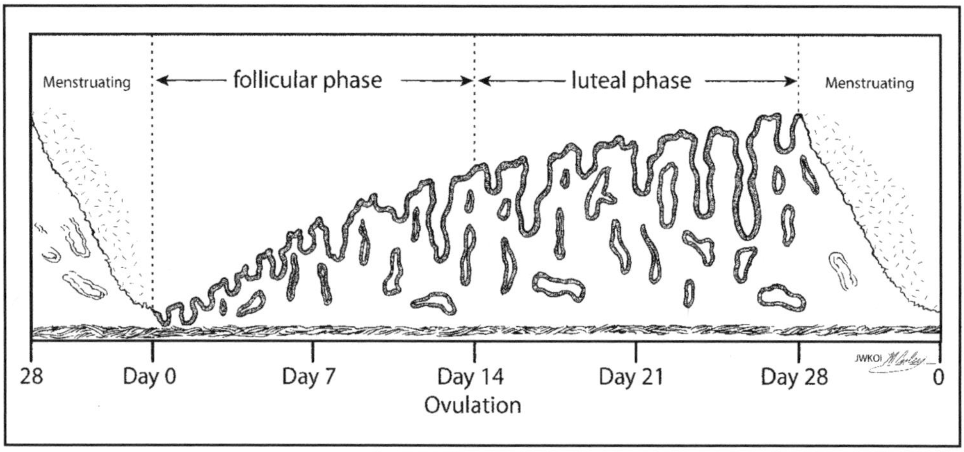

Figure 9-4. Hormonal regulation of menstruation.

growth, as well as enlargement of the breasts, breast ducts, and vagina—although many of the secondary female characteristics (narrow shoulders, broader hips, higher-pitched voice, less body hair) depends at least as much upon the absence of testosterone and other androgens as upon the presence of estrogen. Estrogen also increases libido (sexual motivation) in both sexes.

Several hormones produced by the hypothalamus regulate menstruation. The hypothalamus hormones also stimulate the pituitary gland to release hormones that affect estrogen and progesterone production in the ovaries (Figure 9-4).[5,6] Estrogen and progesterone interact to produce endometrial development in the presence of *ovulation*, the release of an ovum from the ovaries that occurs approximately 2 weeks before menses. Thickening of the endometrium is needed to nuture a fertilized ovum in the event of pregnancy. When estrogen and progesterone levels decrease, the thick, blood-rich endometrium is expelled (menses) to prepare the uterus for the next cycle. The menstrual cycle is very sensitive to hormonal levels and nutrition. *Amenorrhea*, the absence of menses, occurs with pregnancy, endocrine disorders, and malnutrition.

Finally, the urogenital system also has a musculoskeletal component. The organs of the pelvis are supported by a horizontal sling of muscles that form a sling within the pelvic ring. These muscles suspend the organs within the pelvic cavity and assist in urinary and sexual function. Impairment of these muscles can cause urinary or sexual disability.

SIGNS AND SYMPTOMS

Hematuria

Blood in the urine is a sign of kidney or bladder pathology. Gross hematuria after a blow to the back or abdomen suggests kidney, ureter, or bladder injury and is therefore a medical emergency. Infection of the kidney or bladder produces subtle hematuria.

Exertional or "sports" hematuria develops from either exercise-induced renal ischemia during long duration, high intensity exercise, or repetitive microtrauma of the kidney or bladder during running or other vigorous activity ("heel strike hemolysis").[7] Treatment is rest, medical referral, and gradual return to activity. Activities can resume 24 hours after urine returns to normal.[7]

Change in Urinary Habit

Changes in an individual's urinary frequency, particularly if sudden or progressive, can indicate a urogenital disorder. *Dysuria* (difficult urination), *nocturia* (frequent waking from sleep to urinate), unusual urgency, and *incontinence* (inability to control urinary excretions) are symptoms of urogenital pathology. *Oliguria* (very infrequent urination) and *anuria* (absence of urination) result from serious renal, urinary, or metabolic disorders.

Nipple Discharge

Serous (watery), sanguineous (bloody), or serosanguineous (mixed) discharge may occur with breast cancer and other more benign breast conditions, such as gland infection and hormonal imbalances.[8]

Hypertension

High BP may be associated with kidney pathology due to the kidneys role in regulating BP.

Anemia

Kidney pathology may affect the production of erythropoietin, a hormone that regulates red blood cell production. The decrease in erythropoietin decreases the number of red blood cells, leading to anemia.

Sexual Dysfunction

Impotence, painful intercourse, blood in the semen (*hematospermia*), unusual vaginal bleeding during intercourse, or loss of *libido* (psychoemotional sex drive) are symptoms of urogenital pathology. Individuals reporting these symptoms should see a physician.

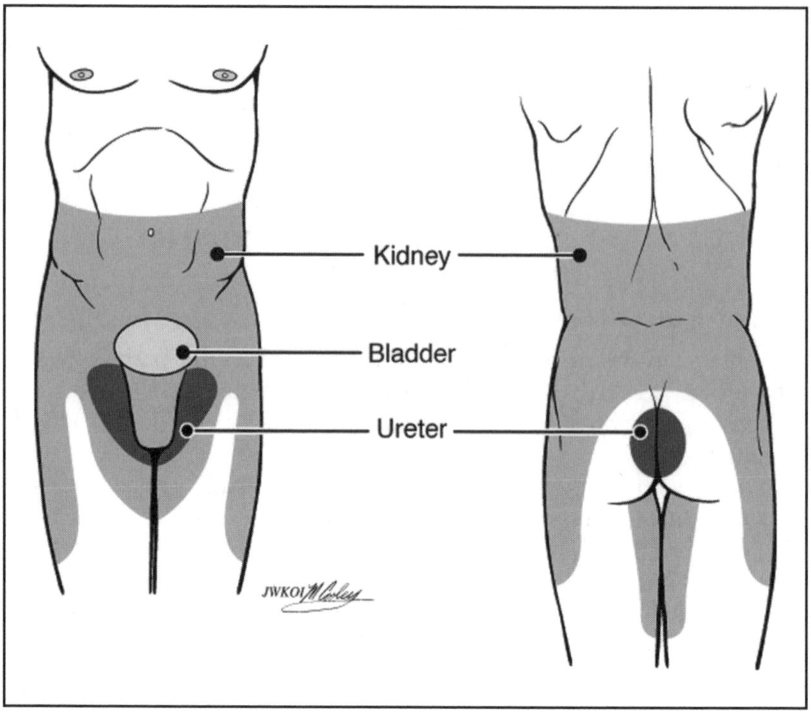

Figure 9-5. Referred pain patterns for the organs of the urogenital system.

Menstrual Irregularities

Amenorrhea and other changes in the menstrual cycle can occur with pathology of the female urogenital system. Amenorrhea, defined as less than three cycles per year or lack of menstruation for three consecutive months,[5,6] is most commonly caused by pregnancy, but may occur with severe dietary restriction, hormonal imbalance, or excessive exercise. Adolescents display a wide variation in regularity and intensity of menses, but amenorrhea in young, healthy females is not normal and requires a medical evaluation.[9] Other irregularities of the menstrual cycle can occur. *Oligomenorrhea,* defined as three to six menstrual cycles per year, is infrequent menstruation, with cycles lasting longer than 35 days.[5,6] *Dysmenorrhea* is disabling pain or discomfort that occurs with menstruation. *Premenstrual syndrome* is a complex of physical and psychological signs and symptoms that occur several days before menstruation. In premenstrual syndrome, the specific signs and symptoms, as well as their intensity and duration, varies from woman to woman. Treatment focuses on identifying the underlying etiology in addition to diet and lifestyle changes.

Pain Patterns

Kidneys, Ureters, and Bladder

The kidneys refer pain to the ipsilateral lower back at the costovertebral angle or to the abdomen, or can cause general lower abdominal pain (Figure 9-5).[10] The ureters usually cause severe pain in the groin, thigh, and abdomen.[10] Bladder pain occurs in the suprapubic region with referral to the lower back or thighs.[10]

An obstruction in the kidney or ureter, as occurs with kidney stones, produces acute intermittent pain in the abdomen and unilateral lower back that radiates to the ipsilateral lower abdominal quadrant, groin, or perineum. An obstruction in the bladder or urethra produces an aching pain in the lower abdomen.

Male Urogenital System

Testicular trauma produces a distinct, temporarily incapacitating pain. Pain persisting longer than ten minutes suggests more serious urogenital injury. Testicular disease may refer a deep, aching pain to the lower abdomen or sacrum.[10] The prostate gland refers pain to the lower back, scrotum, or perineum.[10]

Female Urogenital System

The uterus refers pain to the middle and lower back, whereas the ovaries and fallopian tubes refer pain to the lower abdomen (suprapubic) and sacrum. Breast pain is usually localized to the affected breast, but may refer symptoms into the ipsilateral axilla and upper arm.

Medical History and Physical Examination

Family and Personal History

A history of an untreated urinary infection or sexually transmitted disease can cause significant long-term health problems. A family history of renal disease such as kidney stones or personal history of systemic disorders such as diabetes, hypertension, or sickle cell disease increases risk of urogenital system pathology. Exposure to certain toxins may also affect renal function, including heavy metals, radioactive substances, and medications such as anti-inflammatories, antibiotics, and narcotics.[2] The use of contraceptives, including birth control pills, should also be ascertained. An absence or lack of function of one of the kidneys, testicles or ovaries may preclude participation in certain collision sports; the athletic trainer should be aware of the local, regional, and state policies and laws regarding participation in such cases.

For young females, age of *menarche* (first menses) and menstrual history (pain, difficulty, regularity, etc), including the date of the last period, should be obtained if a urogenital condition is suspected.[5] A history of a family member with breast cancer, particularly with onset at an early age, is important with complaints of breast pain, mass, or discharge.[8]

Both males and females should be asked whether they perform regular self-examinations when they have symptoms related to the urogenital systems. Sexual dysfunction, urethral discharge, or abnormal menses, as discussed above, are symptoms requiring medical referral.

Inspection

Edema in the extremities usually occurs in the late stages of kidney disease. Other urogenital conditions present few signs that would be noticeable upon gross inspection.

Palpation

The kidneys, particularly the right kidney, can sometimes be palpated in the posterior thorax, near the vertebral column just below the costal border of the 12th rib, at the costovertebral angle. Tenderness to palpation at this location is abnormal. Pain reproduced by percussion (or "hammering") directly over the kidney indicates inflammation or injury.

The athletic trainer relies on history, symptoms, and other signs to raise suspicion of pathology in the genital system. If necessary, the person can be instructed to perform a self-examination and report the findings.

Urinalysis

Hematuria (blood in urine), *proteinuria* (protein in urine), and *glucosuria* (glucose in urine), can be detected through a urinalysis performed microscopically in a laboratory or clinically using chemical test strips. Although athletic trainers are not trained in performing laboratory urinalyses, they can use urine test strips to perform screening urinalyses to identify persons with possible pathology, such as during preparticipation physical exams. (Lab Exercise 9-1 provides the opportunity to perform screening urinalyses using chemical test strips and to interpret the test results.) A screening urinalysis can also be used to check for ketones or glucose in a diabetic athlete who is having difficulty regulating the disease.

Urinalysis test kits can be purchased to test urine concentration levels of a variety of substances. Table 9-1 provides a summary of the more common substances tested and their associated pathology. The test strips are thin plastic strips that contain square pads impregnated with specific chemicals that are designed to react with specific substances in urine. Although these test strips are not as accurate as microscopic tests, they are convenient and easy to use in screening patients for pathology such as diabetes, urinary tract infections, or kidney injuries. A *clean catch (midstream) urine sample* provides the most accurate test results as it avoids the collection of contaminants or bacteria that might be present on the skin. To obtain a clean catch urine sample, male patients should wipe the head of the penis and female patients should wipe between the labia (front to back) with a prepackaged sterile wipe. Patients should be instructed to urinate a small amount into the toilet and then place the sterile urine cup into the urine stream. After collecting 1 to 2 ounces of urine, the cup is removed from the stream without stopping the flow. The patient then secures the lid on the urine cup.

The athletic trainer should apply gloves prior to handling the urine specimen. The cup should be placed on a flat, firm surface to prevent spilling. The chemically treated end of the reagent test strip is inserted fully into the urine specimen for 1 second and then promptly removed. The test strip should be tapped on the edge of the urine cup to remove any extra drops of urine and then blotted with a paper towel or other absorbent material to further remove excess urine. Excess urine on the test strip can cause mixing of the reagent chemicals from the different test pads affecting the accuracy of the test. After 60 seconds, the color of the pads on the test strip should be compared to the color indicator chart on the bottle. Leukocytes require a wait of 120 seconds before color comparison. Minor traces of blood in the urine are normal in females during their menstruation cycles.

In addition to the urinalysis test values, changes in color, odor, or volume of urine may also indicate a urinary disorder. Urine is normally a pale yellow, but will darken considerably as fluid content decreases or relative concentration of solute

Table 9-1

Urinalysis Test Substances and Associated Pathology

Test	Possible Pathology
Specific gravity	Normal levels range from 0.002 to 0.028 Increased specific gravity is associated with increased concentration of solutes and dehydration Decreased levels are associated with excessive fluid intake
pH	Urine pH ranges from 4.5 to 8 with 7 being considered neutral pH >7 is considered alkaline, pH <7 is considered acidic Alkaline urine associated with: urinary tract obstruction hyperventilation chronic renal failure salicylate (aspirin) intoxication Acidic urine associated with: acidosis uncontrolled diabetes dehydration vomiting diarrhea
Leukocytes	Presence of leukocytes in the urine suggests possible infection
Protein	The presence of greater than trace amounts of protein in the urine is associated with kidney disease
Glucose	Associated with excessive levels of glucose in the blood (hyperglycemia)
Ketones	Ketones are by-products of fat metabolism and can be present in urine as a result of: diabetic ketoacidosis anorexia (or other form of starvation) excessive vomiting high protein/low carbohydrate diets The presence of ketones in a diabetic patient warrants an injection of insulin
Blood (hemoglobin)	The presence of greater than trace amounts of blood is associated with kidney or bladder injury
Nitrite	Positive test for nitrite indicates the presence of bacteria
Urobilinogen	Normal values range from 0 to 8 mg/dL Increased values suggest liver pathology (eg, infection, cirrhosis) Decreased values suggest blockage of bile passage or decreased bile production
Bilirubin	Bilirubin is a yellowish pigment found in bile Positive test indicates possible liver or gallbladder pathology such as: gallstones cirrhosis of the liver hepatitis liver tumor

increases. Red or brownish urine usually indicates the presence of blood, hemoglobin, myoglobin, bilirubin, or other metabolic proteins and is therefore never normal.[2] A clouded or milky appearance indicates infection, which is usually accompanied by a foul or strong odor.[2] Any abnormal test values or discoloration should be followed up by a physician.

Pathology and Pathogenesis

Renal and Bladder Trauma

A direct blow to the middle or lower back, a sudden deceleration of the trunk, or a fractured rib can injure the kidney. The hallmark of renal injury is hematuria, as bleeding in the kidney passes into the urine.[11] Tenderness or swelling may appear in the back, over ribs 10 through 12. Grossly observable blood in the urine after a blow to the back or other abdominal trauma requires emergency medical imaging and diagnostic studies.

Most kidney trauma can be treated without surgery, but needs close medical monitoring. Return to sports is slow, usually taking at least 6 to 8 weeks before evidence of healing is observable on medical imaging.[11] Collision sports are contraindicated for persons who have only a single kidney.

The urethra and bladder may also sustain trauma during physical activity; however, significant bladder injuries are rare in athletics. The bladder is more commonly injured in high-energy trauma, such as a car accident. Hematuria and pain in the lower abdomen usually occur with bladder injuries.

Urethral bleeding happens with traumatic impact of the genitals or perineum. If inflammation obstructs the urethra, surgery to drain urine and hospitalization until healed are indicated.[11] The immediate course of action includes application of ice packs and emergency transport.

Renal, Bladder, and Genital Infections

Urinary Tract Infection

Urinary tract infection (UTI) by bacteria, fungi, or parasites are very common. Bacterial infection is by far the most prevalent type of UTI. Regardless of the type of invading organism, possible consequences include urethritis (inflamed urethra), cystitis (inflamed bladder), prostatitis (inflamed prostate), and pyelonephritis (inflamed kidney) as the organism progresses up the urinary tract. Symptomatic infection with yeast (*Candida albicans*), which causes vulvular irritation, is very common in women. Men can carry and transmit yeast infections while remaining asymptomatic, so sexual partners may also need to be treated to prevent repeat infection. Signs and symptoms of UTI depend on the primary site of colonization in the urinary tract (Table 9-2) Treatment consists of antibiotics or antifungal medications, as well as analgesics or antipruretics (inhibit itching) to control symptoms.

Sexually Transmitted Infections

Sexually transmitted infections (STI) are communicated to sexual partners by direct contact with genital wounds or body fluids. These diseases can infect the rectum, eyes, and mouth in addition to the genitals. Use of condoms reduces the

Table 9-2
Signs and Symptoms of Urinary Tract Infection by Site of Colonization

Site	Signs and Symptoms
Urethra	Dysuria, discharge
Bladder	Dysuria, urgency, decreased urine volume, nocturia, back pain, pyuria or hematuria
Prostate	Fever, urgency, back pain, dysuria, nocturia, hematuria
Kidney	Fever, back pain, vomiting, costovertebral tenderness

risk of contracting a STI, although they do not guarantee prevention. Contact of any mucous membrane with contaminated fluids or lesions greatly increases the probability of infection. There are several common sexually transmitted infections including gonorrhea, Chlamydia, syphilis, genital warts, and herpes. Each of these conditions is discussed below.

Gonorrhea

Bacteria (*Neisseria gonorrhoeae*) that cause *gonorrhea* incubate for 1 to 3 weeks, then induce purulent urethral discharge and painful dysuria. Other mucous membranes (mouth, throat, eyes, rectum) may be infected, producing pain, erythema, edema, or purulent exudate in those areas. A significant portion of infected persons experience no symptoms themselves, but are contagious and can transmit the organism to others. Gonorrhea often coexists with other STI, such as chlamydia and syphilis (see below). Vigorous and meticulous medical care is necessary to address gonorrhea and all comorbid infections. Sexual contact with others must be strictly avoided until the infection is eliminated. Recent (previous 3 to 6 months) sexual partners should be contacted, examined, and treated if necessary.

Chlamydia

Chlamydia (*Chlamydia trachomatis*), estimated to be the most common STI, is a bacterial infection with an incubation period of 1 to 4 weeks in men. Infected women, although usually asymptomatic, transmit the bacteria to their sexual partners. Symptoms include painful dysuria and clear or purulent urethral discharge. Similar to gonorrhea, other mucous membranes may be affected. Treatment is by antibiotics and screening for comorbid STI. Abstention from sexual activity is required until infection resolves. Recent (3 to 6 months) sexual partners should be contacted, examined, and treated.

Syphilis

Syphilis is caused by yet another bacteria (*Treponema pallidum*) that invades the urogenital system during sexual contact, although the organism ultimately infects other systems, including the nervous and cardiovascular. Symptoms may not occur for up to 3 months after initial exposure. A painless epithelial lesion on the region exposed to the bacteria, called a chancre, does appear and spontaneously resolve within 2 months. Inguinal lymphadenitis may occur, but the nodes are usually not tender and may not be noticed. A skin rash erupts within 2 months and may persist for 2 to 3 additional months. Low-grade fever, fatigue, headache, loss of appetite, and myalgia may also appear during this stage.

If untreated, the disease goes into remission, becoming asymptomatic sometimes for decades. Invasion of bone, skin, myocardium, or the central nervous system eventually occurs, leading to serious and irreversible changes to those systems. Cardiac and central nervous system complications are the most severe, disabling, and ultimately fatal. Treatment begins with early recognition and consists of appropriate antibiotic therapy and identification of coexisting STI.

Genital Warts

Various papillomaviruses cause *genital warts.* External warts, cauliflower-like in appearance, appear on the genitals 1 to 6 months after infection. Internal warts may appear on the rectum, vagina, or cervix, but require physical examination by a physician to identify them. Treatment is by surgical removal and topical medications, although recurrences are common and, in some cases, total resolution may not be possible. During exacerbation, sexual abstinence is required to prevent communicating the virus. One papillomavirus (*human papillomavirus*) has been implicated as a cause of cervical cancer.

Herpes

Genital herpes, caused by herpes simplex viruses type 1 and type 2, occurs after contact with the genital lesions of an infected person. These viruses can infect any mucous membrane. Once infected, the virus remains in the ganglia of the associated nerves for the remainder of the host's lifetime. Periodically, the virus reactivates and causes recurrence of the characteristic lesions.

Small vesicles appear within a week of the initial infection. These lesions are circular, painful, appear in clusters, and generally heal in 1 to 2 weeks. Dysuria, paresthesia, and other neurological signs may appear. General systemic signs, including fever, malaise, and inguinal lymphadenitis, may be present after initial infection. Subsequent recurrences usually have shorter duration and are less symptomatic. Diagnosis requires medical laboratory tests. Treatment involves medications to control symptoms during outbreaks and to limit recurrent episodes. Abstention from sexual activity when lesions are present is essential to prevent spreading the virus.

Pelvic Inflammatory Disease

Pelvic inflammatory disease (PID) results from infection of the cervix, uterus, or fallopian tubes. Chlamydia and gonorrhea, usually contracted during sexual intercourse, are the most common organisms that infect these organs in PID. Signs and symptoms include abdominal pain, high-grade fever, nausea, and purulent or bloody vaginal discharge. PID can cause infertility, ectopic pregnancy, chronic pelvic pain, or death. Once the organism is identified, immediate antibiotic treatment begins. Clinically, the signs and symptoms of acute PID are difficult to discern from ectopic pregnancy, thus requiring an emergency medical examination.

911

Renal Disorders

Urolithiasis

Urolithiasis, commonly known as kidney stones, results when excess insoluble salts, calcium, or uric acid enter the kidney filtrate. Since these substances cannot be excreted in the urine, they collect in the kidney and form solid masses. When these stones grow large enough to block the flow of urine or irritate the urinary tract, sudden severe pain appears as the renal tubules or capsule becomes distended with urine.

History will be negative for trauma. The characteristic clinical presentation is severe, unilateral pain in the lower back and abdomen that radiates into the anterior thigh.[4] Vomiting, pallor, and tachycardia may also be noted. Signs of shock (decreased BP and rapid, weak pulse) will not be present since no internal hemorrhaging occurs.

Small kidney stones are treated with pain medication and intravenous hydration; the hydration increases urine output, which helps to pass the stones out of the body. Large stones may need to be fragmented by sound, shock (lithotripsy), or light (laser) treatments. Recovery is usually complete, although recurrences are not uncommon. Risk of kidney stones decreases with proper diet and hydration.[4]

Renal Failure

Acute renal failure occurs as a result of toxins or acute obstruction of the ureter.[4] Signs include sudden weight gain, generalized edema, hypertension, and signs of left-sided heart failure (see Chapter Six).[2] These signs are the result of the kidneys failing to remove water and waste products from the bloodstream. Water and waste products accumulate in the blood, producing hypertension and left-sided heart failure, and eventually have to be moved from the blood into the interstitial tissues, producing edema and weight gain.

Chronic renal failure is unlikely among physically active persons. As a complication of diabetes, hypertension, or other kidney disease, however, chronic renal failure is not uncommon among the American population. Diabetes and hypertension irreparably damage the nephrons, as does chronic kidney disease. Once the nephrons are damaged, the function of the kidney is permanently impaired and chronic renal failure results. In early stages, chronic renal failure may be asymptomatic. As the disease progresses, nocturia, hypertension, gastrointestinal symptoms, impaired cognitive function, neurological changes (decreased reflexes, paresthesias), bone degeneration, muscle dysfunction, and cardiovascular complications gradually occur as waste products normally filtered out by the kidney accumulate and damage other organs.[4] Chronic renal failure is not curable since damaged kidney cells cannot regenerate.

Male Urogenital Disorders

Monorchidism

Monorchidism, or the absence of one testicle, congenitally occurs in 0.02% (1 in 5000) of males, but can also be traumatically acquired.[12] Monorchidism often excludes a male from contact sports. More rarely, complete absence of both testicles or the presence of more than two testicles occur.[12] Decisions regarding sports participation in these conditions should be deferred to a urologist or endocrinologist.

Prostate Disorders

Prostate disorders often gradually produce symptoms that are related to chronic or acute inflammation (*prostatitis*). The prevalence of prostate disorders increases with age. The most frequent cause of prostatitis is infection, although it can occur with cancer or other urogenital disease.[4] Dysuria, painful urination, an increase in urinary urgency and frequency, and nocturia are common symptoms.[4] In addition, a dull ache may develop in the lower back or sacrum. The gland also enlarges with age (benign prostatic hypertrophy), causing the signs and symptoms to recur chronically.[4]

Prostate Cancer

Prostate cancer is primarily a disease of aging males, becoming progressively more prevalent each decade after age 50. Prostate cancer causes the second most cancer deaths among men, after lung cancer; the lifetime risk of prostate cancer is 1 in 6 men, and 1 in 34 men will die of the disease. Over 230,000 cases are diagnosed each year, and prostate cancer causes over 30,000 deaths per year. Although the etiology is unknown, prostate cancer is more prevalent in African Americans than in any other races. Also, males with a history of a first-degree relative (father or brother) with prostate cancer are twice as likely to develop the disease.

Metastases to the spine, pelvis, hips, lung, and liver are very common and are often the first indication of prostate cancer. As tumor size increases, the urethra becomes progressively obstructed and urinary function becomes impaired. Pain in the low back, hips, and upper thighs, along with dysuria, and nocturia suggests prostate enlargement in middle-aged men, which may be a result of prostate cancer or benign prostate changes with age (benign prostatic hypertrophy). The American Cancer Society recommends annual prostate screening tests, *prostate specific antigen* (PSA) and *digital rectal exam* (DRE), in males 50 years of age and older. A history of diagnosed prostate cancer increases the probability of vertebral metastasis. If history is suspicious for prostate involvement, the person should be referred to his physician for x-rays and medical testing. A diagnosis of prostate cancer is made through biopsy. The 5-year survival rate for prostate cancer which has not metastasized is nearly 100%; 5-year survival rate drops to 34% once the cancer has metastasized.

Scrotum and Testicular Trauma

The scrotum is vulnerable to trauma in sports, necessitating the use of a protective cup. Unfortunately, male athletes often refuse to use a cup consistently. Most scrotum trauma is relatively benign, however more significant injury can occur, such as testicular torsion (see below).[11] Scrotal or testicular pain that does not improve in 10 minutes is highly suspicious for more serious injury.

Testicular Torsion

Testicular torsion occurs primarily during late childhood or adolescence because the still-developing scrotum may allow rotation of the testicle and its connective tissue capsule.[12] When this rotation occurs, the spermatic cord twists, compressing arteries and veins and causing ischemia of the affected testicle.[4]

A history of trauma or previous torsion may or may not be present.[11] Table 9-3 compares benign scrotum trauma with the clinical presentation of testicular torsion. Nausea and vomiting are also common.[12] The twisted spermatic cord elevates the affected testicle from its normal position; the athlete can perform a self-examination to detect this change. Emergency surgery is necessary to save the testicle, even if spontaneous or manual "derotation" occurs.[12]

Table 9-3
Simple Scrotum Trauma vs Testicular Torsion

	Scrotum Trauma	Testicular Torsion
Pain	Bilateral, <10 minutes	Unilateral, >10 minutes
Scrotum swelling	None	Progressive
Nausea/vomiting	None or very brief nausea	Increasing nausea and eventual vomiting
Testicular position	Normal	Unilateral elevation

Varicoceles

Varicose veins in the scrotum (*varicoceles*) occur most commonly in adolescents and cause a sensation of heaviness or tenderness.[4,12] Varicoceles are a result of incompetent vein valves and an acute angle of confluence between the spermatic veins and the renal vein (left testicle) and inferior vena cava (right testicle). Varicoceles range in diameter from 1 cm to 2 cm, are more prominent when standing, and may be described as a "bag of worms."[12] Surgical correction may be necessary since varicoceles do not spontaneously regress and may lead to fertility problems.[12] Trauma may produce a testicular *hydrocele*, or a fluid-filled sac, which produces similar signs and symptoms to varicocele, but with sudden onset after trauma. Medical referral is appropriate.

Testicular Cancer

Testicular cancer is the most common cancer among males aged 15 to 35; approximately 8,000 new cases are diagnosed each year. Although primarily genetic in nature, a history of cryptorchidism, significant testicular trauma or infection, or infertility are risk factors for developing testicular cancer. Although usually detectable upon regular self-exam as a progressive, unilateral testicular swelling or nodule, the disease may go unrecognized until metastases to the spine cause back pain or other symptoms such as abdominal pain, fatigue, weight loss, or nausea. The American Cancer Society recommends that males perform monthly testicular self-exams (TSE) starting at 15 years of age (Figure 9-6). Table 9-4 summarizes the steps for correctly performing a TSE.

Testicular cancer is curable. Early detection is critical for long-term survival; the 5-year survival rate for non-metastatic testicular cancer is over 99%. Metastases to the spine has a worse prognosis, with survival rates dropping below 75%.

Table 9-4
Testicular Self-Examination

- The TSE should be performed right after a hot bath or shower when the skin of the scrotum is relaxed and soft.
- Become familiar with the normal size, shape, and feel of each testicle.
- Standing in front of a mirror, check for swelling of the scrotum.
- Using both hands, cup the index and middle fingers under each testicle with the thumbs on top.
- Gently roll each testicle between the thumb and fingers. (One testicle may be larger than the other; however, this is normal.)
- Identify the epididymis, which will feel like a rope- or tube-like structure on the top and back of each testicle. (This structure is normal and should not be mistaken for a lump.)
- Feel for any abnormal lumps. This tissue will feel like a piece of uncooked rice or small peanut.
- Any lump or swelling detected on self-exam should be reported to a physician.

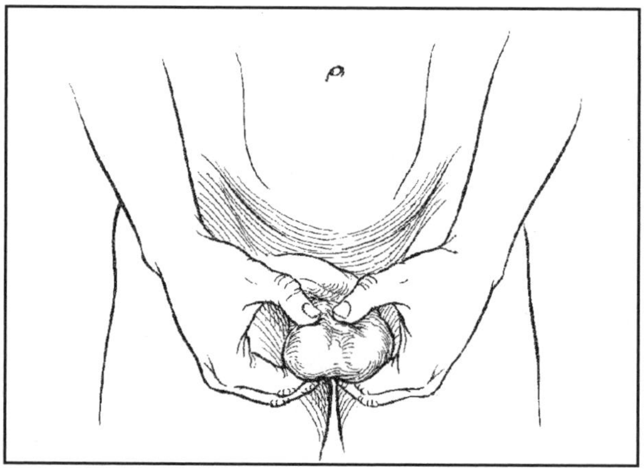

Figure 9-6. Testicular self-exam.

Female Urogenital Disorders

Endometriosis

Endometriosis occurs when endometrial tissue grows outside of the uterus and is most common between 30 and 40 years of age.[4] The etiology is unknown. Menstruation becomes painful and the volume of menstrual discharge increases. Painful intercourse and pain in the lower back is also usually reported. Fibrosis and infertility can result, so prompt referral is important. Treatment consists of hormone therapy or surgery.[4]

Pregnancy

Pregnancy occurs when a fertilized ovum attaches to the endometrium. Signs and symptoms are often the first indication of pregnancy; most initial symptoms are caused by higher than normal levels of estrogen and progesterone in the bloodstream. Amenorrhea, weight gain (5 to 10 pounds a month), recurrent nausea and vomiting, and abdominal pain in a female beyond menarche require a physician referral. Other signs and symptoms appear as pregnancy advances and the size of the fetus increases, including frequent urination, hypotension in the supine position, peripheral neurovascular occlusion syndromes (from fluid retention and edema), and breast enlargement and tenderness. A weight gain of 25 to 30 pounds during the course of a pregnancy is normal, but may cause fatigue and musculoskeletal strain syndromes.[13]

Resting heart rate increases early in pregnancy and increases to as much as 15 bpm over normal throughout the pregnancy.[13] BP, however, progressively decreases and is lower by 8 to 10 mmHg by the 20th week. The decrease in BP is exacerbated in supine, so exercise in this position should be avoided after the fourth month.[13] As a precaution, pregnant women should be taught the symptoms of rapidly decreasing BP, including dizziness, syncope, and nausea so they can change positions to restore BP.

The physician who is managing the woman's prenatal care should be consulted before recommending any type of exercise program. Conditions such as diabetes, hypertension, history of miscarriage, and presence of multiple fetuses usually render exercise contraindicated.[14,15] If exercise is recommended, 15-minute intervals of regular, low-impact aerobic exercise keeping the HR below 140 bpm are usually indicated.[13,15] Duration and intensity of exercise sessions should be adjusted to avoid elevating body temperature, injury, exhaustion (i.e., depletion of blood glucose), or dehydration.[14,15] In addition, environment (temperature and safety) and adequate nutrition (an additional 300 kcal/day usually recommended throughout pregnancy) should be considered.[13-15] The NCAA has a published guideline that recommends avoidance of contact and collision sports and urges the pregnant athlete in noncontact sports to continue at subcompetitive intensities; it also recommends that if a pregnant athlete chooses to compete, she should sign an informed consent about the risks and her institution should obtain approval from her personal physician, the team physician, and an institutional official.[16]

The circulating concentration of the hormone relaxin increases substantially during pregnancy. Relaxin increases the extensibility of connective tissues, such as ligaments, which will allow for expansion of the pelvic girdle during labor and delivery. Relaxin also makes skeletal joints susceptible to injury during physical activity and thereby prohibits vigorous sports participation. Precaution is also needed during manual therapy techniques, such as joint mobilization.

Returning to a "regular" exercise regimen may take several months after delivery. Physical changes of pregnancy often persist up to 6 weeks postpartum (after giving birth).[14] Activities to avoid in the immediate postpartum stage include: exercise in hot, humid weather (dehydration); high-impact or high-intensity exercise; excessive stretching or joint motions (due to relaxin); and sudden changes in posture (orthostatic hypotension).[13] An additional 400 to 600 kcal/day may be required for women who are breast feeding to meet their basic metabolic demands.[13]

Ruptured Ectopic Pregnancy

An ectopic pregnancy occurs when a fertilized ovum attaches outside the uterus, usually in a fallopian tube. The usual signs of pregnancy are initially present. When the embryo grows large enough, it ruptures the tube and causes severe internal hemorrhaging. Ruptured ectopic pregnancy produces acute, lacerating lower abdominal pain with lower quadrant tenderness, vaginal bleeding, syncope, and shock.[17] Syncope associated with abdominal pain in a female of childbearing age always requires prompt medical attention.[17] An embryo implanted ectopically has no chance of surviving. The condition is fatal to the mother unless emergency surgery is performed.[17]

Female Athletic Triad

Female athletic triad describes the simultaneous presence of disordered eating, amenorrhea, and osteoporosis in an otherwise healthy woman.[5,6] Each condition can occur independently (eg, most athletes with amenorrhea do not have an eating disorder[18]), but in this syndrome they are causally related. Restricted caloric intake and abstention from high-fat or high-calorie foods to reduce or maintain body weight are the most common manifestation of disordered eating among athletes (see Chapter Fourteen). Poor nutrition may also result from disordered eating.[5]

Athletes with disordered eating have increased pituitary gland activity, due to the combined effects of intense exercise and restricted caloric intake. The increase in pituatary activity inhibits hypothalamic hormone release, which inhibits pituitary hormone release, resulting in inadequate estrogen and progesterone production from the ovaries. The decrease in estrogen and progesterone causes amenorrhea or oligomenorrhea.[5,6]

Low body fat, once thought to contribute to amenorrhea, is no longer considered a cause. Low overall body weight, including both low body fat and low lean body weight, is thought to be a factor in amenorrhea.[18] Restricted caloric intake alone induces amenorrhea, even in athletes who have normal levels of body fat.[5,14] Amenorrhea is caused by an interaction of hormone imbalances and inadequate nutrition, both of which can be consequences of disordered eating.[5,9,14,19] The underlying cause of amenorrhea should be medically identified.

Hormone changes and amenorrhea then contribute to development of osteoporosis, a condition involving inadequate bone formation and premature bone loss.[19] Estrogen inhibits the activity of a cell in bone called an osteoclast, which functions to resorb minerals in the bone matrix. When erratic or irregular menstruation causes low estrogen levels, osteoclast activity increases and, consequently, bone density decreases.[5] This biological mechanism is the same as that of postmenopausal osteoporosis, common in women over 50 years of age.

Osteoporosis can occur in young women who have amenorrhea. Osteoporosis among young female athletes can decrease bone mass between 2% and 6% per year. Recovery of bone mass with treatment may not be complete.[5,6] Since 60% to 70% of bone mass is acquired before age 20, adolescent females with osteoporosis may be at increased risk for fractures and other orthopedic complications later in life.[14]

The definitive management of the female athletic triad depends strongly on early recognition. Signs of disordered eating (see Table 14-5) may be the first detectable indication. Disordered eating alone is associated with high rates of morbidity (illness) and mortality (death) and should be addressed promptly and appropriately. Amenorrhea in athletes, particularly when disordered eating or decreased bone density is detected, requires a decrease in exercise intensity and an increase in caloric intake, as well as a daily calcium intake of 1200 to 1500 mg.[6]

Breast Disorders

Breast masses in an adult woman, changes in breast shape or resiliency, tenderness, or discharge, require urgent referral to a physician, particularly if the woman has a positive family history of breast cancer. However, most cases of breast cancer are diagnosed in women without a family history.

In adolescents, however, some breast changes, including tender lumps detected during self-examination, are often benign.[8] The proper term for these benign breast changes is "proliferative breast changes," formerly called "fibrocystic breast disease." Small multiple lumps accompanied by cyclic pain (pain associated with the menstrual cycle) are common with proliferative breast changes. Genetic and hormonal factors are linked to the development of these changes.[8] Most cases of proliferative breast changes have no adverse long-term health consequences; however, any new lump found on self-exam should be evaluated by a physician. Treatment of benign breast lesions is usually observation, aspiration or core biopsy, or surgical excision.[8]

Breast pain may be a result of direct trauma or repetitive strain from activities such as running with poor support.[11] Ice is recommended following a painful blow to the breast. Anti-inflammatories should be avoided since they may increase bleeding and subsequent scarring. Use of a sports bra can prevent repetitive strain injuries caused by sprain of the suspensory (Cooper's) ligaments of the breast.[11]

Breast Cancer

Breast cancer is the most common malignancy among women. One in seven women will be diagnosed with breast cancer at some point in their lifetime. Approximately 210,000 cases are diagnosed each year, nearly 1700 of which are among men, and over 40,000 deaths a year are attributable to breast cancer. A positive family history increases risk and is associated with an earlier age of onset.[20] Hormonal factors are also involved since women who experienced an early onset of menarche, have never been pregnant, or who have a first child after age 35, all of which affect estrogen and progesterone levels, are at increased risk.[20] Breast cancer typically occurs in women over age 40, but appearance at an earlier age usually indicates greater severity of the disease.

The first physical sign of breast cancer is a palpable lump in the breast tissue.[20,21] In addition, the breast may be unusually tender, display dimpling or produce discharge from the nipple.[21] Common sites of metastasis from breast cancer include the bones of the ribs, vertebrae, or hips.[20] The American Cancer Society recommends monthly breast self-examinations (BSE) beginning by age 20 (Figures 9-7a and 9-7b). Table 9-5 summarizes the proper steps for performing a BSE. Approximately 90% of breast lesions are discovered in this manner. Regular mammography (radiographic imaging of the breast) should begin between ages 35 and 40 years and be repeated biannually until age 50, and repeated annually thereafter. Mammography and other imaging tests may be able to identify breast cancer before it becomes a palpable tumor. Definitive diagnosis of breast cancer requires a biopsy to obtain sample tissue.

Depending on the stage of the disease, breast cancer is generally treated with either a lumpectomy (removal of the tumor) or a mastectomy (removal of the entire

Figure 9-7a. Breast self-exam: supine.

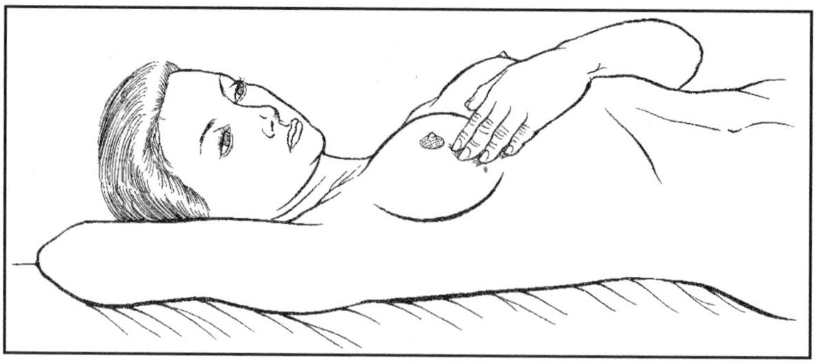

Figure 9-7b. Breast self-exam: standing.

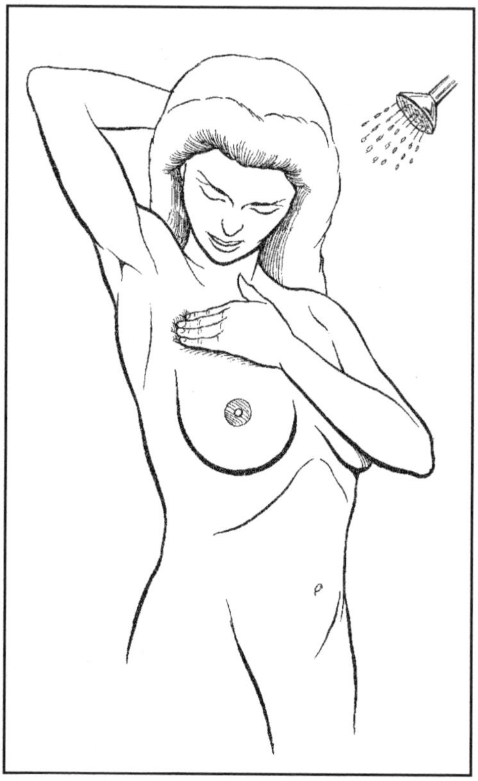

breast and underlying muscle tissue). Also depending on the stage of the cancer, chemotherapy and radiation therapy are often part of the overall treatment plan. If the tumor is estrogen and progesterin positive (ER/PR+; meaning the tumor's growth was stimulated by estrogen and progesterin hormones), breast cancer patients will also be treated with estrogen suppressants such as tamoxifen. Unfortunately for these patients, maintaining low levels of estrogen can lead to other health complications such as decreased bone density and osteoporosis.

Breast cancer in early stages is curable, with 5-year survival rates exceeding 98%, but in later stages the 5-year survival falls below 50%.

Table 9-5

Breast Self-Examination

- Lie supine with a pillow under the right shoulder and the right arm behind the head.
- Use the finger pads of the three middle fingers on the left hand to feel for lumps in the right breast.
- Press firmly enough to feel the tissue below the skin.
- Check the entire breast area following either a vertical or circular pattern (be consistent with each evaluation).
- Repeat the evaluation on the left breast, using the finger pads of the right hand.
- Repeat the evaluation of both breasts while standing, with one arm again placed behind the head. The upright position makes it easier to check the upper outer part of the breasts (toward the axilla). Approximately 50% of breast cancers are found in this area. The standing examination can be performed in the shower. Soapy hands allow the hands to glide over the wet skin making it easier to detect abnormal lumps.
- After completing the BSE, inspect the breasts by standing in front of a mirror looking for any changes in appearance, such as dimpling of the skin, changes in the nipple, changes in contour, redness, or swelling.

Ovarian Cysts

Fibrous cysts (vascularized, fluid-filled sacs) can form within the female urogenital system, including the ovaries.[4] Although usually asymptomatic and benign, occasionally they cause significant health problems. *Ovarian cysts* may cause unusual bleeding or interfere with the menstrual cycle. If ovarian cysts are large or numerous (polycystic ovary syndrome), they may interfere with normal estrogen production, causing course hair to grow on the chest and face (*hirsutism*).[4] Although many ovarian cysts will resolve on their own, others may require surgical removal. Furthermore, ovarian cysts can also rupture, producing sudden and severe internal hemorrhaging. Ruptured ovarian cysts lead to lower quadrant abdominal pain, peritonitis, shock, and, occasionally, death.[4,22,23]

Cervical, Ovarian, and Uterine Cancers

Cancers of the female reproductive system occur primarily in women over age 45 and are typically asymptomatic until metastases exist. These cancers vary with respect to prevalence and survival rates. *Cervical cancer* is diagnosed in about 10,000 women and causes over 3700 deaths each year. Five-year survival in the early stages are over 90%, and the rate drops to about 70% for advanced disease. *Ovarian cancer* is diagnosed in about 22,000 women and causes 16,000 deaths each year. Five-year survival early in the disease is 90%, but falls to 20% in the most advanced stage. *Uterine cancer* is diagnosed in 40,000 women and causes over 7000 deaths each year. Five-year survival rate is 50% in the earliest stage and drops below 10% for advanced uterine cancers.

Unusual vaginal bleeding or discharge may be the only indication of cancer in these organs. Early precancerous changes of the cervix can be detected during routine annual medical examination with a medical test called a Pap smear, which has lead to much higher survival rates than were observed in the mid-20th century. Risk factors for these cancers include a history of numerous sexual partners, postmenopausal estrogen supplementation, endocrine disorders, never becoming pregnant, family history, and an age of 40 years or greater.[21,24] Presence of the human papilloma virus (HPV) is also associated with cervical cancer.

Pediatric Concerns

Primary Amenorrhea

Primary amenorrhea is when menarche (first menses) fails to occur by age 16. The most common causes are hormonal imbalance, genetic disorders, and reproductive organ diseases.[14,19] If not already receiving medical care, referral to a pediatrician or gynecologist is appropriate.

Kidney Trauma

Among children, kidney injuries resulting from traumatic blows to the abdomen or trunk are more frequent than spleen or liver injuries.[11] The kidneys are exposed below the costovertebral angle until adolescence. Hence, a child who has received trauma to the trunk or back should be screened for signs (hematuria, shock) and symptoms (flank pain) of renal damage.

Cryptorchidism

Cryptorchidism, which describes an undescended testicle, is the most common congenital abnormality of the male genitalia.[12] Normally, both testicles descend from the abdomen into the scrotum just before birth or during the first year of life.[4] Usually detected in infancy during regular pediatric care, cryptorchidism occasionally persists into early childhood. The undescended testicle has a high rate of malignancy and infertility if uncorrected.[4,12] There is also a high rate of inguinal hernia that is associated with cryptorchidism.[12] Although such hernias are usually surgically corrected before the age of 2 years, a history of cryptorchidism may be an indication of a recurrent hernia when assessing groin pain.

Summary

The renal and urinary systems remove metabolic wastes from the blood and have a major role in regulation of body fluid levels, electrolyte levels, and BP. The signs of renal damage include hematuria, an abnormal dipstick test (proteinuria, glucosuria), and hypertension. Symptoms include pain in the back and abdomen, tenderness to percussion at the costovertebral angle, and change in urinary habit (frequency, urgency, volume). The genital or reproductive system contains the organs of procreation specific to each gender. The male genitals are prone to traumatic injury, most of which is temporary and benign. Unilateral scrotum pain or swelling, however, may indicate an emergency condition. The menstrual cycle is an indication of female reproductive system function. If menses is unusually heavy or painful, or very infrequent or absent, pathology may exist in the uterus or ovaries.

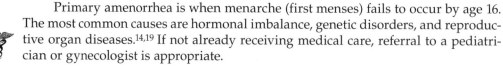

Pregnancy produces certain characteristic signs and symptoms and requires precautions both during and after pregnancy to prevent injury to the mother or fetus. Female athletic triad is the simultaneous presence of disordered eating, amenorrhea, and osteoporosis. Early recognition and intervention are necessary to prevent long-term complications. Any sign of renal or genital pathology accompanied by shock indicates internal bleeding and is an emergency. Cancers commonly involve both male and female genital structures. Self-examinations and regular physician examinations are important in the prevention and early detection of these diseases.

Case Study

You are asked by the women's athletic director to develop an education and prevention program for the female athlete triad. The goals of the program are to educate the female athletes on the causes and the short-term and long-term consequences of the triad and to provide the coaches with a simple way to screen athletes for signs of potential female athlete triad.

Critical Thinking Questions

1. What are the important points to include in your presentation to the athletes?
2. What advice are you going to provide to the coaches to help them screen for the female athlete triad among their athletes?

References

1. National Athletic Trainers' Association. *Athletic Training Educational Competencies.* 4th ed. Dallas, TX: National Athletic Trainers' Association; 2005.
2. Andreoli TE, Culpepper RM, Thompson CS, Weinman EJ. Section III-Renal disease. In: Andreoli TE, Carpenter CCJ, Plum F, Smith Jr. LH, eds. *Cecil Essentials of Medicine.* 2nd ed. Philadelphia, PA: WB Saunders Co; 1990:176-252.
3. Ganong WF. *Review of Medical Physiology.* 22nd ed. New York, NY: McGraw-Hill Medical; 2005.
4. Gould BE. Urinary system disorders. *Pathophysiology for the Health-Related Professions.* Philadelphia, PA: WB Saunders Co; 1997:299-319.
5. Putukian M. The female athlete triad. *Clin Sports Med.* 1998;17(4):675-696.
6. West RV. The female athlete: the triad of disordered eating, amennorrhea, and osteoporosis. *Sports Med.* 1998;26(2):63-71.
7. Abarbanel J, Benet AE, Lask D, Kimche D. Sports hematuria. *J Urol.* 1990;143:887-890.
8. Neinstein LS. Breast disease in adolescents and young women. *Pediatr Clin North Am.* 1999;46(3):607-629.
9. Wilson CA, Abdenour TE, Keye WR. Menstrual disorders among intercollegiate athletes and non-athletes: perceived impact on performance, preventative medical care for the female athlete. *Athletic Training.* 1991;26(2):170-177.
10. Stopka CB, Zambito KL. Referred visceral pain: what every sports medicine professional needs to know. *Athl Ther Today.* 1999;4(1):29-36.
11. Amaral JF. Thoracoabdominal injuries in the athlete. *Clin Sports Med.* 1997;16(4):739-753.
12. Pillai SB, Besner GE. Pediatric testicular problems. *Pediatr Clin North Am.* 1998;45(4):813-830.
13. Artal R. Exercise and pregnancy. *Clin Sports Med.* 1992;11(2):363-377.
14. Teitz CC, Hu SS, Arendt EA. The female athlete: evaluation and treatment of sports-related problems. *J Am Acad Orthop Surg.* 1997;5(2):87-96.
15. Kelly AKW. Practical exercise advice during pregnancy: guidelines for active and inactive women. *Physician Sportsmed.* 2005;33(6):24-30.

16. NCAA Committee on Competitive Safeguards and Medical Aspects of Sport. *Guideline 3B: Participation by the Pregnant Student-Athlete.* Indianapolis, IN: National Collegiate Athletic Association; June 2002.
17. Stone R. Primary care diagnosis of acute abdominal pain. *Nurse Practitioner.* 1996;21(12):19-20, 23-26, 28-30, 35-41.
18. Harmon KG. Evaluating and treating exercise-related menstrual irregularities. *Physician Sportsmed.* 2002;30(3):29-35.
19. Worthington G. Athletic amenorrhea: updated review. *Athletic Training.* 1991;26(3):270-273.
20. Randall T, McMahon K. Screening for musculoskeletal system disease. In: Boissonnault WG, ed. *Examination in Physical Therapy Practice: Screening for Medical Disease.* 2nd ed. New York, NY: Churchill-Livingstone Inc; 1995:223-255.
21. Gould BE. Reproductive system disorders. *Pathophysiology for the Health-Related Professions.* Philadelphia, PA: WB Saunders Co; 1997:428-452.
22. Giudice L. Menstrual abnormalities and abnormal uterine bleeding. In: Beers MH, Berkow R, eds. *The Merck Manual of Diagnosis and Therapy.* 17th ed. Whitehouse Station, NJ: Merck Research Laboratories; 1999:1932-1942.
23. Hendrix S. Pelvic pain. In: Beers MH, Berkow R, eds. *The Merck Manual of Diagnosis and Therapy.* 17th ed. Whitehouse Station, NJ: Merck Research Laboratories; 1999:1944-1948.
24. Gould BE. Neoplasms. *Pathophysiology for the Health-Related Professions.* Philadelphia, PA: WB Saunders Co; 1997:54-69.

Online Resources

American Cancer Society
www.cancer.org

National Cancer Institute
www.cancer.gov

Prostate Cancer Foundation
www.prostatecancerfoundation.org

Susan G. Komen Breast Cancer Foundation
www.komen.org
www.breastcancer.org

Lab Exercise 9-1
Urinalysis

Objectives

After completing this lab activity, students will be able to:

1. Measure urine values with Chemstrips.
2. Record urine values obtained from Chemstrips.

Competencies

This lab exercise addresses the following psychomotor competencies from the NATA's *Athletic Training Educational Competencies, 4th ed*:

- Medical Conditions and Disabilities: 4f

Equipment Needed

- Urinalysis reagent strips
- Color chart on bottle or color chart poster to match reagent strips
- Sterile urine cups
- Watch with second hand
- Gloves
- Paper towels or other absorbent cloth

Instructions

1. Instruct your lab partner to collect a clean catch (midstream) urine specimen, cover the cup with the lid, and wipe any spills from the outside of the specimen container.
2. Follow the instructions for performing a urinalysis as outlined in the physical examination section of the chapter.
3. Record the results for each substance tested. (Each brand of reagent strips may have a slightly different test result chart. The chart provided on the next page may need to be revised to match the test reagent strips provided by your lab instructor.)

Lab Exercise 9-1 (continued)
Urinalysis

Athletic Training Student: ________________________________ Date:____

Subject Name or Number:________________________________

Analysis Results—Chemstrip 10

Urobilinogen 60 sec (mg/dL)	___ neg	___ 2	___ 4	___ 8		
Glucose 60 sec (mg/dL)	___ neg	___ 50	___ 100	___ 250	___ 500	___ 1000
Ketones 60 sec (mg/dL)	___ neg	___ trace 5	___ + 15	___ ++ 40	___ +++ 80	___ ++++ 100
Bilirubin 60 sec	___ neg	___ neg	___ +	___ ++	___ +++	
Protein 60 sec (mg/dL)	___ neg	___ trace	___ + 30	___ ++ 100	___ +++ 500	
Nitrite 60 sec	___ neg		___ +	___ ++		
Leukocytes 120 sec	___ neg	___ trace	___ +	___ ++		
Blood 60 sec	___ neg	___ trace	___ small	___ mod	___ large	
pH 60 sec	___ 5	___ 6	___ 7	___ 8	___ 9	
Specific Gravity 60 sec	___ 1.005	___ 1.010	___ 1.015	___ 1.020	___ 1.025	___ 1.030

Interpretation of Results:

Chapter Ten

Endocrine and Metabolic Systems

Chapter Outline and Objectives

Introduction

Review of Anatomy, Physiology, and Pathogenesis

- Describe basic endocrine system structures and their functions.
- Review pathophysiological mechanisms of the endocrine system, including contributions to homeostasis and metabolism.
- Explain how the endocrine system contributes to the regulation of body energy.
- Explain how the endocrine system contributes to the regulation of body temperature.
- Explain how the endocrine system contributes to the regulation of body fluid.
- Describe the response of the endocrine system to exercise.
- Describe basic metabolic responses to exercise.
- Identify signs and symptoms of endocrine pathology.
- Identify signs and symptoms of metabolic pathology.

Signs and Symptoms

- Skin Changes
- Diaphoresis-Hyperhydrosis
- Body or Breath Odor
- Polydipsia and Polyuria
- Arthralgia and Myalgia
- Muscle Atrophy and Weakness
- Amenorrhea and Impotence
- Confusion or Change in Mental Status
- Paresthesia
- Edema and Pitting Edema
- Polyphagia
- Postural (Orthostatic) Hypotension
- Lethargy and Fatigue

Pain Patterns

Medical History and Physical Examination

- ❖ Discuss medical history findings relevant to endocrine and metabolic pathology.
- ❖ Perform physical examination tasks relevant to the endocrine system and normal metabolism.

Pathology and Pathogenesis

- ❖ Differentiate between common endocrine and metabolic disorders.
  - Diabetes Mellitus
  - Disorders of the Pituitary Gland
  - Disorders of the Thyroid and Parathyroid
  - Disorders of the Adrenals
  - Thermoregulation and Environmental Conditions
  - Metabolic Disorders

Pediatric Concerns

- Osteogenesis Imperfecta

This chapter addresses the following competencies from the *Athletic Training Educational Competencies, Fourth Edition*[1]:

Domain	**Cognitive**	**Psychomotor**
Acute Care of Injuries and Illnesses	4, 10, 16, 27b, 29	4c, 4j
Medical Conditions and Disabilities	1–3, 13	4
Orthopedic Clinical Examination and Diagnosis	1, 6, 16	
Pathology of Injuries and Illnesses	2, 4–6	
Risk Management and Injury Prevention	8, 9, 20	

Introduction

The endocrine system works in concert with the nervous system to maintain homeostasis. Through the release of hormones, the endocrine system regulates the functions of many other organ-systems including reproduction, growth and development, mobilization of defenses against stressors, blood glucose levels, core body temperature, and water, electrolyte, and nutrient levels. One of the primary functions of the endocrine system is the regulation of metabolism.

Metabolism describes the biochemical functions and interactions of the organ-systems of the body. Metabolic processes respond to the normal cyclic increases and decreases in organ activity, internal energy demands, environmental factors, and nutrition. Metabolic activity is regulated internally by hormones and organs and externally by environmental factors and intake of calories, carbohydrates, protein,

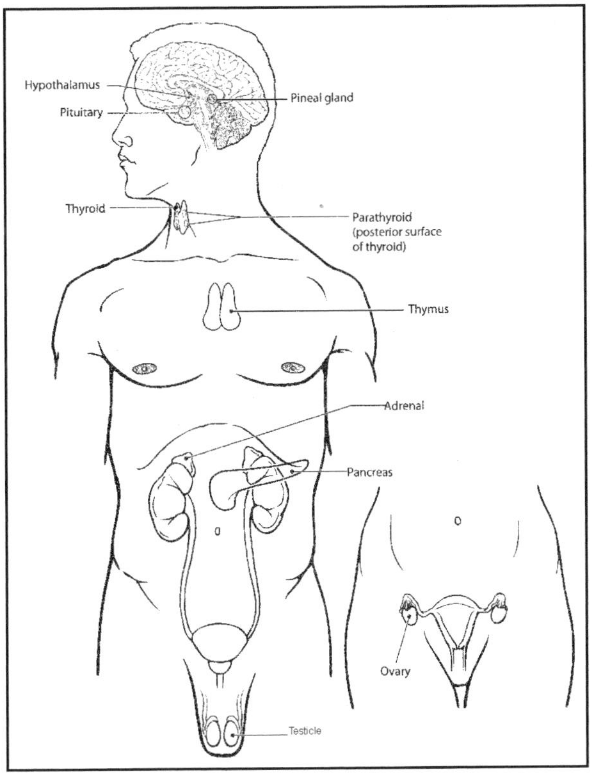

Figure 10-1. Glands of the endocrine system.

fat, water, minerals, and vitamins. Thus, metabolism is the manifestation of the endocrine system's attempt to maintain homeostasis. When the delicate balance of homeostasis is disturbed, acute and chronic diseases can develop involving one or more of the glands within the endocrine system, which in turn affects many other systems and bodily functions.

Review of Anatomy, Physiology, and Pathogenesis

The endocrine system consists of several small glands located throughout the body (Figure 10-1). These glands secrete chemical substances called hormones into the blood to stimulate activity in the organ-systems of the body, including inhibition or stimulation of other hormones. The endocrine system also interacts with and receives input from the nervous, gastrointestinal, cardiovascular, hepatic, and renal systems.

Almost all of the hormones produced by the endocrine system can be categorized as amino acid derivatives, peptides, or steroids; however, the majority of them fall into the first category. Although hormones are widely circulated throughout the body, they will only produce a response with their specific target cells. Each hormone has a specific relationship with its target cells. For a hormone to affect the cell, the cell must have a specific protein receptor. Table 10-1 lists the endocrine glands, their primary hormones, and the targets of their hormones.[2-4]

The hypothalamus serves as a communication link between the nervous system and the endocrine system. It regulates the endocrine system in three key ways.

Table 10-1

Endocrine Glands, Selected Associated Hormones, and Hormone Functions

Gland	Hormone(s)	Targets	Hormone Function
Hypothalamus	Antidiuretic hormone (ADH) Oxytocin (OT)	Posterior pituitary	Stimulate release of hormones by posterior pituitary
Anterior pituitary	Growth hormone (GH)	All cells	Growth and development; protein synthesis; breakdown of fats for energy
	Adrenocorticotropic hormone (ACTH)	Adrenal cortex	Cause adrenals to release cortisol
	Thyroid-stimulating hormone (TSH)	Thyroid gland	Increase thyroid function; stimulate release of thyroid hormones (T3 and T4)
	Follicle-stimulating hormone (FSH)	Ovaries	Increase estrogen release
		Testes	Increase sperm production
	Luteinizing hormone (LH)	Ovaries	Stimulate ovulation
		Testes	Increase testosterone release
	Prolactin (PRL)	Mammary glands in females	Production of milk
Posterior pituitary	Antidiuretic hormone (ADH)	Kidneys	Reabsorption of water; increased blood volume; increased blood pressure
	Oxytocin (OT)	Uterus, mammary glands (females)	Labor contractions, milk secretion
		Ductus deferens, prostate glands (males)	Contractions of ductus deferens and prostate; ejection of secretions
Thyroid	Thyroxine (T4)	Most cells	Increase metabolism, protein synthesis, growth and development
	Triiodothyronine (T3)	Most cells	Increase metabolism, protein synthesis, growth and development
	Calcitonin (CT)	Bones, kidneys	Decrease demineralization of bone
Parathyroid	Parathyroid hormone (PTH)	Bones, kidneys	Increase calcium in blood by demineralizing bone

continued

Table 10-1 (continued)

Endocrine Glands, Selected Associated Hormones, and Hormone Functions

Gland	Hormone(s)	Targets	Hormone Function
Thymus	Thymosins	Lymphocytes	Increase effectiveness of immune system
Adrenal	Aldosterone	Kidneys	Increase reabsorption of water and sodium ions in kidneys
	Cortisol	Most cells	Anti-inflammatory effects, tissue catabolism, respond to stress; increases synthesis of glucose and glycogen formation
	Epinephrine	Most cells	Respond to stress (increase heart rate, increase blood flow to muscle, decrease blood flow to internal organs), increases glycogen breakdown and release of lipids from adipose tissue
	Norepinephrine	Most cells	Vasoconstriction
Pancreas (endocrine)	Insulin	All cells (except those of brain, kidneys, GI, epithelium, RBCs)	Increase glucose transport out of blood and into cells
	Glucagon	Liver, adipose tissues	Breakdown of glycogen in liver, release glucose from liver into blood, release of fat stores
Testes	Testosterone	Most cells	Produce secondary male sex characteristics, increase protein synthesis, increase sperm production, inhibit luteinizing hormone release
Ovaries	Estrogen	Most cells	Produce secondary female sex characteristics, regulate menstrual cycle, inhibit luteinizing hormone release
	Progesterone	Uterus, mammary glands	Prepares uterus for egg implantation; secretory function of mammary glands
	Relaxin	Pubic symphysis, uterus, mammary glands	Relaxes uterine muscles and pubic symphysis
Pineal	Melatonin	All cells	Inhibits release of FSH and LH, slows maturation of reproductive organs, assists in regulation of circadian rhythms, works as antioxidant to protect CNS and boost immune system

First, the hypothalamus stimulates the adrenal medullae to release epinephrine and norepinephrine in response to sympathetic activation. Second, the hypothalamus produces two hormones, antidiuretic hormone (ADH) and oxytocin (OT), which are then transported to the posterior pituitary where they are released into the bloodstream. Third, the hypothalamus stimulates the anterior pituitary to release hormones that in turn regulate all of the other endocrine glands.

The pituitary gland is divided into two lobes: an anterior and a posterior. As just mentioned, the posterior lobe receives ADH and OT from the hypothalamus and then releases these hormones into the bloodstream. The anterior lobe of the pituitary gland secretes growth hormone (GH), an anabolic hormone, which stimulates protein synthesis and tissue growth. GH also promotes the use of fats for fuel, providing a glucose sparing effect. The anterior lobe of the pituitary also produces several other hormones that are responsible for regulating other endocrine glands. As the name implies, thyroid-stimulating hormone (TSH) stimulates the thyroid gland to produce thyroid hormones. Adrenocorticotropic hormone (ACTH) stimulates the adrenal cortex to release glucocorticoids and androgens. Follicle-stimulating hormone (FSH) and luteinizing hormone (LH) both regulate the secretion of hormones from the ovaries and testicles.

The thyroid, the largest of the endocrine glands, is a butterfly-shaped gland located on the trachea along the anterior aspect of the neck. This gland secretes two hormones, thyroxine (T4) and triiodothyronine (T3), which regulate the basal metabolic rate (BMR), and are therefore considered to be the body's major metabolism regulating hormones. These two hormones also work together to affect the normal functioning of almost every system in the body including the nervous, cardiovascular, muscular, skeletal, gastrointestinal, reproductive and integumentary. For this reason, as will be discussed later, dysfunction or pathology of the thyroid leads to dysfunction within many other systems.

The parathyroid secretes parathyroid hormone (PTH) which functions primarily to regulate the level of calcium in the blood. Calcium blood levels are important for the conduction of nerve impulses, normal muscle contraction, and blood clotting. High or low levels of PTH are associated with hyperparathyroidism and hypothyroidism, respectively.

The adrenal glands are actually a set of paired glands located just above the kidneys. The adrenal medulla, or inner part of each adrenal gland, secretes epinephrine and norepinephrine and is associated with the sympathetic nervous system. The outer portion of the adrenals, or adrenal cortex, secretes many corticosteroid hormones including aldosterone, cortisol, and testosterone. Aldosterone functions to increase blood levels of sodium while decreasing levels of potassium. The regulation of these and other electrolytes in the blood affects blood volume and blood pressure. Cortisol has many functions including raising blood glucose levels through the stimulation of gluconeogenesis, which is the production of glucose from noncarbohydrate sources (ie, fats and proteins). Cortisol also suppresses the immune system and produces anti-inflammatory effects, which can decrease cartilage and bone formation. Dysfunction of the adrenals is associated with two disorders: Addison's disease and Cushing's disease.

The pancreas is located behind the stomach and is made up of both endocrine and exocrine gland cells. Injuries and illnesses involving the exocrine pancreas were discussed in Chapter Eight. The endocrine portion of the pancreas secretes glucagon and insulin. Glucagon is considered a hyperglycemic hormone and functions to raise blood glucose levels. Glucagon stimulates the breakdown of glycogen to glucose in the liver and assists with gluconeogenesis. Insulin is a hypoglycemic hormone that works to lower blood glucose levels by promoting the transport of glucose from the blood to the cells.

The ovaries secrete estrogen and progesterone. These hormones are responsible for the development of the female reproductive organs, secondary sex characteristics, and the menstrual cycle. The testicles secrete testosterone which promotes the maturation of the male reproductive organs, secondary sex characteristics, sperm production, and sex drive. Pathological conditions involving the ovaries and testicles were addressed in Chapter Nine.

Regulation of Body Energy

Glucose is the body's primary energy source. The endocrine system is responsible for maintaining normal blood glucose levels to meet the body's energy needs. This delicate balance is achieved through the functions of multiple hormones including insulin and glucagon from the pancreas, epinephrine, norepinephrine, and cortisol from the adrenal glands, and growth hormone from the pituitary.

As mentioned previously, insulin lowers blood glucose levels by transporting glucose from the blood into the cells for energy. When glucose levels exceed the body's need for fuel, insulin sweeps the excess glucose out of the blood to be stored as either glycogen in the liver and the muscles, or fat in the adipose tissues. Glucagon, epinephrine, norepinephrine, cortisol, and growth hormone all function as insulin antagonists, working to increase blood glucose levels. These hormones stimulate the release of glucose from glycogen stores and promote gluconeogenesis, both of which increase blood glucose levels.

During exercise, insulin levels decrease as metabolic demand for glucose increases. Glucose is released in response to this increased fuel demand, primarily through the function of glucagon.[5,6] Simultaneously, insulin receptors on muscle cells become more sensitive; this change increases the muscular uptake of glucose despite decreases in blood insulin level.[5] Epinephrine and norepinephrine released as exercise begins, and growth hormone and cortisol during extended exercise, inhibit insulin production, thereby further aiding release of glucose from the liver.[5]

Regulation of Body Temperature

Normal metabolic processes produce excess energy at rest. Most of this energy is released as heat, which maintains the body's temperature within a narrow range. The body can also regulate heat loss or heat production in response to environmental conditions.[7]

At the start of exercise, core body temperature rises slightly and the physiological heat-dissipating mechanisms begin to function, primarily evaporation of water from the skin (ie, sweating) and radiation of heat from the head and neck. Ideally, a steady state is reached where heat production and heat dissipation stabilizes body temperature.[7]

The hypothalamus, which is sensitive to blood temperature, increases or decreases thyroid-stimulating hormone (TSH) in the pituitary gland. In response to decreases in body temperature, increased TSH increases the production of thyroid hormone, which causes metabolism to increase. Higher metabolism requires more energy-producing biochemical reactions, which then increases body temperature. Through opposite reactions, increased body temperature decreases TSH, lowering metabolism and body temperature (more accurately, it does not further increase body temperature).

Table 10-2

Hormones That Are Released During Exercise

Hormone	Response to Exercise
Growth hormone	Mobilizes free fatty acids; increases glycogenolysis (release glucose from the liver into the blood); inhibits uptake of glucose by the liver; stimulates release of insulin-like growth factor 1, which stimulates tissue growth
Adrenocorticotropic hormone	Stimulate cortisol release, which increases gluconeogenesis (increases blood glucose); increases protein synthesis; inhibits uptake of glucose by the liver
Follicle-stimulating hormone and luteinizing hormone	Men: stimulate testosterone release, which increases protein synthesis Women: stimulate estrogen release, which inhibits uptake of glucose
Epinephrine	Increases glycogenolysis (release glucose from the liver into the blood); stimulates lipolysis (breaks down fat for conversion into glucose via gluconeogenesis)

Regulation of Body Fluid

Antidiuretic hormone (ADH) forms in the hypothalamus and is secreted by the pituitary gland. ADH retains water in the body by increasing water reabsorption in the kidneys, thus decreasing urine volume. Exercise increases ADH secretion when baroreceptors, which are sensitive to pressure, detect a decrease in blood pressure from a decrease in blood volume and the hypothalamus detects an increase in blood solutes.[8] Maintaining hydration during activity inhibits this secretion of ADH since, when properly hydrated, there is no need to retain water.

Hormonal Response to Exercise

Exercise, or any other physical stress, causes a release of hypothalamic, pituitary, and adrenal hormones (Table 10-2).[8] As an adaptation to regular exercise, the release of these hormones decreases with successively higher levels of conditioning.

Relatively intense exercise stimulates the release of growth hormone, which increases with higher levels of fitness.[8] The intensity of exercise rather than duration or frequency appears to be the most important factor stimulating growth hormone release. By contrast, endurance exercise increases the level of cortisol, which decreases growth hormone secretion.[8] Thus, a potential effect of overtraining is a net decrease in growth hormone. Adverse effects, such as stunted height and physical development problems, can occur with combined overtraining and nutritional deficiencies among young female athletes.

Secretion of the catecholamines, epinephrine and norepinephrine, occurs with onset of exercise, and does not appear to adapt with conditioning. Frequent, intense exercise decreases follicle-stimulating hormone and lutenizing hormone and, subsequently, decreases secretion of estrogen and, to a lesser extent, testosterone. Decreased estrogen levels can produce amenorrhea among young female athletes, but usually only when excessive exercise is accompanied by a nutritional deficiency.

Although circulating testosterone also decreases with endurance exercise, delay of male puberty is very rare, possibly because a much higher exercise intensity is needed in males to depress testosterone release through this mechanism. Occasionally, highly active males report depressed *libido* (psychoemotional sex drive) and decreased semen volume, although these effects may be caused by dehydration, immune system depression, or undetected systemic illness rather than exercise-induced hormone changes.

Neurotransmitters known as endorphins, or endogenous opiods, are released during exercise of moderate to high intensity. Endorphins are thought to have a mild analgesic effect to alleviate muscle pain during exercise. Endorphins also counteract the rise in cortisol that occurs with exercise. Additionally, endorphins stimulate *lipolysis*, the breakdown of stored fat, in order to provide carbohydrate to working muscles.

Signs and Symptoms

The signs and symptoms listed below represent the general signs and symptoms associated with endocrine pathology. The clinical presentation of specific endocrine conditions or disorders may not include all of these signs and symptoms.

Skin Changes

Some endocrine disorders produce changes in the color, texture, or appearance of the skin. Hormones control the activity of melanin, a skin pigment, and can thus affect skin color. Changes in skin thickness, flexibility, texture, and integrity may appear in response to pathological conditions of the endocrine system.

Diaphoresis-Hyperhydrosis

Diaphoresis (sweating) or hyperhydrosis (excessive sweating) occur as metabolism increases. Diaphoresis is a normal response to exercise or increased body temperature. Metabolic imbalance or endocrine disorders, however, can cause hyperhydrosis at rest. Release of epinephrine and norepinephrine can also cause profuse sweating.

Body or Breath Odor

High blood glucose levels, as occurs with an absence of insulin (diabetes mellitus), produces a very sweet odor on the breath and from the body. Metabolic breakdown of toxins and other organic substances (eg, alcohol, drugs) can be exhaled or secreted in breath, sweat, and urine, where they can often be detected by smell.

Polydipsia and Polyuria

Excessive thirst (polydipsia) or excessive urination (polyuria) can be caused by inadequate secretion of ADH or thyroid disorders.

Arthralgia and Myalgia

Pain in joints (arthralgia) and muscles (myalgia) is common with disturbance of endocrine function or metabolism. Usually multiple joints or muscles are involved and the pattern is symmetric bilaterally.

Muscle Atrophy and Weakness

Changes in muscle function and structure are results of insufficient nutrition, from either starvation or disease, or the chronic presence of hormones that increase metabolic demand (eg, cortisol, epinephrine). Many endocrine disorders also affect muscle energy metabolism, causing unusual weakness and atrophy.

Amenorrhea and Impotence

Function of the reproductive organs can be affected by disorders affecting the hypothalamus, pituitary gland, ovaries, or testes since these glands control the activity of those organs.

Confusion or Change in Mental Status

Cognitive function can be affected by many endocrine-metabolic disorders, including hypoglycemia, dehydration, abnormal body temperature, or insufficient nutrition.

Paresthesia

Long-term endocrine or metabolic disorders can cause damage to nerve cells, axons, or myelin, causing progressive peripheral paresthesias.

Edema and Pitting Edema

Extracellular fluid can accumulate with certain endocrine or metabolic system disorders that cause water retention.

Polyphagia

Excessive intake of food without weight gain suggests overactive thyroid production, nutritional deficits, or metabolic imbalances that create a large caloric deficit.

Postural (Orthostatic) Hypotension

The endocrine system regulates fluid levels in the blood. If blood volume decreases through excessive urination or dehydration, blood pressure decreases rapidly with a change in posture from lying or sitting to standing.

Lethargy and Fatigue

Since the endocrine system regulates metabolism, disorders in this system affect availability and utilization of oxygen and energy. Fatigue and lethargy (abnormal sluggishness, drowsiness, or indifference) result either from an overactive metabolism requiring large energy expenditures, or from an underactive metabolism that does not provide the body with enough energy. In addition, many endocrine conditions directly or indirectly (eg, through nocturia) affect sleep quality and duration, leading to fatigue from sleep deprivation.

Pain Patterns

The endocrine glands rarely produce pain directly. The signs and symptoms of hormonal imbalances are usually more relevant than reports of pain. Large tumors in the hypothalamus and pituitary glands may produce headache or visual disturbances by compressing the brain. Pathology of the thyroid or parathyroid glands may cause tenderness in the anterior, inferior aspect of the throat and neck, especially during extension of the head and neck. Adrenal disorders can produce widespread myalgia and arthralgia (see below). As discussed in Chapter Eight, the pancreas produces upper left quadrant or generalized epigastric pain. Unfortunately, extensive pancreatic disease is usually present before pain is noticed.

Medical History and Physical Examination

Family and Personal History

Certain metabolic disorders, such as diabetes mellitus, have a strong genetic component that may be evident in a family history. Metabolic disturbances can also be caused by environmental factors (eg, temperature, toxins, physical stress), so these should be investigated during the medical history. Many endocrine disorders produce a characteristic pattern or progression of symptoms detected through a careful medical history.

Physical Examination

Skin or hair changes, secondary sex characteristics, muscle atrophy, hyperhydrosis, odor of breath or perspiration, edema, postural hypotension, and paresthesia may all be related to endocrine system disorders. Depending on the condition, observation, palpation, and the assessment of vital signs may be the only physical examination procedures that indicate potential endocrine pathology. An enlarged thyroid can be seen and palpated lateral to the trachea, just above the clavicles.[9] An abnormally enlarged thyroid, called a goiter, is a sign of thyroid toxicity, iodine deficiency, or thyroid pathology. Most endocrine diseases require medical laboratory testing to confirm the diagnosis.

A glucometer can be used by an athletic trainer to monitor or quickly assess a patient's blood glucose level (Figure 10-2). These units are easy to use and can play a vital role in the management of patients with diabetes. When purchased, each glucometer kit includes test strips and lancets, and replacement strips and lancets can be purchased when needed. The units run on batteries and many of them contain a memory chip that allows the storage of multiple glucose values, which can be helpful in tracking an individual's control over their diabetes. Although each glucometer may differ slightly, the steps for measuring blood glucose levels are very similar across the different brands. Table 10-3 provides a list of the general step-by-step instructions for measuring blood glucose levels using a glucometer. Normal random blood glucose levels should be between 70 and 126 mg/dL. Normal fasting (nothing to eat or drink other than water for at least 8 hours) levels should be between 70 and 100 mg/dL and postprandial (2 hours after a meal) levels should be between 100 to 140 mg/dL. (Lab Exercise 10-1 provides the opportunity to practice using a glucometer to assess blood glucose level.)

Table 10-3

Measuring Blood Glucose Levels Using a Glucometer

Step 1.	Check that the glucometer's battery is good.
Step 2.	Check that the glucometer is coded correctly for the test strips to be used. (The test strip bottle will have a code that should match the code displayed by the glucometer. If you purchase different test strips, you can change the code within the glucometer.)
Step 3.	Wipe the fingertip with an alcohol prep pad.
Step 4.	Insert the lancet in the automatic lancet device.
Step 5.	Stick the fingertip with the lancet device.
Step 6.	Squeeze a small drop of blood onto the test strip.
Step 7.	Insert the test strip into the glucometer.
Step 8.	Read the digital display of the blood glucose level.
Step 9.	Remove lancet from the lancet device and dispose of in appropriate sharps container.

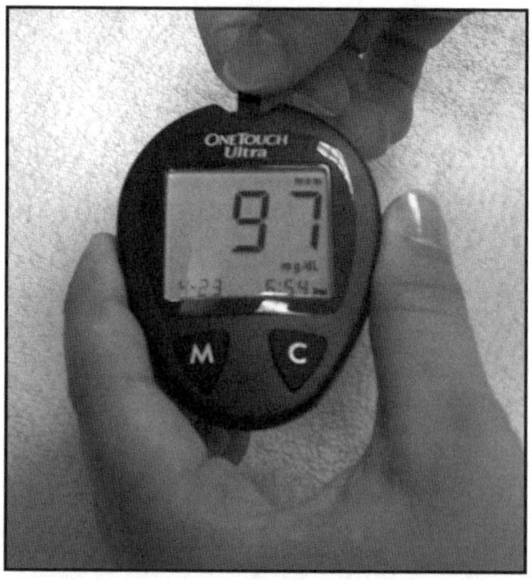

Figure 10-2. Glucometer.

A routine urinalysis can be used by the athletic trainer to screen for glucose and ketones. When blood glucose levels become excessively high (>250 mg/dL), glucose spills over into the urine (glucosuria). The presence of ketones in the urine is a sign of impending ketoacidosis, a potentially life-threatening condition. The procedures for performing a urinalysis were described in Chapter Nine.

Pathology and Pathogenesis

Diabetes Mellitus

There are three types of diabetes mellitus: *type 1,* formerly called insulin dependent diabetes mellitus (IDDM) or juvenile diabetes; *type 2,* formerly known

Table 10-4
Diagnostic Criteria for Diabetes Mellitus

Test	Normal	Prediabetes	Diabetes
Random (taken anytime) plasma glucose	70 to 126 mg/dL	127 to 199 mg/dL	≥200 mg/dL with symptoms*
Fasting plasma glucose	70 to 100 mg/dL	100 to 125 mg/dL	≥126 mg/dL with symptoms*
2-hour postpranidal (after a meal) test	100 to 140 mg/dL	>140 mg/dL	>140 mg/dL
Oral glucose tolerance test (OGTT)	<140 mg/dL	140 to 199 mg/dL	≥200 mg/dL

mg/dL=milligrams of glucose in 1 deciliter (100 millimeters) of blood.
**Symptoms of diabetes include polydipsia, polyurea, polyphagia, and weight loss.*

as noninsulin dependent diabetes mellitus (NIDDM) or adult onset diabetes; and *gestational*, which can occur during pregnancy. Athletic trainers are more likely to encounter patients with type 1 than type 2; they will rarely encounter gestational diabetes. Therefore this chapter will only address type 1 and type 2 diabetes.

Type 1 Diabetes Mellitus

Type 1 diabetes mellitus is an autoimmune disease that destroys the insulin-producing cells of the endocrine pancreas.[10] This condition affects approximately one in 500 children and adolescents[5,6] and represents approximately 10% of the cases of diabetes. Without insulin, the body cannot regulate blood glucose and, as a result, blood glucose levels become very high. Since there is no cure for this condition, persons with type 1 diabetes mellitus must learn to maintain a delicate balance between insulin, diet, and exercise. Inability to maintain this balance can lead to both acute life-threatening complications (hypoglycemia and hyperglycemia) and long-term health concerns (cardiovascular disease, delayed wound healing, and peripheral neuropathies).

Type 1 diabetes is typically diagnosed in individuals prior to age 25. In most cases, individuals will present clinically with polydipsia, polyphagia, polyuria, and weight loss. It should be noted, however, that some individuals with type 1 diabetes, particularly young children, may experience no signs or symptoms prior to an initial presentation of ketoacidosis. Definitive diagnosis of diabetes mellitus requires a laboratory blood test. Table 10-4 outlines the types of blood glucose tests and criterion values for normal, prediabetes, and diabetes. The diagnosis is made when a patient's lab results are positive for at least two of the criteria, and these results are then reconfirmed on a second test day.

Type 1 diabetes is treated with insulin. There are several types of insulin available for use, ranging from fast-acting to slow-acting. Fast-acting insulin will generally produce effects within 5 to 30 minutes, with a peak effect occurring between 1 and 4 hours and a duration of 4 to 8 hours. Long acting insulin will produce effects within 2 to 4 hours, with a peak level obtained somewhere between 8 and 14 hours. The effects produced by long acting insulin may last up the 24 hours.

Persons with type 1 diabetes require several injections of insulin each day. Many physicians will recommend their patients use alternating injections of short- and long-acting insulin or use a short- and long-acting insulin mix. These injections are administered subcutaneously and are usually given before breakfast and dinner.[11] It is generally recommended that athletes inject their insulin into a nonexercising body part such as the abdomen. Some individuals may use an insulin pump to administer their insulin. The pump is a pocket-sized device that administers continuous insulin subcutaneously in varying doses depending on the individual's meal times and activity schedule. The pump provides more flexibility and consistency for those individuals who have difficulty balancing their insulin doses with meals and exercise.[11] Although small in size, the pump can still be somewhat cumbersome for athletes during practice and competition. The pump may need to be removed prior to swimming or some contact sports[11]; however, decisions regarding its use during athletic competition should be left to the individual's physician.

Persons who have difficulty regulating glucose levels through insulin and diet have a higher risk of severe complications.[12] Long-term health consequences of type 1 diabetes mellitus include peripheral and autonomic neuropathy, retinopathy leading to blindness, cardiovascular disease, hypertension, kidney disorders, chronic skin ulcers, and poor healing capability.[10] Regular aerobic exercise indirectly inhibits the development or advancement of some complications among people with type 1 diabetes, such as cardiovascular disease. Generally, significant health problems do not occur for at least 10 years after onset of the disease in patients who can maintain good glucose control. The risk for complications increases with age.

Athletic trainers should be aware of which, if any, of their patients suffer from diabetes. The preparticipation examination is the ideal time to identify diabetic athletes and to determine the level of control they have over their disease. The frequency of *hypoglycemia* (low blood sugar) or *hyperglycemia* (high blood sugar) bouts can provide a clear indication of the patient's level of control over his or her diabetes. As mentioned previously, both of these conditions can be potentially life-threatening; therefore athletic trainers must be able to recognize and treat these emergencies. Table 10-5 compares and contrasts the signs and symptoms of hypoglycemia and hyperglycemia.

Hypoglycemia is much more common than hyperglycemia among persons with type 1 diabetes.[13] Hypoglycemia occurs during physical exertion when there is a high level of circulating insulin. This commonly occurs when an individual injects insulin before exercise and then fails to eat.[14,15] Athletes must learn to estimate the correct insulin dosage based on the expected intensity and duration of the practice or competition. Injecting too low of an insulin dose prior to a high intensity workout or failing to take in carbohydrates during an extremely long event can lead to hypoglycemia due to the depletion of glucose. Athletes should use a glucometer to monitor their blood glucose levels two to four times a day. Most individuals will begin showing signs and symptoms of hypoglycemia when their blood glucose levels drop to 50 to 60 mg/dL. If an individual recognizes an impending hypoglycemic attack, he should stop activity immediately and consume 30 to 40 g of carbohydrate. Table 10-6 provides examples of snacks that contain approximately 30 to 40 g of carbohydrate.

Table 10-5

Signs of Hyperglycemia (Diabetic Ketoacidosis) and Hypoglycemia in Person With Diabetes Mellitus

Hyperglycemia (diabetic ketoacidosis, diabetic "coma," or diabetic hyperosmolar state)

- Blood glucose >200 mg/dL
- Gradual onset
- Abdominal pain
- Thirst but not hunger
- Fruity odor on breath (acetone)
- Dehydration
- Lethargy
- Confusion
- Loss of consciousness (coma)

Hypoglycemia (insulin shock)

- Blood glucose <70 mg/dL
- Sudden onset
- Headache
- Hunger but not thirst
- Blurred vision
- Dizziness
- Decreased performance
- Autonomic signs (pallor, diaphoresis, tachycardia, tremors)
- Fatigue
- Slurred speech
- Confusion

Table 10-6

Samples of Snacks Containing Approximately 30 to 40 gm of Carbohydrate

- Apple juice (10 oz) unsweetened
- Orange juice (12 oz)
- Cola (12 oz)
- Gatorade (8 oz)

Hypoglycemia can progress very quickly, therefore, athletic trainers, coaches, and parents should watch closely for signs of a problem. Individuals suffering from hypoglycemia will often times exhibit changes in behavior such as mood swings, increased frustration, agitation, or increased aggression.

Hyperglycemia is caused by excessively high levels of glucose, which is associated with low levels of insulin. There are a number of factors which can increase glucose levels including emotional stress, illness or injury, a change in activity level, addition of a new medication that might stimulate glucose release, or a missed insulin dose. Hyperglycemia will usually develop rather slowly and can lead to a dangerous state of metabolic acidosis referred to as diabetic ketoacidosis (DKA). DKA occurs with extreme depletion of insulin and can result in coma and possible death.

When the body is unable to move glucose from the blood to the cells, it turns to fats as an energy source. Ketones are then produced as a by product of the breakdown of fats for fuel. These toxic acids build up in the blood and eventually spill over into the urine. Ketones are responsible for the fruity odor noticed on the breaths of persons suffering from extreme hyperglycemia and DKA.

A glucose reading over 200 mg/dL should prohibit exercise and requires a urinalysis to screen for ketones. The presence of ketones in the urine is a sign of impending diabetic ketoacidosis. Insulin should be administered immediately and the person should be transported for medical examination and monitoring.[6,10,15] Treatment involves rehydration and restoration of electrolyte balance to correct the acidosis.

Type 2 Diabetes Mellitus

Type 2 diabetes mellitus is characterized by normal or high levels of insulin, but decreased insulin receptor sensitivity. Glucose uptake by the liver and muscles is substantially impaired because the insulin receptors do not respond to circulating insulin.[5,6] As a result, blood glucose levels remain higher than normal. Until recently, type 2 diabetes was primarily a disease of adults, but the disorder has been gradually increasing among children. Type 2 diabetes is nine or ten times more common than type 1 diabetes, affecting at least 10 to 20 million people in the United States, many of whom are unaware they have the condition.[6]

The chronically elevated blood glucose level eventually produces hyperlipidemia (increased fat in blood), arteriosclerosis (hardening of arteries), peripheral neuropathy, chronic infections, and bone changes (eg, osteoporosis).[9] A positive family history of type 2 diabetes and the presence of obesity are strong predictors of this condition.[6] Polydipsia and polyuria are the most common symptoms of type 2 diabetes mellitus.[9] Increased fluid intake (polydipsia) occurs to dilute blood glucose concentration, but the increased fluid intake causes an increase in fluid excretion by the kidneys (polyuria).

The most severe metabolic consequence in type 2 diabetes mellitus is hyperosmolar hyperglycemic nonketotic coma; this potentially fatal complication occurs most often in older patients who have a concurrent illness, such as influenza or gastroenteritis, that predisposes them to dehydration.[13] This condition is a result of an extreme hyperglycemic state (>600 mg/dL) that results in the blood being hyperosmolar—meaning that it has too many particulates relative to the amount of fluid. The hyperosmolarity causes a flow of fluids from the tissues into the blood in an effort to dilute the particulate level. The result is a severe state of dehydration that is self-perpetuating; clinical signs include seizure, coma, delirium, lethargy, and vision changes.[13] Treatment involves hydration, restoring electrolyte balance, insulin to reduce hyperglycemia, and addressing any underlying illness.

Exercise and a controlled diet are mainstays in the prevention and treatment of type 2 diabetes.[6,12] Exercise directly affects blood glucose level by increasing metabolic demand of muscle, which burns more glucose as fuel, and increasing the effectiveness of insulin receptors. Low to moderate intensity exercise thus facilitates muscle glucose uptake among persons with type 2 diabetes.[12,16] In contrast to type 1 diabetes, hyperglycemia is more common than hypoglycemia in type 2 diabetes[13]; in type 2 diabetes, the person's resting state is hyperglycemic and exercise causes a further release of glucose into the blood. Exercise may lead to hypoglycemia if the person is using hypoglycemic agents to control their high glucose levels.[13]

Diabetes and Exercise

Aerobic exercise has certain advantages for persons with diabetes: no increase in blood pressure, which would increase the risk of retinopathy or nephropathy; a decreased potential for skin wounds; increased insulin receptor sensitivity; cardiovascular benefits (eg, lowering blood lipids); and weight control (particularly for type 2).[5,12] Children and adolescents who maintain a good regimen and controlled diet can participate in most sports with few or no precautions.[6,12] Adults with poorly controlled type 1 diabetes mellitus are at substantial risk for cardiovascular pathology and should exercise only under medical advice and guidelines.[14]

Since exercise affects glucose levels, athletes with type 1 diabetes should discuss adjustment of insulin type, dose, or regimen with their physician.[12,14] Preparticipation meals and insulin should be adjusted for both expected exercise intensity and blood glucose level at the time of the meal.[14] Immediately before exercise, a blood glucose level below 100 mg/dL requires a carbohydrate snack to raise blood glucose.[17] Approximately 15 to 30 g of carbohydrate per half hour of athletic exercise may be needed to prevent hypoglycemia.[6,10,17] A source of quick glucose, such as fruit juice, glucose tablets or gel, cola, sectioned oranges, or hard candy, should be available during practice and competition to counteract acute hypoglycemia during exercise.[6,10,12,15] A plan for glucagon and insulin availability and administration in the event of hypoglycemia or hyperglycemia should be established between the patient, patient's parents (if the patient is a minor), athletic trainer, and physician.[10] Table 10-7 outlines the management of patients with diabetes mellitus.

Any athlete or patient who has diabetes should be allowed to stop activity at the first sign of a hypoglycemic attack. Should the individual lose consciousness or begin to have a seizure, the athletic trainer must quickly administer glucagon. All athletic trainers should be familiar with their patient's glucometers and emergency glucagon kits should they need to use them in an emergency situation. Most emergency glucagon kits will include a glucagon powder and dissolving liquid to produce a single dose of 1 mL of glucagon. Once dissolved completely, the glucagon is injected IM or subcutaneously. Unconscious individuals suffering from hypoglycemia will usually regain consciousness within 5 to 20 minutes after a glucagon injection.[11] Once conscious, the athlete should eat a small snack made up of CHO and proteins.

In addition, persons with type 1 diabetes may have a significant hypoglycemic response 6 to 24 hours after strenuous exercise.[5,6,14,15] After exercise, the body's muscle and liver glycogen stores must be restored. This process, which uses existing blood glucose to synthesize glycogen, leads to a further depletion of blood glucose levels. Postexercise insulin dose may need to be decreased and the postexercise meal should ensure adequate caloric intake.[6] Conversely, failure to inject insulin after exercise causes hyperglycemia since glucose released during exercise is not countered by insulin secretion. Additional potential risks for patients with diabetes

Table 10-7

Managing the Athlete With Diabetes Mellitus

- Obtain frequency of hypoglycemia episodes in preparticipation examination.
- Communicate with doctor relative to adjusting insulin dose and schedule specific to type of exercise.
- Take blood glucose before practice or competition and take appropriate action:
  <100 mg/dL=eat a carbohydrate snack before practice (30 to 40 gm)
  >200 mg/dL=no practice, urinalysis for ketones (ketones=emergency), insulin injection
- Communicate with athlete and coach to be excused from practice immediately at the first sign of hypoglycemia.
- Have a ready source of simple carbohydrate (hard candy, fruit juice) available at all times.
- Establish an emergency plan for severe hypoglycemia with athlete and athlete's physician or team physician, including injection of glucagon or intravenous glucose if available.

are orthostatic hypotension and dehydration, both consequences of polyuria and a decrease in blood volume.[6,15]

Competitive athletes must adhere to specific regimens to maintain blood glucose control, including injection schedules, frequent blood glucose monitoring, and strict diet.[6,10,12,14] With awareness and simple precautions, most patients with diabetes mellitus can participate in sports without restriction or complications.[6,14] Again, the athlete's physician should guide any medical or dietary adjustments.

Disorders of the Pituitary Gland

Diabetes Insipidus

Inadequate secretion of ADH from the pituitary gland causes diabetes insipidus. Decreased ADH level prevents water from being reabsorbed in the kidneys; the result is large amounts of dilute urine. Polyuria and polydipsia in the presence of normal blood glucose level characterize this disorder. Most cases are *idiopathic* (no discernable cause), but can be caused by tumors, infection, or vascular problems that affect the hypothalamus or pituitary gland. Medical examination to find an explanation is warranted.

Acromegaly

Overproduction of growth hormone causes a condition called acromegaly.[9] Excess growth hormone causes continual growth of bones and soft tissues. Persons with acromegaly are usually tall, have a thick prominent mandible, protruding frontal bone, large thick hands and feet, a "barrel" chest, and thoracic kyphosis.[9] Some organ systems, including cardiovascular, renal, and digestive, are affected by both the excess growth hormone and the metabolic stress of maintaining a large, continually growing body. The lifespan is shortened and the most common causes of death are cardiovascular disease (from cardiomyopathy, hypertension, and hyperlipidemia) and cancer (from overstimulation and overproduction of organ cells). Abuse of human growth hormone as an ergogenic aid can produce similar physical characteristics and clinical syndromes.

Disorders of the Thyroid and Parathyroid

Hyperthyroidism

An excess of thyroid hormone impairs glucose metabolism by interfering with insulin function and changing glucose absorption rate; the result is that muscles may have difficulty maintaining exercise.[18] In addition, core body temperature increases to above normal both at rest and with exercise as a result of thyroid hormone increasing overall body metabolism. Monitoring for signs of hyperthermia during exercise is warranted.[18] Heart rate response to exercise may also be greater than normal. Hyperthyroidism is treated with medication, radiation, or surgery to inhibit or remove the thyroid gland, depending on the severity and stage of disease.

Graves' disease is the most common form of hyperthyroidism and is eight times more common in women than men. Graves' disease causes tremors, weakness, difficulty swallowing or speaking, fatigue, and facial or eye motor disorders called tics.[9] Other signs and symptoms include an enlarged thyroid gland (goiter), heat intolerance, nervousness, sweating, weight loss, and protrusion of the eyes. Diagnosis is made based on symptoms, laboratory blood tests, and a thyroid scan. Treatment is similar to that discussed for hyperthyroidism.

Hypothyroidism

After diabetes mellitus, hypothyroidism is the second most common endocrine disorder and affects the functioning of multiple organ-systems. Hypothyroidism is caused by a deficiency of thyroid hormones T3 and T4, although T4 is the primary hormone involved. Inadequate thyroid hormone decreases cardiac output by limiting heart rate (bradycardia) and left ventricle contractility.[18] Furthermore, the normal peripheral vasodilation during exercise may not occur. The net effect is decreased oxygen and glucose available to exercising muscle, thus limiting endurance.[18] Signs and symptoms of hypothyroidism include dry skin, weakness, myalgia, bilateral paresthesias, peripheral non-pitting edema, bradycardia, constipation, poor peripheral circulation,[9] a thickened tongue that may cause slurred speech, memory problems, and slowed cognition.

Hypothyroidism is diagnosed based on symptoms and the results of laboratory blood tests measuring the hormone blood levels of TSH and T4. Elevated TSH levels with lowered T4 values indicate primary hypothyroidism. High TSH levels demonstrate that the pituitary is functioning normally by continuing to secrete TSH; however, the thyroid is unable to produce normal levels T4. Low TSH levels with normal T4 levels indicate that the pituitary gland may not be functioning properly, causing secondary hypothyroidism.

Hypothyroidism is treated with levothyroxine (Levothroid [Lloyd, Shenandoah, Iowa], Synthroid [Abbott Laboratories, Abbott Park, Ill]), a synthetic thyroid hormone. Because there is no cure for hypothyroidism, persons with this disorder must take thyroid hormone for the rest of their lives. It may take 6 months to a year to effectively regulate the thyroid hormone levels.

Parathyroid Hormone

Hyperparathyroidism and hypoparathyroidism, or excess or inadequate secretion of parathyroid hormone, respectively, are rarely encountered in athletes. Parathyroid hormone regulates calcium metabolism. Hyperparathyroidism causes excess calcium release, primarily from bone, into the bloodstream. The most obvious consequences are muscle weakness, arthralgia in the hands and feet, and hyperactive reflexes. Untreated, kidney stones, peptic ulcers, and cognitive changes occur.[9] Hypoparathyroidism, conversely, creates a deficiency of blood calcium, leading to muscle spasms during activity, cardiac arrhythmia, thin hair, and brittle nails. Hyper- and hypoparathyroidism also cause symptoms in the gastrointestinal, neurological, and urogenital systems. Surgical removal of the glands is the treatment of hyperparathyroidism, whereas calcium and vitamin D supplementation are used for hypoparathyroidism.[9]

Disorders of the Adrenals

Addison's Disease

Addison's disease is the inadequate production of the adrenal hormones aldosterone and cortisol. Hyperpigmentation ("bronzing") of the skin, fatigue, hypotension, weakness, GI symptoms, and joint pain are common. Fluid and electrolyte imbalances from decreased aldosterone causes dehydration and impaired cardiac output. Tolerance for physical or emotional stress decreases, coordination declines, and hypoglycemia may occur between meals.

If untreated, Addison's disease is fatal. Lifetime pharmacological corticosteroids are usually prescribed as treatment. Fluid and electrolyte levels should be maintained, particularly during exercise. The side effects of long-term corticosteroid therapy (see Cushing's Syndrome below) become more prominent with age. Persons with Addison's disease should have ready access to hydrocortisone to counteract acute adrenal crisis, which exhibits signs of shock and hypoglycemia.

Cushing's Syndrome

Cushing's syndrome, in contrast to Addison's disease, occurs as a result of overproduction of cortisol. This syndrome can also occur in individuals who must take glucocorticoids for extended periods of time, such as prednisone for the treatment of asthma, lupus, rheumatoid arthritis, or other chronic inflammatory condition. Classic signs and symptoms include: "moon face," upper body obesity, a pendulous abdomen with stretch marks (sometimes called "central obesity"), muscle atrophy, easy and frequent bruising, fatigue, and impaired wound healing. Cortisol acts as a very potent anti-inflammatory and may mask signs of infection or tissue damage. In addition, emotional disturbances, decreased libido, and type 2 diabetes mellitus (from inhibition of insulin receptors) eventually occur.[9]

Diagnosis is usually made based on the patient's history, physical examination, and the results of laboratory tests. Surgery, radiation, and adrenal suppression medication are the courses of treatment.[9] If extended use of glucocorticoids were the cause of the Cushing's syndrome, the patient's dose will be reduced to obtain controlled levels of cortisol. The patient's glucocorticoid dose will then be increased, with dosing every other day rather than every day.

Thermoregulation and Environmental Conditions

Thermoregulatory mechanisms are less effective in very young and very old persons. In addition, nutrition, drugs and alcohol, and fitness level affect the ability of the body to disperse or retain heat.[7,19] Persons with seizure disorders or sickle cell anemia may also be predisposed to conditions caused by thermoregulatory disorders.[19]

During exercise in hot and humid environments, large amounts of sweat are produced to cool the body by evaporation. Simultaneously, peripheral vasodilation supplies muscles with additional oxygen and glucose and provides an increased surface area to dissipate heat through the skin by convection. These mechanisms, sweating and vasodilation, create a relative hypovolemia, which decreases the heart's stroke volume. As a result, heart rate increases to maintain cardiac output.

If hypovolemia continues to increase as a result of dehydration, vasoconstriction occurs in the periphery, thus impairing heat dissipation mechanisms. Central ("core") body temperature rises as a consequence. If hydration is not restored, further vasoconstriction and a further rise in body temperature results; heart rate increases as cardiac output decreases and blood pressure falls, eventually producing shock and, in extreme cases, death.[20] Several stages of this pathological process, called heat illness (heat cramps, heat exhaustion, and heat stroke), theoretically exist, and there are other heat-related conditions that include heat syncope and exertional hyponatremia.

Heat Cramps

Heat cramps occur in the leg and trunk muscles during exercise in hot weather after mild dehydration. Associated signs and symptoms include fatigue, thirst, and profuse sweating.[21] Athletes who are accustomed to exercising in heat ("acclimatized") produce very dilute sweat, which preserves salt. Unacclimatized athletes, however, secrete a relatively high concentration of salt in their sweat. Attempts by unacclimatized athletes to replace fluid loss with plain water may further dilute the blood and cause muscle spasms as a result of lowered electrolyte (sodium and potassium) levels.[7]

Gradual acclimatization is usually preventative. During an attack of heat cramps, cooling, rehydration, and a dilute (0.1% to 1.0%) saline solution can be used.[21] Adding ¼ teaspoon of table salt to a sports drink can be very effective. Ice, stretching, and massage can help to alleviate the pain associated with heat cramps. Return to play decisions should be based on the individual's ability to perform at the necessary level and the individual's hydration status.[22] Increased dietary salt intake is not necessary, and may actually contribute to heat cramps by stimulating sweat glands to secrete even more salt.[7]

Heat Syncope

This condition typically occurs within the first few days of returning to exercising in hot, humid conditions. The combined effects of peripheral vasodilation, hypovolemia, and dehydration decrease cardiac output, depriving the brain of blood.[21,23] When the blood flow to the brain is inadequate, syncope results. Precipitating actions include standing for a long time, stopping strenuous exercise suddenly, and rapidly standing up from sitting. The person usually recovers consciousness within minutes and may report feeling dizzy or having tunnel vision just before fainting. Skin may be pale or sweaty, heart rate is generally slowed, and body temperature is elevated from exercising, but is not excessive. Treatment is moving the person into the shade, elevating the legs, and rehydrating. Vital signs should be monitored to ensure that the condition does not progress.

Heat Exhaustion

Advanced dehydration, usually from a failure to adequately replace fluid or sodium, produces heat exhaustion.[19,23] The signs and symptoms, although variable, include profuse sweating, rising body temperature (100°F to 103°F), tachycardia, hyperpnea, hypotension, headache, fatigue, and nausea.[7,19] The person may report muscle cramping, weakness, or dizziness.[21] Changes in mental status are usually not present, although the athlete may physically collapse.[7]

Rapid cooling with cool towels, cool shower, removing excess clothing, resting in shade or air conditioning, and rehydration with a very dilute electrolyte drink (0.1% saline content) usually precipitate recovery.[7] Rehydration with large amounts of plain water may dilute the blood, thus accentuating electrolyte depletion.[19] Transport to a physician for intravenous rehydration is recommended if recovery does not progress rapidly.[21] Avoiding extreme heat, a reasonable acclimatization period, and proper rehydration during exercise can prevent heat exhaustion. Individuals should be fully hydrated and free of symptoms before returning to activity.[22]

Exertional Heat Stroke

Heat stroke, a medical emergency with a very high rate of mortality, occurs with body temperatures over 104°F (*hyperthermia*).[21,23] It is the third leading cause of sport-related death, after head and neck trauma and cardiac failure.[19] Severe dehydration and hypovolemia inhibits the sweating mechanism, which causes the peripheral vascular system to collapse in an attempt to preserve blood pressure to the vital organs.[7] When this occurs, the body has no mechanism to dissipate heat and central body temperature increases very quickly. Lactic acid and potassium levels build in the blood, and the muscles begin to degenerate, flooding the bloodstream with proteins that eventually block the kidneys and cause acute renal failure (rhabdomyolosis). Cardiac output eventually falls so low it cannot maintain blood flow to the brain and kidneys, which produces a reflex systemic vasodilation in a vascular system that does not have enough fluid volume. Vasodilation greatly increases cardiac demand in a now insufficient cardiovascular system, which results in heart failure. Loss of consciousness, convulsions, coma, and death can result.[7]

An individual exercising in a hot environment who has tachycardia, very high core body temperature, lack of coordination, physical collapse, and altered cognitive ability (ie, disorientation, confusion, seizure, hallucination) suggests heat stroke. These central nervous system symptoms, as well as the core temperature, help to distinguish exertional heat stroke from heat exhaustion. The NATA recommends that athletic trainers assess rectal temperatures to obtain the most accurate measure of core temperature. When exertional heat stroke is suspected, drastic measures should be undertaken immediately. Rapid cooling by immersion in cold water (35°F to 58°F) is the preferred method for reducing core temperature. Once core temperature reaches 101°F to 102°F, the individual should be transported immediately to the closest emergency room. If on-site cooling is not available, then the individual should be transported immediately with cooling performed in route to the hospital using cold towels or ice bags.[7,21] Intravenous fluids need to be administered under medical direction since overhydration can cause pulmonary or cerebral edema. Return-to-play decisions should be made by the treating physician. Once clearance is obtained, the individual should begin a gradual return to activity, allowing time for reacclimatization.

Exertional Hyponatremia

The final type of heat-related illness has signs and symptoms that are similar to exertional heat stroke. Exertional hyponatremia is a dangerous condition in which the sodium level in the blood falls below 130 mmol/L.[21,24] Exercise lasting 4 hours or longer during which a person drinks a large amount of water, much more than they have lost through sweat (water intoxication; the person may actually gain weight during exercise), or fails to replace sodium lost through sweat, or both, lead to this condition.[23] The result of low blood sodium is a flow of water from the vascular system into the tissues. The cells in the tissues swell to the point of bursting, causing a severe alteration in cell function. Fluid in the lungs and brain can quickly cause death.

Exertional hyponatremia produces headache, nausea, impaired cognition, loss of consciousness, seizures, and swollen extremities. The central nervous system signs and symptoms of hyponatremia are similar to those of exertional heat stroke; however, the core body temperature is typically not elevated above 104°F. The person with exertional hyponatremia should never be given fluids until a physician has properly diagnosed the condition and an appropriate hypertonic saline solution is determined. Suspicion of hyponatremia warrants immediate referral to the hospital. Return-to-play decisions should be made by the treating physician.

Prevention of Heat Illness

Deaths during exercise or activity that are attributable to environmental heat are preventable, in contrast to most cardiac incidents and head injuries. Preparticipation examinations can be used to identify people at risk for heat illness, such as a history of previous exertional heat illness. Coaches, participants, and others involved in organized outdoor activities should be educated regarding the prevention and recognition of heat illness. The NATA position statements on exertional heat illness and fluid replacement for athletes lists several other preventative measures.[21,25]

First, a period of acclimatization should be allowed, during which the cardiovascular system and sweating mechanism can adapt.[7,21] Usually physiological acclimatization begins within several days, but takes 2 weeks or longer to become effective.[19,21] Second, and most obvious, vigorous exercise during the hottest part of the day should be avoided, or drills and practice moved indoors whenever feasible.[21] For over 50 years, sports medicine practitioners have been issuing guidelines for exercise in hot, humid conditions. Most of these recommendations are unheeded since they effectively prohibit exercise for large portions of outdoors sports seasons in the southern United States.[26] Reasonable precautions, however, are usually available, such as modifying activities, frequent breaks in shade, and shorter pratices.[21] Third, appropriate clothing, avoidance of diuretics such as alcohol and caffeine, and continuous monitoring of athletes during practice can prevent many heat illnesses.[7]

Proper hydration maintains thermoregulatory and cardiovascular function.[25] Individuals should begin exercise fully hydrated. Prehydration guidelines recommend the consumption of 17 to 20 oz of water or sports drink 2 to 3 hours before exercise and an additional 7 to 10 oz 10 to 20 minutes before exercise.[25] Fluid intake during exercise is also essential for preventing dehydration.[7,20] During shorter, less intense events (up to 1 hour), plain water can be used to rehydrate. Replacement of electrolytes, and to some extent carbohydrates, in addition to water becomes more important as intensity and duration of exercise increases.[7,20] During endurance events and in between practices, however, plain water increases urine output even when mildly dehydrated. Thus, a carbohydrate-electrolyte drink (solute content between 3% and 6%) may be preferred.[20,25] An athlete who has lost 3% or more of his or her body weight during exercise in heat should be held from subsequent practices until body weight is restored.

Exposure to Cold

Prolonged exposure to cold environmental temperatures can also cause medical problems, some of which are life threatening, particularly if moisture and wind are also present. Water has 25 times the heat conductance of air, so wet clothes, rain or sleet, or immersion in cold water quickly removes body heat.[7] Wind chill, the effect of convection on the skin, can substantially reduce body temperature, which is compounded if running or moving against the wind.[7] In addition, at least half of the body's expelled heat radiates through the head and neck during exercise. Appropriate clothing or protective gear should protect against rain, snow, and wind, and cover the head and neck to prevent excessive heat loss during prolonged exposure.

Frostbite

Frostbite, although rarely fatal, can cause severe tissue damage or limb loss.[27] As exposed skin temperature decreases, a transient blanching and paresthesia called frostnip occurs. This condition is quickly reversible with rewarming (moving indoors) and protecting the area from further exposure.[27]

With prolonged exposure, superficial frostbite, which is limited to the upper layers of the skin, occurs as ice crystals form in extracellular spaces.[23,27] The skin appears waxy, dry, or cyanotic, and becomes hardened over the joints.[7] Ice in the tissues draws fluid from the cells, causing permanent damage to epithelial cells and blood vessels.[27] Once blood supply is disrupted, hypoxic necrosis occurs unless blood can be delivered through adjacent vessels. This tissue hypoxia is the primary cause of tissue damage in frostbite.[19]

Continued exposure progresses to deep frostbite, which involves freezing in the deep layers of skin and possibly muscle or other underlying tissues.[27] The mechanism of tissue damage is the same as superficial frostbite; ice formation and hypoxia from vascular destruction. The appearance of cyanosis, blood blisters, or completely frozen skin indicate extensive, irreversible tissue damage.[19]

Once frostbite is recognized, prompt removal from the cold should be undertaken. Weight bearing, pressure, or friction of the frostbitten area should be avoided. Wet clothing can be removed if it is not frozen to the skin, and replaced with dry, soft blankets or other cloth. The area should not be thawed if refreezing is a possibility, since refreezing increases the extent of tissue damage. Rapid rewarming of the frostbitten limb can be performed by warm water (104°F to 108°F, 40°C to 42°C) immersion.[7,27] During rewarming, intense pain, bright erythema, edema, and eventually blistering occur as blood supply returns.[7] With large regions of frostbite, transport to a medical facility is required since limb-threatening compartment syndromes and infection are common.

Hypothermia

Prolonged exposure to cold environmental temperatures can produce a potentially fatal condition called hypothermia, a central body temperature of 94°F (34.4°C) or less.[23,27] As central body temperature decreases, metabolism decreases, blood viscosity (resistance to flow) increases, and heart rate and cardiac output decrease.[7,27] Uncontrollable shivering may occur and changes in cognitive function occur, such as confusion, psychosis (loss of reasoning), lethargy, or coma.[7,19] Physical signs include facial erythema and edema, ataxia (incoordination of gait), bradycardia, and hypotension.[19]

Treatment of hypothermia takes precedence over frostbite.[27] Passive rewarming, or placing the victim in a warm environment (indoors with blankets) is preferred to applying heating pads or immersion in warm baths. Rapid reheating can cause a paradoxical reaction known as "afterdrop," wherein peripheral vasodilation and subsequent rush of cold fluids from the extremities actually causes core temperature to decrease even further.[19,27] For severe cases of hypothermia, emergency department techniques are required to prevent cardiac fibrillation.[19] Prevention of hypothermia primarily involves avoidance of cold, wet environments and wearing appropriate clothing. Clothes should be layered, with a light, wicking material near the skin, insulating materials in the layers in between, and a water-resistant layer on the outside.[7] 911

Altitude Sickness

Exercise in altitude can cause several pathological conditions due to decreased barometric pressure, hypoxia, decreased ambient temperature, higher intensity sunlight, and dehydration.[23] Within 6 to 24 hours of ascent to over 12,000 feet, headache, loss of appetite, nausea, irritability, and mild confusion characterizes acute altitude sickness.[28] Although bothersome, this condition is seldom serious at altitudes below 15,000 feet. Most cases resolve in a few days with rest and hydration. Slow ascent to altitude may prevent or substantially decrease symptoms.

Some people experience pulmonary or cerebral edema in high altitude, particularly with rapid ascent to at least 8000 feet.[28] Pulmonary edema is recognized by dyspnea, cough, cyanosis, tachycardia, hyperpnea, and rales upon auscultation.[23] Cerebral edema impairs cognitive and other central nervous system functions, causing confusion, ataxia, and loss of consciousness. Early recognition of these serious conditions allows descent from altitude in a timely manner. Oxygen supplementation and corticosteroids may be needed in more severe cases.[28]

At very high altitude (over 15,000 feet), retinal hemorrhage and retinopathy may occur. Exercise may exacerbate this situation, which is recognized by blurring vision and aching in the orbits. The condition is usually self-limiting with no permanent complications if descent occurs quickly.[28]

High altitude also increases the risk for sickle cell crisis in individuals with sickle cell trait. The increased oxygen demand at altitude leads to an increased rate of RBC production, which in turn leads to an increased viscosity of the blood. This thickened blood increases the risk for clumping or clotting of the abnormally shaped red blood cells associated with sickle cell trait. Anyone relocating to a high altitude environment should allow time for gradual acclimatization.

Metabolic Disorders

Gout

Gout is caused by a defect in the breakdown of an amino acid called purine, which causes accumulation of uric acid in the blood. As uric acid concentration increases, it cannot be efficiently excreted by the kidneys and forms crystals in the joints and other tissues. The typical first manifestation of gout is sudden, severe pain and swelling in one or more joints. Over 90% of patients with gout have symptoms in the great toe. The foot, knee, and wrist are also commonly involved. Surgery, fatigue, rich diet, stress, infection, or certain medications can precipitate gout attacks. Chalky crystal deposits may erupt through the skin of a gouty joint. Unless treated, the attacks recur with increasing frequency and severity, although remissions lasting years are not uncommon. Treatment is through medication and dietary lifestyle changes.

Metabolic Bone Diseases

Osteoporosis

A pathological decrease in bone density is called osteoporosis.[29] Many factors contribute to the development of osteoporosis, including hormonal disturbances (decreased estrogen), nutritional deficiencies (primarily of calcium), and age.[29] The bones eventually become very fragile and fracture easily. Frequently, compression fractures of the vertebrae cause permanent deformities such as severe thoracic spine kyphosis ("Dowager's hump"), loss of height, and back pain.[29] Simple falls fracture the femur, tibia, humerus, or radius. For persons at risk for osteoporosis (female, postmenopausal, over age 75 years), precautions should be taken when applying manual mobilization techniques, exercising the spine, or performing load-bearing exercises. As mentioned in Chapter Nine, osteoporosis can also occur in females with an eating disorder and amenorrhea (female athletic triad syndrome).

Paget Disease

Paget disease (osteitis deformans) is an abnormality of bone remodeling, with alternating excess deposition or resorption of bone during various stages of the disease. The etiology is unclear, but the pathophysiology involves a deposition-resorbtion cycle that happens many times faster than normal. The disease begins in a destructive phase, in which bone resorption dominates. The second phase displays an acceleration of bone formation to counter the high rate of resorbtion. The final phase involves osteosclerotic changes in which the bone becomes thickened and dense. The disease may affect one bone or many. Although many patients are asymptomatic or have minor aching pains, in others the thickening of bone leads to neural compression, particularly of the cranial nerves. The abnormal bone is also prone to deformity, particularly in the spine (kyphosis) and long bones of the legs (bowing), and fracture.

The condition occurs most frequently in the flat and long bones of elderly men.[29] Over time Paget disease produces bony deformities, functional disability, head or face pain, and pathological fractures.[29] Treatment involves control of symptoms with anti-inflammatory medications and administration of hormones that control bone metabolism. Treatment precautions, such as avoiding heavy loads or extreme motions, are necessary to lower the risk of fracture.

Pediatric Concerns

Osteogenesis Imperfecta

Osteogenesis imperfecta (OI) is an inherited, autosomal dominant (in most cases) condition that interferes with bone formation by affecting the synthesis of type I collagen.[30] OI makes the bones very brittle and suseptible to fracture, even during normal activities. Persons with OI are nearly always diagnosed in early childhood and rarely participate in athletics. Several variants of OI, from mild to severe, exist and there is no cure.[30] Signs are due to the collagen defect, and include heart valve disorders, stunted growth, blue eye sclera, dental problems, joint laxity, and scoliosis. Fractures may be surgically stabilized or casted. Most patients become progressively disabled by multiple fractures and their lifespan is shortened. Treatment is limited to prevention and management of fractures and bony deformities.

Summary

The endocrine system regulates the functions of many organ-systems including normal metabolism and homeostasis. Pathology of the endocrine glands can produce signs and symptoms in many organs, including those of the gastrointestinal, cardiovascular, neurological, urogenital, and musculoskeletal systems. The personal medical history, which can reveal distinct patterns of endocrine dysfunction, is the most important aspect of assessment for endocrine or metabolic disorders. Diabetes, thyroid hormone imbalance (hypo- and hyper-), and Cushing's syndrome (either primary or a result of long-term corticosteroid use) are the most common endocrine disorders. Treatment of endocrine disorders is complicated and may involve many side effects that impair physical activity. Pathological metabolic conditions frequently encountered include adverse environmental exposure (heat, cold, and altitude) and bone diseases. Pathology caused by environmental conditions are treated by prevention (avoiding extreme environments) or removal from the dangerous environment.

Case Study

Part 1

Scott, one of your high school junior varsity football athletes, has recently been diagnosed with type 1 diabetes. He is having trouble regulating his blood glucose levels, particularly now during two-a-day practice sessions. You notice during the second workout of the day that Scott is starting to look a little sluggish. You ask him how he feels and he insists that he is fine. Still suspecting a problem, you continue to watch him closely. Just before the next water break, you see Scott stumble and then collapse on the field. As you reach him, you find that he is pale, clammy, confused, and slurring his words.

Critical Thinking Questions

1. Based on Scott's medical history and the current signs and symptoms, what condition(s) do you suspect?
2. How would you treat the condition(s), both on the field and after removing Scott from the field?
3. What could you have done differently to prevent the condition(s) from occurring?

Part 2

Scott's physician has decided to have him use an insulin pump in an effort to better regulate his blood glucose levels. For the next 3 weeks, he wants Scott wearing his pump during all practices and games.

Critical Thinking Questions

1. How would you modify Scott's football equipment to accommodate and protect the insulin pump?

References

1. National Athletic Trainers' Association. *Athletic Training Educational Competencies.* 4th ed. Dallas, TX: National Athletic Trainers' Association; 2005.
2. Ganong WF. *Review of Medical Physiology.* 22nd ed. New York, NY: McGraw-Hill Medical; 2005.
3. Gould BE. Endocrine disorders. *Pathophysiology for the Health-Related Professions.* Philadelphia, PA: WB Saunders Co; 1997:377-395.
4. Martini FH, Timmons MJ, McKinley MP. The endocrine system. *Human Anatomy.* 3rd ed. Upper Saddle River, NJ: Prentice-Hall; 2000:499-521.
5. Hough DO. Diabetes mellitus in sports. *Med Clin North Am.* 1994;78(2):423-437.
6. Landry GL, Allen DB. Diabetes mellitus and exercise. *Clin Sports Med.* 1992;11(2):403-418.
7. Thein LA. Environmental conditions affecting the athlete. *J Orthop Sports Phys Ther.* 1995;21(3):158-171.
8. Allen DB. Effects of fitness training on endocrine systems in children and adolescents. *Adv Pediatr.* 1999;46:41-66.
9. Boissonnault JS, Madlon-Kay D. Screening for endocrine system disease. In: Boissonnault WG, ed. *Examination in Physical Therapy Practice: Screening for Medical Disease.* New York, NY: Churchill Livingstone; 1995:155-173.
10. Jimenez CC. Diabetes and exercise: the role of the athletic trainer. *J Athl Training.* 1997;32(4):339-343.
11. Landry GL, Burnhardt DT. Diabetes mellitus. *Essentials of Primary Care Sports Medicine.* Champaign, IL: Human Kinetics; 2003:37-53.
12. Bell DS. Exercise for patients with diabetes: benefits, risks, precautions. *Postgrad Med.* 1992;92(1):183-184, 187-190, 195-198.
13. Jimenez CC. Recognizing and managing diabetes-related emergencies. *Athl Ther Today.* 2004;9(2):6-10.
14. Fahey PJ, Stallkamp ET, Kwatra S. The athlete with type I diabetes: managing insulin, diet and exercise. *Am Fam Physician.* 1996;53(5):1611-1617.
15. Martin DE. Glucose emergencies: recognition and treatment. *J Athl Training.* 1994;29(2):141-143.
16. Petrella RJ. Exercise for older patients with chronic disease. *Physician Sportsmed.* 1999;27(11):79-104.
17. Fincher AL. Managing diabetic emergencies. *Athl Ther Today.* 1999;4(4):45-46.
18. McAllister RM, Delp MD, Laughlin MH. Thyroid status and exercise tolerance: cardiovascular and metabolic considerations. *Sports Med.* 1995;20(3):189-198.
19. Bracker MD. Environmental and thermal injury. *Clin Sports Med.* 1992;11(2):419-436.
20. Murray R. Dehydration, hyperthermia, and athletes: science and practice. *J Athl Training.* 1996;31(2):248-252.

21. Binkley HM, Beckett J, Casa DJ, Kleiner DM, Plummer PE. National Athletic Trainers' Association position statement: exertional heat illnesses. *J Athletic Training.* 2002;37(3):329-343.
22. Interassociation Task Force on Exertional Heat Illness. Consensus statement. Available at www.nata.org. Accessed 2003.
23. Seto CK, Way D, O'Connor N. Environmental illness in athletes. *Clin Sports Med.* 2005;25(3):695-718.
24. Hew-Butler T, Almond C, Ayus JC, et al. Consensus statement of the 1st International Exercise-Associated Hyponatremia Consensus Development Conference, Cape Town, South Africa 2005. *Clin J Sport Med.* 2005;15(4):208-213.
25. Casa DJ, Armstrong LE, Hillman SK, et al. National Athletic Trainers' Association position statement: fluid replacement for athletes. *J Athletic Training.* 2000;35(2):212-224.
26. Francis K, Feinstein R, Brasher J. Optimal practice times for the reduction of the risk of heat illness during fall football practice in the southeastern United States. *Athletic Training.* 1991;26(1):76-80.
27. Grace TG. Cold exposure injuries and the winter athlete. *Clin Orthop.* 1987;216:55-62.
28. Mountain RD. High-altitude medical problems. *Clin Orthop.* 1987;216:50-54.
29. Boissonnault WG, Bass C. Pathological origins of trunk and neck pain: part III-diseases of the musculoskeletal system. *J Orthop Sports Phys Ther.* 1990;12(5):216-221.
30. Myers GJ. Congenital anomalies: musculoskeletal abnormalities. In: Beers MH, Berkow R, eds. *The Merck Manual of Diagnosis and Therapy.* 17th ed. Whitehouse Station, NJ: Merck Research Laboratories; 1999:2218-2222.

ONLINE RESOURCES

American Diabetes Association
www.diabetes.org
Centers for Disease Control and Prevention—Division of Diabetes Translation
www.cdc.gov/diabetes
Cushing's Syndrome and Cushing's Disease
http://cushings.homestead.com
Juvenile Diabetes Research Foundation International
www.jdrf.org
National Diabetes Education Program
www.ndep.nih.gov
National Heart, Lung, and Blood Institute
www.nhlbi.nih.gov
National Institute of Diabetes and Digestive and Kidney Diseases
www.niddk.nih.gov

Lab Exercise 10-1
Assessment of Blood Glucose Levels

Objectives

After completing this lab activity, students will be able to:

1. Measure blood glucose levels with a glucometer.
2. Interpret blood glucose levels in response to administration of glucose or other form of sugar.
3. Identify the effect of exercise on blood glucose levels.

Competencies

This lab exercise addresses the following psychomotor competencies from the NATA's *Athletic Training Educational Competencies, 4th ed:*

- Medical Conditions and Disabilities: 4

Equipment Needed

- Glucometer
- Lancets
- Test strips
- Watch, clock, or other timing device
- Glucose tablets or gel (15 gm)
- Two additional forms of glucose/sugar (fruit juice, hard candy, sports drink, soda, etc)
- Students should wear workout clothes (ie, shorts, t-shirt, tennis shoes)
- Treadmill, stationary bicycle, or other fitness machine

Instructions

This lab exercise involves the assessment of both fasting and non-fasting blood glucose levels. When completing the lab exercise during a class, students should determine prior to the lab who will eat breakfast (or other meal) and who will fast for at least 6 hours prior to the lab. At least four students will need to fast prior to the lab. When completing the lab exercise outside of class, each student will need to test four subjects who have fasted and one who has not.

Part 1: Blood Glucose Response to Sugar Intake

1. Measure fasting blood glucose level of at least three separate individuals (no food for at least 6 hours).
2. Give each subject 15 gm of some form of sugar (glucose tablets or gel, soda, fruit juice, sports drink, hard candy). Have each subject completely ingest sugar before you start timing.
3. Measure each subject's blood glucose level at 2 minutes post-ingestion.
4. Measure each subject's blood glucose level at 5 minutes post-ingestion.

Lab Exercise 10-1 (continued)
Assessment of Blood Glucose Levels

Subject #1:__________________ Form of sugar:____________________
Fasting glucose level ______________mg/dL
2 minutes post-ingestion____________mg/dL
5 minutes post-ingestion____________mg/dL

Subject #2:__________________ Form of sugar:____________________
Fasting glucose level ______________mg/dL
2 minutes post-ingestion____________mg/dL
5 minutes post-ingestion____________mg/dL

Subject #3:__________________ Form of sugar:____________________
Fasting glucose level ______________mg/dL
2 minutes post-ingestion____________mg/dL
5 minutes post-ingestion____________mg/dL

Part 2: Blood Glucose Response to Exercise

1. Measure the blood glucose level of one subject that has eaten breakfast (or other meal) and one subject who has fasted for at least 6 hours. Measure the results below.
2. Have each subject exercise for 20 minutes at 70% to 85% HR max (see calculation instructions below).
   a. Select a workload and have the subject begin exercising.
   b. Monitor his or her HR until he or she reaches an intensity that requires the target HR.
   c. Have him or her continue to exercise for 20 minutes at the intensity while monitoring his or her HR.
3. Immediately post-exercise, check blood glucose level.
4. Have him or her ingest 15 gm of some form of glucose or sugar.
5. Wait 5 minutes and recheck blood glucose level.

Karvonen Method for Determining Target Heart Rate

[(220 – age – HR resting) x target intensity] + HR resting
Heart rate max (HR max) = 220 – age = __________
Heart rate reserve (HRR) = HR max – HR rest = _______ - _______ = ______
Target HR = (HRR x intensity) + HR rest = (________ x 0.85) + ______ = ______

Lab Exercise 10-1 (continued)
Assessment of Blood Glucose Levels

Subject #4:__________________

Fasting glucose level__________________mg/dL
Target heart rate_____________________bpm
Exercise start time__________________mg/dL
(once target heart rate reached)
Exercise stop time________________________

Post-exercise glucose levels:
Immediately post-exercise____________mg/dL
5 minutes post-ingestion______________mg/dL

Subject #5:__________________

Non-fasting glucose level_____________mg/dL
Target heart rate_____________________bpm
Exercise start time__________________mg/dL
(once target heart rate reached)
Exercise stop time________________________

Post-exercise glucose levels:
Immediately post-exercise____________mg/dL
5 minutes post-ingestion______________mg/dL

Part 3: Analysis

1. Based on the results from Part 1, which form of glucose administration is the most effective in raising blood glucose levels? What are the implications for these findings in planning an emergency action plan for managing a diabetic athlete?
2. Based on the results from Part 2, what are the implications for not eating prior to a morning workout or competition?

Chapter Eleven

Eye, Ear, Nose, Throat, and Mouth Disorders

Chapter Outline and Objectives

Introduction

Review of Anatomy, Physiology, and Pathogenesis

- ❖ Describe the basic anatomical structures of the eye and their functions.
- ❖ Describe the basic anatomical structures of the ear and their functions.
- ❖ Describe the basic anatomical structures of the nose and their functions.
- ❖ Describe the basic anatomical structures of the throat and their functions.
- ❖ Describe the basic anatomical structures of the mouth and their functions.

Signs and Symptoms

- ❖ Identify the general signs and symptoms of eye pathology.
- ❖ Identify the general signs and symptoms of ear pathology.
- ❖ Identify the general signs and symptoms of nose pathology.
- ❖ Identify the general signs and symptoms of throat pathology.
- ❖ Identify the general signs and symptoms of mouth pathology.

Pain Patterns

- ❖ Identify the referred pain patterns associated with pathology of the eye, ear, nose, throat, and mouth.

Medical History and Physical Examination

- ❖ Describe medical history findings associated with eye, ear, nose, throat, and mouth pathology.
- ❖ Describe the physical examination procedures associated with eye, ear, nose, throat, and mouth pathology.
  - Palpation
  - Inspection
  - Physical Exam

  - Visual Acuity
  - Pupillary Shape and Reaction
  - Eye Movements
  - Peripheral Vision
  - Fluorescein Strips and Cobalt Blue Light
  - Ophthalmoscope
  - Otoscope

Pathology and Pathogenesis

- Discuss the signs, symptoms, management, and medical referral guidelines for eye pathology.
  - Eye Injuries
    - Subconjunctival Hemorrhage
    - Foreign Body in the Eye
    - Corneal Abrasions
    - Hyphema
    - Ruptured Globe
    - Orbital Fracture
    - Detached Retina
  - Eye Infections
    - Conjunctivitis
    - Stye
  - Glaucoma
- Discuss the signs, symptoms, management, and medical referral guidelines for ear pathology.
  - Ear Injuries
    - Auricular Hematoma
    - Ruptured Tympanic Membrane
  - Ear Infections
    - Otitis Externa
    - Otitis Media
    - Impacted Cerumen
- Discuss the signs, symptoms, management, and medical referral guidelines for nose pathology.
  - Nose Injuries
    - Epistaxis (Nosebleed)
    - Nasal Fracture
  - Nasal Allergies and Infections
    - Allergic Rhinitis
    - Sinusitis and Sinus Infections
- Discuss the signs, symptoms, management, and medical referral guidelines for throat pathology.
  - Throat Infections
    - Laryngitis, Pharyngitis, and Tonsillitis
- Discuss the signs, symptoms, management, and medical referral guidelines for mouth pathology.
  - Mouth Disorders
    - Gingivitis
    - Periodontitis
    - Dental Caries
    - Oral Candidiasis
    - Oral Cancer

This chapter addresses the following competencies from the *Athletic Training Educational Competencies, Fourth Edition*[1]:

Domain	Cognitive	Psychomotor
Acute Care of Injuries and Illnesses	4, 11, 16, 30	
Medical Conditions and Disabilities	1–7, 21	3, 4e
Orthopedic Clinical Examination and Diagnosis	1, 6, 16	
Pathology of Injuries and Illnesses	4–6	

INTRODUCTION

Regardless of their setting, athletic trainers may encounter injuries or illnesses involving the eye, ear, nose, throat, and mouth. Although most of these conditions are relatively benign in nature, others have the potential for serious complications (loss of sight or hearing) if not managed properly. This chapter will review the pertinent anatomy, signs and symptoms, evaluation procedures, and referral guidelines for the common injuries and illness involving the eye, ear, nose, throat, and mouth.

REVIEW OF ANATOMY, PHYSIOLOGY, AND PATHOGENESIS

Eye

The eye globe, or eyeball, is made up of many individual structures, some of which can be easily viewed by the naked eye, and others which require an opthalmascope to view (Figure 11-1). The sclera, also referred to as "the white of the eye," forms the outer protective layer of the eye. It covers the posterior 5/6 of the globe with openings in the front and back for the cornea and optic nerve, respectively. The clear cornea is located in the center of the most anterior portion of the eye. The conjunctiva is a thin mucous membrane that covers the anterior eye and lines the eye lids. The iris contains pigment cells which give the eye its color and includes muscles that work to constrict or dilate the pupil. Located in the center of the iris, the pupil is often compared to the aperture lens of a camera, controlling the amount of light allowed into the eye. The anterior chamber is formed by the space between the cornea and the iris and is filled with aqueous humor. The lens is a clear, biconvex structure located just posterior to the pupil and the iris. It is surrounded by the ciliary body, a ring of muscular tissue, which through contraction and relaxation controls the shape of the lens and the degree of focus on near and far objects. The ciliary body also produces the aqueous humor that fills the anterior chamber of the eye. The retina is a multi-layer tissue that lines the inner, posterior portion of the eye. The space within the globe is made up of a gelatinous substance called vitreous humor. The macula is located in the center of the retina and provides detailed central vision. Located within the center of the macular, the fovea is responsible for the sharpest detail in central vision. Located at the back of the eye, the optic nerve transmits nerve impulses from the eye to the brain. A portion of the optic nerve, the optic disc, is visible when viewed with an ophthalmoscope.

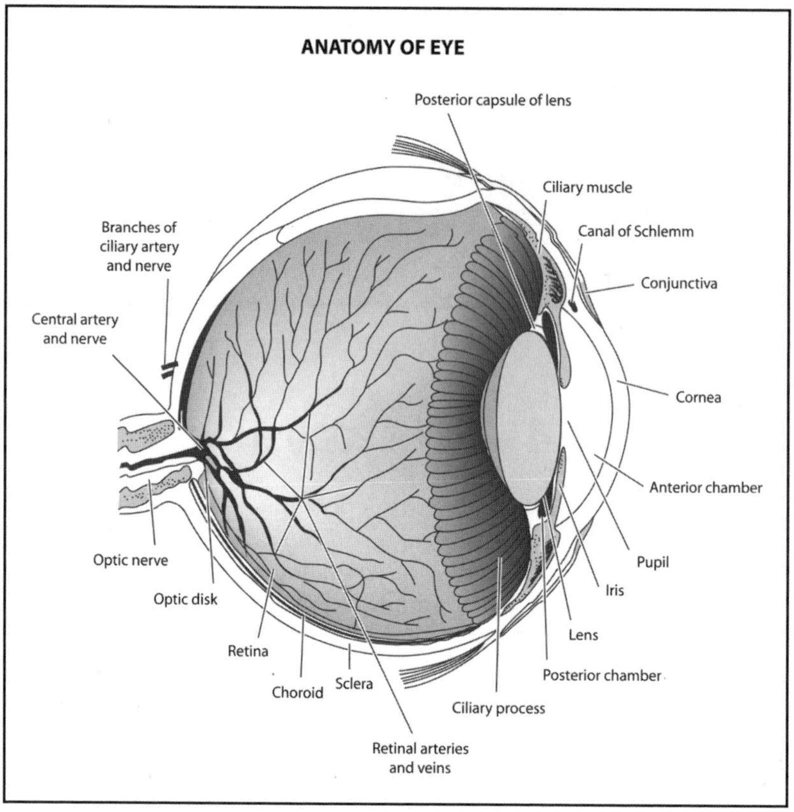

Figure 11-1. Anatomy of the eye.

The paired orbits, or eye sockets, that surround and protect the eyes are formed by seven bones: frontal, zygomatic, maxillary, ethmoidal, sphenoid, lacrimal, and palatine (Figure 11-2). The orbital floor and medial walls are the weakest portion of the bony socket and are therefore often fractured with external periorbital forces (blow-out fractures). Movement of the eyes is controlled by the six extraocular muscles. These muscles include four rectus muscles, which function to adduct, abduct, elevate, and depress the eye globe, and two oblique muscles which control circular movements (Figure 11-3). The lacrimal apparatus, which functions to produce, distribute, and collect tears, can also be damaged with lacerations involving the medial portion of the eye lids.

Ear

The ear is divided into three main sections: the external ear, the middle ear, and the inner ear. The external ear includes the auricle (Figure 11-4), which is visible to the naked eye, and the external auditory canal. The outermost portion of the external canal is funnel shaped which helps to move sound waves toward the tympanic membrane (ear drum). The tympanic membrane forms the outermost border of the middle ear, separating the external canal from the three tiny ossicle bones: the malleus, incus, and stapes. The tympanic membrane vibrates when sound waves strike it initiating the process of converting sound waves to electrical nerve impulses. Damage to the membrane can result in some degree of hearing loss. The inner ear contains the cochlea and semicircular canals which function to continue

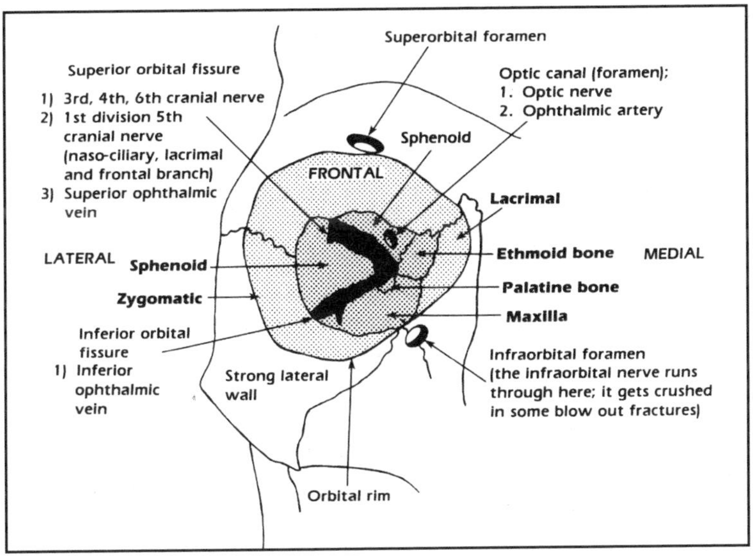

Figure 11-2. Bony orbit. (Reprinted with permission from Nemeth SC, Shea CA. *Medical Sciences for the Ophthalmic Assistant.* Thorofare, NJ: SLACK Incorporated; 1988.)

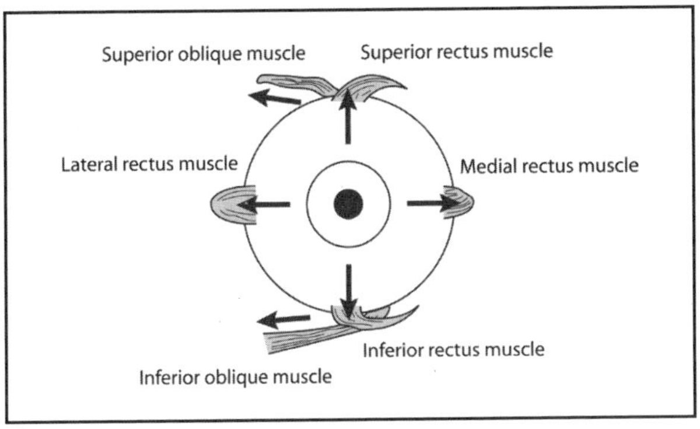

Figure 11-3. Extraocular muscles.

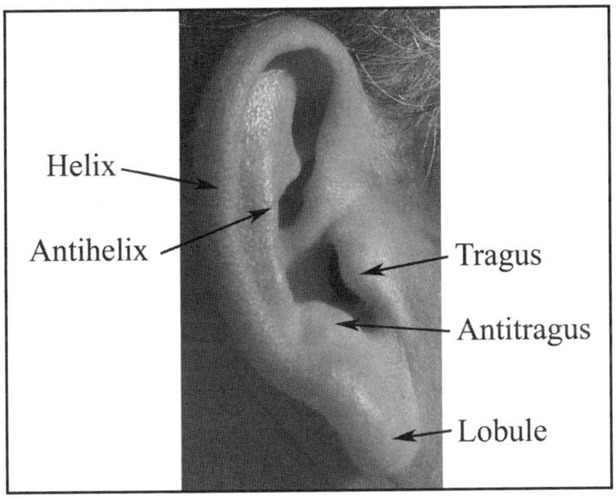

Figure 11-4. Auricle.

the conversion of sound waves to nerve impulses for the brain to interpret and to maintain balance, respectively. The eustachian tube connects the middle ear to the nasal passages and regulates the amount of pressure within the middle ear.

Nose

The nasal complex is made up of the bones and cartilage that form the nasal cavity and the paranasal sinuses (frontal, sphenoid, ethmoidal, maxillary). The upper third of the nose is formed by the nasal bones, while the lower two-thirds is supported by cartilage. The nasal cavity includes three curved bony structures called turbinates which are covered in a highly vascularized mucous membrane. Air enters the nose through the paired nares (nostrils), vestibule, and nasal cavity where it is filtered, warmed, and humidified before passing on to the nasopharynx, trachea, and lung.

Throat

The throat, or pharynx, includes the tonsils, adenoids, uvula, epiglottis, and esophagus. The tonsils are located on both sides of the back of the mouth and the adenoids are on the back of the nasal cavity. Both structures are made up of lymphoid tissue and function to help fight infection. The uvula hangs at the back of the throat between the two tonsils. Functionally, the pharynx provides the pathway for food and fluids to pass from the mouth to the esophagus and for air to pass to the lungs. The pharynx is divided into three sections: the nasopharynx, the oropharynx, and laryngopharynx. Like the nose and mouth, the pharynx is also lined with mucous membranes and cilia to warm, filter, and humidify inspired air. Below the laryngopharynx, the pharynx becomes the esophagus. The epiglottis lies between the oropharynx and laryngopharynx and functions to prevent food from entering the larynx. The larynx has three main functions: (1) prevent food and fluids from entering the trachea, (2) produce sound vibrations, and (3) to assist in the cough mechanism.

Mouth

The oral cavity is lined with mucous membranes and in the adult contains 32 teeth: 16 in the upper jaw and 16 in the lower jaw. The visible portion of each tooth is referred to as the crown and is made of enamel. The dentin forms a layer just below the enamel and is harder than bone. The tooth fits into an individual socket in the jaw bone and is surrounded at its based by the gums. The root of the tooth, which sits below the gum line in the bony socket, contains the blood vessels and nerves that provide circulation and sensation to the tooth.

Signs and Symptoms

Eye

Pain

Eye pain can occur periocular, ocular, or retrobulbar (behind the globe). The location of the pain along with the intensity, onset, and duration can provide clues regarding the possible pathology. Severe eye pain accompanied by systemic symptoms (eg, nausea) or significant changes in vision (ie, severe photophobia, blurring, flashing, "floaters," partial loss of visual field) suggest serious pathology, such as acute glaucoma (increased pressure in the eye). In such situations, a risk of permanent loss of vision exists, and therefore, emergency medical care is indicated.

Discharge

With eye allergies and infections, the eye will often present with a discharge or drainage. This discharge can range from a clear, watery substance to a white or yellowish pus.

Double Vision

Patients with double vision (*diplopia*) will see two images of the same object, one from each eye. Normally the images seen by both eyes are fused into a single image. Double vision can result from a variety of disorders including a head injury. Systemic conditions associated with double vision include multiple sclerosis, diabetes, and myasthenia gravis. Patients complaining of diplopia should be referred to an ophthalmologist.

Itching

Itching of the eyes is commonly associated with allergy; however, some eye infections may also cause itching.

Photophobia

Photophobia, or sensitivity to light, is a common symptom reported with corneal abrasions.

Ptosis

Drooping of the eye lid, or *ptosis*, can occur with some eye pathologies.

Tearing

Increased tearing can occur due to an irritation of the anterior eye surface. Injury or illness involving the lacrimal apparatus can cause either increased or decreased tearing.

Halos

Halos around lights at night are often reported by patients with glaucoma, corneal edema, corneal scarring, or a dislocated intraocular lens.

Light Flashes and Floaters

Brief light flashes (photopsia) or a sudden increase in "floaters" are common symptoms reported by patients who have suffered some form of retinal tear or detachment.

Anisocoria

Unequal pupils are referred to as *anisocoria*. Differences in pupil size less than 0.5 mm are found normally in approximately 20% of the general population. Differences greater than 0.5 mm, particularly when accompanied by abnormal papillary reactions and a history of head or eye trauma, are considered abnormal.

Nystagmus

Nystagmus can occur with neurological pathology and presents as a rhythmic oscillation of the eyes.

Protruding Eyes

Retraction of the eye lids can cause the appearance of protruding eyes (*exophthalmos*) and is a common sign associated with Graves' disease (see Chapter Ten).

Curtain Over Vision

Patients may report having a curtain suddenly drop down blocking either their direct vision or their peripheral vision. This curtain is associated with a detached retina or detached vitreous and warrants immediate referral.

Ear

Tinnitus

A sensation of ringing in the ears is referred to as *tinnitus*. Patients may report tinnitus when they suffer a ruptured tympanic membrane.

Pain

Pain is a common symptom with most ear pathologies. The typical "ear ache" can occur with ear infections and is difficult for the patient to localize (ie, middle ear or external ear). Both palpation of the tragus and traction of the ear lobe will often cause ear pain in patients with otitis externa (see below). A blocked Eustachian tube or middle ear infection (otitis media) can result in increased pressure behind the tympanic membrane which can cause a sensation of pressure or pain.

Loss of Hearing

Damage to middle and inner ear structures can result in partial to complete hearing loss. The degree of hearing loss is usually related to the severity of injury.

Nasal Cavity

Runny Nose

Inflammation of the mucous membranes within the nasal cavity can lead to the production of a clear, watery drainage (*coryza*).

Congestion and Pressure

Accumulation of mucous and drainage within the nasal cavity and sinuses can lead to congestion and a feeling of pain and pressure within the sinuses.

Throat

Pain

Throat infections are associated with throat pain.

Difficulty Swallowing

Throat pain can make it difficult for patients to swallow.

White or Red Spots

Throat infections can produce white or red spots on the tonsils and soft palate.

Mouth

Pain

Pain is one of the most common symptoms of mouth disorders. Mouth pain can be local and specific to the disorder (cavity, tooth fracture, infection, etc) or be referred from one area (sinuses) or to another area (ear).

Swollen, Red, or Bleeding Gums

Inflammation and infection from gingivitis can produce swollen and red gums that may bleed when brushed.

Sensitivity to Hot and Cold Beverages

Demineralization of the teeth secondary to plaque or cavities can lead to sensitivity to hot or cold beverages.

Bad Breath (Halitosis)

Poor dental hygiene and periodontal disease lead to bad breath.

White or Yellow Plaques

Plaques may develop on the tongue, buccal mucosa (inside of check), and palate with fungal infections of the mouth such as oral candidiasis.

Pain Patterns

The pain associated with most eye, ear, nose, throat, and mouth pathology is very localized. Sinus infections can involve referred pain to the teeth and some tooth disorders can refer pain to the ipsilateral ear.

Medical History and Physical Examination

Medical History

With the exception of glaucoma, most disorders involving the eye, ear, nose, throat, and mouth do not have a genetic factor associated with them. Findings from a personal history, however, can be very important in the assessment of these disorders, especially eye and ear conditions.

Palpation

Palpation of the bony orbit and surrounding facial bones is an essential part of a thorough eye or nose exam. Also, when evaluating the ear, pain with palpation of the tragus or traction of the ear lobe is associated with otitis media.

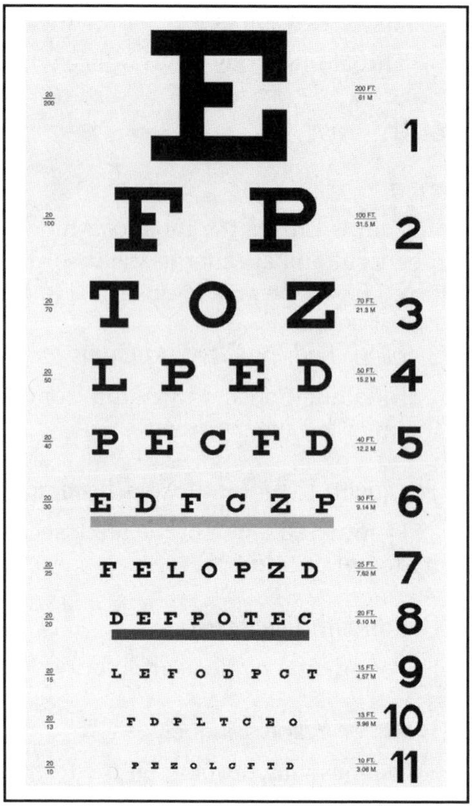

Figure 11-5. Snellen eye chart. (Reprinted with permission from Scheiman M, Scheiman M, Whittaker S. *Low Vision Rehabilitation: A Practical Guide for Occupational Therapists.* Thorofare, NJ: SLACK Incorporated; 2007.)

Inspection

Unlike many of the other systemic disorders within this text, injuries and illnesses involving the eye, ear, nose, throat, and mouth require close visual inspection. Inspection of the facial anatomy is critical for detecting deformity or abnormalities.

Physical Exam

Eye

Visual Acuity

Examination of the eye typically begins with an assessment of visual acuity. This assessment should include testing the patient's ability to see an object at 20 feet and the ability to focus and read text at 14 to 16 inches. In the clinical setting, visual acuity is most often tested using a *Snellen eye chart* (Figure 11-5) to test distant vision and the *Rosenbaum pocket card* to test near vision. The eye chart is hung on a wall at eye level, and a mark is then made on the floor 20 feet from the wall. Each eye should be tested separately by covering the opposite eye. If the patient wears glasses or contacts, then he or she should be tested with these on. The patient should start at the smallest line on the eye chart and move upward until he or she is able to correctly read over half of the letters. If the patient is unable to read the top line at 20 feet, then he or she is placed closer to the chart (15, 10, or 5 feet) and the test is repeated. Distant visual acuity is recorded as a fraction, with the numerator containing the patient's distance from the chart and the denominator representing the distance that

Table 11-1

Ocular First Aid Kit

- Penlight with cobalt blue filter
- Fluorescein strips
- Rosenbaum pocket eye card or similar near vision chart
- Sterile irrigation fluid (squeeze bottle of saline works well)
- Sterile eye cups
- Sterile-tipped applicators
- Sterile eye patch (soft) or Fox Eye Shield (hard)
- Contact case with contact solution
- Visual occluder (to cover opposite eye when testing visual acuity)
- Topical anesthetic
- Topical antibiotic drops or ointment
- Gloves
- Sterile gauze pads
- Tape
- Phone numbers for local hospital, team physican, and team ophthalmologist

a "normal" person would read that line. For example, if a patient reads a line at 15 feet that a normal person could read at 40 feet, this visual acuity would be recorded at 15/40. The Rosenbaum pocket card is used in a similar fashion to test near vision. The card should be held approximately 14 to 16 inches from the face. If a Snellen eye chart or Rosenbaum packet card are not available, other objects can be used to screen visual acuity, although an acuity value will not be obtained. For example, when on the sideline, the athletic trainer can ask the athlete to read the score board or other object in a distance. Also, a game program or magazine can be used to assess near vision. Any loss of visual acuity secondary to an eye injury warrants immediate 911
referral. Athletic trainers should consider having an ocular first aid kit on the sideline of all events and in the athletic training facility. Table 11-1 provides a list of items that should be included in this kit.

Pupillary Shape and Reaction

Following a head injury or isolated ocular injury, the pupils should be inspected for size, shape, and reaction to light. As mentioned above, anisocoria can occur normally in some individuals; however, unequal pupil size following a head or ocular injury suggests neurological involvement and warrants immediate referral. A tear-drop shape or an irregularly peaked pupil suggests possible globe rupture and is considered a medical emergency. The pupils' response to light should be checked 911
for both direct and consensual response. To check direct response to light, the penlight should be directed from an angle lateral to the eye to shine directly into the eye. Normally, the pupil should constrict in response to the light. The opposite eye is then tested in the same fashion. Failure of the pupil to constrict is considered abnormal and warrants referral. To test consensual response, again shine the penlight directly into one eye; however, observe the reaction of the opposite eye. When the penlight is directed into one eye, the other eye should also constrict. Failure of the opposite eye to constrict is considered abnormal. Lastly, the penlight is rapidly swung from

Table 11-2

Fluorescein Dye Test for Corneal Abrasions

- Remove a single fluorescein strip from the package.
- Wet the tip of the strip with sterile saline.
- Pull the lower lid out slightly forming a pouch.
- Touch the wet tip of the strip within the lower lid pouch. (The strip should not be touched directly to the cornea.)
- Instruct the patient to blink several times to spread the orange-colored dye across the eye.
- Dim the lights in the room if possible.
- Attach the cobalt blue filter to the end of the penlight.
- Shine the cobalt blue light in the involved eye.
- Under the blue light, the fluorescein dye will appear yellowish-green.
- Carefully inspect the eye for abrasions or foreign objects.

one eye to the other without allowing time between eyes (Swinging Flashlight Test). Each eye should constrict as the light hits it. If one of the pupils dilates instead of constricts, this is considered a positive test and indicates a problem with the nerve between the eye and the brain (afferent pupil defect).[2]

Eye Movements

Assessment of the extraocular muscles should be performed following any traumatic eye injury. Using a penlight or a finger, the athletic trainer should instruct the patient to follow the object with out moving the head. The patient's ability to look laterally, medially, upward, downward, diagonally up and out, and diagonally down and out should be tested. Orbital blowout fractures can entrap the inferior vastus muscle, preventing the patient from being able to look up. Normal eye movement can also be affected with head injuries or other neurological conditions.

Peripheral Vision

The patient's peripheral field of vision can be tested by asking him or her to cover one eye with his or her hand. The examiner also covers his or her eye (same as the patient's—right or left) so as to compare the patient's peripheral vision with his or her own. On the same side as the eye being tested, the examiner will place his or her hand out laterally to the patient with one or more fingers held up. The examiner slowly brings his or her hand inward toward the patient's direct vision and asks the patient to tell him or her when he or she can see the hand and to state how many fingers he or she sees. This test would then be repeated on the opposite side.

Fluorescein Strips and Cobalt Blue Light

Staining the eye with fluorescein dye can enable the athletic trainer to visualize corneal abrasions or clear foreign objects in the eye such as glass or contact lens fragments. The dye stains the eye orange and highlights areas of abrasion within the cornea or conjunctiva. When viewed with a cobalt blue light, the die appears yellowish green further enhancing the visual identification of abrasions or foreign objects. The proper steps for performing the fluorescein dye test are outlined in Table 11-2. The fluorescein dye is water soluble and can be easily flushed from the eye using saline irrigating solution.

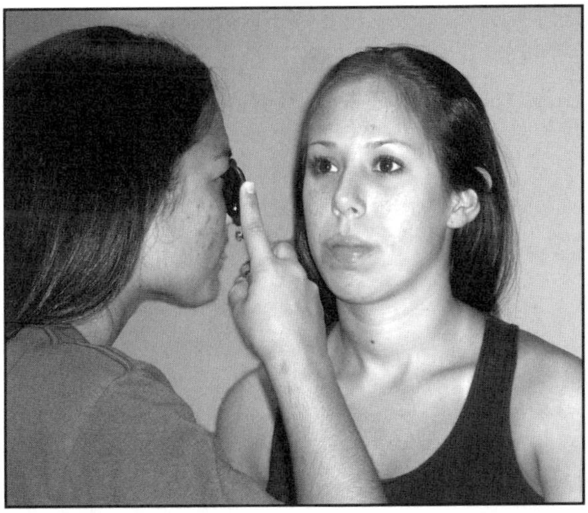

Figure 11-6. Ophthalmoscope.

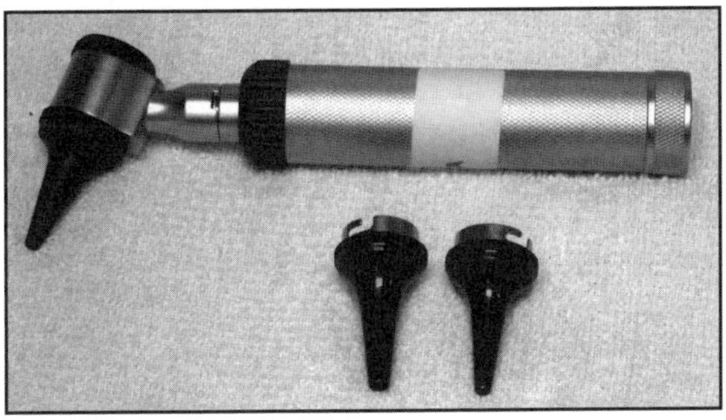

Figure 11-7. Otoscope with additional specula.

Ophthalmoscope

A hand-held direct ophthalmoscope uses a battery powered light source and a series of magnifying lens to look inside the eye to view the cornea, lens, and central portion of the retina (Figure 11-6). This evaluation instrument is easy to use and, with practice, can provide the athletic trainer with valuable information when assessing the eye. The steps for using an ophthalmoscope to evaluate the eye are outlined in Table 11-3. (Lab Exercise 11-1 provides the opportunity to perform an eye examination using an ophthalmoscope.)

Ear

Otoscope

Injuries or illnesses involving the external auditory canal or the tympanic membrane can be evaluated using an otoscope (Figures 11-7 and 11-8a). These hand-held units include a handle, light source, and several specula of varying sizes. Selecting units with halogen bulbs and magnifying lenses provide the most optimal viewing of the tympanic membrane. Table 11-4 outlines the proper steps for using an otoscope. To prevent cross-contamination, the unaffected ear should always be evaluated first. This practice also provides a basis for comparison when viewing the affected ear. The otoscope can also be used to inspect the nose for injury. (Lab Exercise 11-2 provides the opportunity to practice the skill of otoscopic examination.)

Table 11-3

Steps for Using an Ophthalmoscope to Evaluate the Eye

Step 1.	Darken the examination room.
Step 2.	Turn on the ophthalmoscope with the lens disc set on large round beam. Shine the beam of light on your hand to check the level of brightness and the charge of the ophthalmoscope.
Step 3.	Turn the lens disc to the 0 diopter setting, keeping your index finger on the lens disc in order to adjust the setting later.
Step 4.	Hold the ophthalmoscope in the right hand when examining the right eye and the left hand when examining the left eye.
Step 5.	Rest the head of the ophthalmoscope on the medial aspect of your orbit, with the handle tilted laterally approximately 20 degrees.
Step 6.	Instruct the patient to focus on a point on the wall up and over your shoulder.
Step 7.	Start at a position approximately 15 inches away from the patient and in a plane approximately 15 degrees lateral to the patient's line of vision. Shine the light beam into the patient's eye and look for the red reflex, which will appear as an orange glow in the pupil.
Step 8.	While keeping the light beam focused on the red reflex, move slowly toward the patient in the 15-degree plane until you are almost touching the patient's eyelashes.
Step 9.	Keep both eyes open as you begin to look into the eye. If the brightness of the light beam is uncomfortable for the patient, adjust it slightly.
Step 10.	As you look through the eye, locate the optic disc which will appear as a round, yellowish-orange structure. If you are unable to find the optic disc initially, locate a blood vessel and follow it centrally to the disc.
Step 11.	Once you locate the optic disc, adjust the sharpness of the image by turning the lens disc.
Step 12.	Inspect the optic disc for clarity and color. (It is not abnormal to find the edge on the nasal side of the disc to be slightly blurry.) The normal disc is yellowish-orange to creamy pink; however, the outer ring may be white.
Step 13.	Inspect the retina looking for lesions. Move the ophthalmoscope and your head as one unit as you attempt to view all areas of the retina.
Step 14.	In order to view the macula and fovea, instruct the patient to look directly into the light beam. (A light reflection off of the fovea helps to identify these structures.) The macula surrounds the fovea.

Table 11-4

Steps for Using an Otoscope to Evaluate the Ear

Step 1.	Place your patient in a seated position with his or her head turned slightly downward and away from the ear to be examined.
Step 2.	Select the largest possible speculum that can be comfortably inserted into the ear. When inserted, the speculum should fit snugly in the outer third of the canal and rest against the tragus and anterior wall of the canal. Choosing a speculum that is too small will cause movement within the canal. Excessive movement can cause discomfort for your patient.
Step 3.	Hold the otoscope with the same hand as the ear you are examining: Right hand for right ear Left hand for left ear
Step 4.	Stabilize the otoscope by placing the ring and little finger resting on the patient's cheek or temple using one of two grips: Hammer grip (Figure 11-8b) Pencil grip (Figure 11-8c)
Step 5.	Pull the pinna upward and backward to straighten the canal.
Step 6.	While maintaining traction on the pinna, place the speculum of the otoscope at, but not in, the ear canal.
Step 7.	"Watch your way into the ear." Never insert the otoscope blindly. If the patient experiences pain, reposition the canal by adjusting the angle and degree of traction on the pinna. If the patient's discomfort persists even after readjustment of the canal, halt the examination and refer the patient to a physician.
Step 8.	Once the tympanic membrane comes into view, rotate the speculum to view as much of the membrane as possible. This is like trying to view the corners of a room through a keyhole.
Step 9.	Inspect the membrane for color, clarity, and position.
Step 10.	Identify key landmarks. Malleus Manubrium (angles toward 2:00 in right ear, angles toward 10:00 in left ear) Short process Umbo Light reflex Pars flaccida Pars tensa Annulus Stapes Incus
Step 11.	Look for abnormalities: Fluid Perforations

Figure 11-8a. Examining the ear with an otoscope.

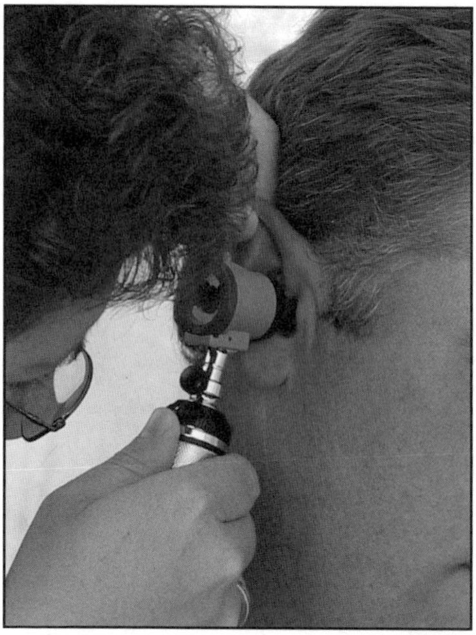

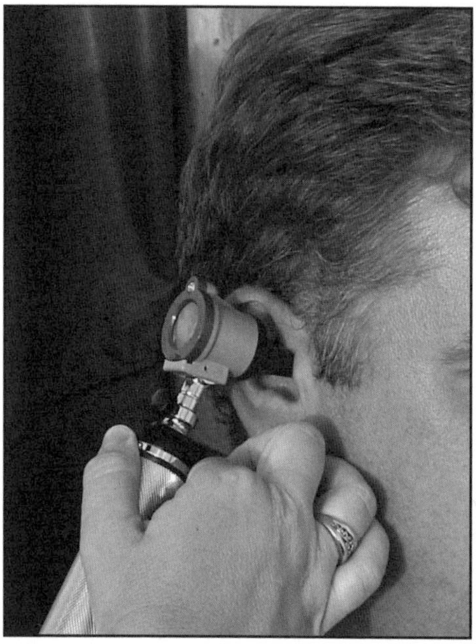

Figure 11-8b. Hammer grip.

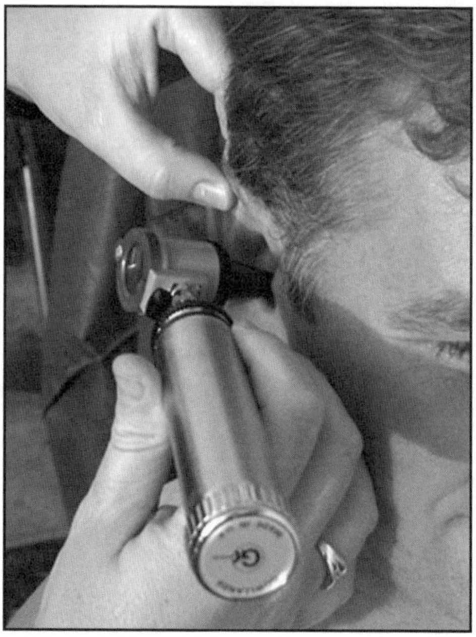

Figure 11-8c. Pencil grip.

Pathology and Pathogenesis

Eye Injuries

Subconjunctival Hemorrhage

Bleeding under the clear conjunctiva can be caused by trauma, forceful coughing, high blood pressure, or some bleeding disorders. In some cases, the etiology is never known. Although this condition may look serious, in the absence of trauma, it is generally benign. Most cases of subconjunctival hemorrhaging will resolve on their own within 1 to 3 weeks.

Foreign Body in the Eye

A foreign object can often enter the eye producing pain and tearing. When inspecting for a foreign object in the lower lid, pull the lower lid away from the eye and instruct the patient to look upward. If a foreign object is visible, it can usually be easily removed by rinsing the eye with saline or other appropriate eye wash, or by touching the object with the corner of moist gauze pad. When a patient reports the sensation of a foreign body under the upper pull lid, the upper lid should be pulled down over the lower lid. This procedure will often times move the foreign body down to the lower lid area where it is more visible and more easily removed. The under surface of the upper lid can also be viewed by inverting the lid onto a cotton-tipped applicator. Again, if visible, the object can be removed by rinsing the eye or using a moist gauze pad. Objects that are imbedded or impaled into the eye should never be removed. Should this occur, the object should be stabilized and the emergency action plan should be activated.

Corneal Abrasions

Corneal abrasions are one of the most common sports-related eye injuries. These injuries are usually the result of a direct blow to the eye by an external object (eg, ball, elbow, hockey stick, finger, etc). Corneal abrasions can also be caused by foreign objects becoming trapped between the upper lid and the cornea, particularly when the eye is rubbed in an attempt to remove the object. Patients with a corneal abrasion will complain of photophobia, eye pain, and a sensation of a foreign body being in the eye. Inspection of the eye may find increased tearing, redness, and possible swelling, depending on the severity of the abrasion. A differential diagnosis can be made using a fluorescein strip and cobalt blue penlight (see Table 11-2). Patients with corneal abrasions should be referred to a physician or ophthalmologist immediately. Deep or large abrasions or lacerations can be very serious and can lead to vision loss. Pre-hospital or pre-physician care of corneal abrasions has typically involved topical antibiotics, an eye patch, and analgesics for pain; however several recent clinical trials have demonstrated that eye patches provided no added effect in the healing of corneal abrasions as compared to no patches,[3-7] and in fact, may decrease oxygen delivery to the abrasion, increase moisture, and increase the infection rate.[8] As a result of these findings, athletic trainers should consult their team physician or ophthalmologist when establishing a protocol for managing corneal abrasions. Patients with a corneal abrasion should be reevaluated by their physician or ophthalmologist at 24 hours. Patients who wear contact lenses should refrain from wearing their lenses during the healing period. These patients should also be reevaluated again 3 to 4 days later. Most corneal abrasions heal within 24 to 72 hours; however, deeper lesions may take 4 to 5 days to heal.

Hyphema

A hyphema injury results from a direct blow to the globe and results in bleeding within the anterior chamber. Patients will usually complain of eye pain and decreased vision. Forces great enough to cause a hyphema can also rupture the globe; therefore, a thorough eye exam should be performed to rule out a ruptured globe. Patients with a hyphema should be immediately referred to the team ophthalmologist or the local emergency room. Hyphema injuries are usually treated with a topical steroid, an eye patch, and decreased activity, which may mean bed rest depending on the severity of the injury. Patients are reassessed daily by their ophthalmologist to check for rebleeding or other complications. Patients are also instructed to avoid the use of nonsteroidal anti-inflammatory drugs (NSAIDs) during this treatment period.

Ruptured Globe

Any eye injury caused by blunt or penetrating trauma to the orbit or globe can result in a *ruptured globe*. The rupture may not be apparent on inspection due to the fact that most ruptures occur at sites which are not visible. Patients will usually complain of eye pain, decreased vision, and possibly diplopia. Key signs to watch for include excessive subconjunctival bleeding, swelling, irregular pupil shape, asymmetry in the depth of the anterior chamber,[9] and enophthalmos (recession of the globe within the orbit) or exophthalmos (protrusion of the globe beyond the orbit).[10] The eye should be protected from any type of pressure or contact; therefore, a hard eye shield should be applied rather than a pressure eye patch.[10] Any penetrating foreign body should be left in place during transport to the emergency room. Ruptured globes are medical emergencies that require surgical repair as soon as possible.

Orbital Fracture

Blunt trauma to the bony orbit can result in an orbital fracture. Because the orbital floor and medial wall are the thinnest and weakest part of the orbit, fracture to this area, referred to as *blow-out fractures,* occur most often. Patients will typically complain of pain and diplopia. Clinical presentation will include periorbital swelling, ecchymosis, and enophthalmos.[11] Palpation may detect a bony step-off and point tenderness along the orbital rim as well as subcutaneous emphysema (air under the skin) and numbness in the upper cheek area. Eye movement may be limited and painful. Entrapment of the inferior rectus muscle often prevents the patient from looking upward.

Detached Retina

As described previously, the retina forms the inner lining of the back wall of the eye and is responsible for sending visual images to the brain. A sudden jarring of the head can cause the retina to pull away from the back wall causing a *detached retina*. In some cases, a sneeze has been the reported cause of a torn or detached retina, while with other cases, there has been no apparent cause. Patients with detached retinas will most commonly report floaters, halos, blind spots, or describe a curtain falling over their field of vision.[2] A suspicion of retinal injury warrants immediate referral to an ophthalmologist. In most cases, the torn retina will need to be repaired surgically.

Eye Infections

Conjunctivitis

Inflammation of the conjunctiva can result from allergens or infection (bacterial or viral). Itching (allergy) or burning (infection) with mucoid (allergy) or purulent (infection) drainage from the eye occurs. The "white" of the eyeball appears swollen and reddened, thus the layman's term "pink eye." Allergic reactions usually affect both eyes, whereas an infection begins unilaterally. Infectious conjunctivitis, however, spreads quickly to the opposite eye, usually after rubbing first the infected eye and then the other. This eye infection can also spread to others; therefore infected individuals should not share towels with anyone else during sports participation.

Allergic conjunctivitis is usually treated with antihistamines or anti-inflammatories. Treatment of infectious conjunctivitis involves antibiotic eyedrops or oral medications. The person must be instructed not to touch the eyedrop applicator to their eye, to avoid rubbing the face, and to practice meticulous hand washing to avoid spreading the disease.

Athletes who wear contacts should have a pair of glasses as a backup should they develop an eye infection. Wearing disposable lenses beyond their recommended time frame can lead to eye infections. Also wearing infected lenses can lead to repeated infections and possible scarring of the cornea.

Eye infections associated with significant pain or photophobia suggest a more serious condition such as corneal injury or a herpes viral infection. Medical referral for definitive diagnosis and treatment is indicated.

Stye

Infection of an eyelid duct or follicle is called a *stye*. Caused most often by staphylococcal bacteria, the stye produces localized pain on the margin of the eyelid. Lacrimation (tears) and a sensation of "something in the eye" also occur. Visual inspection usually reveals a round, red lump on the lid margin. A stye can be treated with warm, moist compresses for 10 minutes a few times a day and should completely resolve in a few days. Lesions observed in other parts of the eyelid or eye require prompt referral to an ophthalmologist.

Glaucoma

Glaucoma is an eye disease that is caused by optic nerve damage secondary to increased intraocular pressure. As discussed in the anatomical section, the anterior chamber is filled with aqueous fluid. The level of fluid in this area is constantly being produced and then drained away to maintain a healthy level of pressure within this chamber. If the draining mechanism becomes damaged, then the intraocular pressure in the eye will rise. This increased pressure is then transmitted to the back of the eye causing damage to the optic nerve. The optic nerve damage first leads to a loss of peripheral sight. Because this loss of sight may occur gradually, glaucoma is sometimes referred to as the "sneaky thief of sight" Risk factors for glaucoma include: (1) positive family history, (2) age (40 or over), (3) nearsightedness, (4) diabetes, (5) hypertension, and (6) African Americans.[2] Although there is no cure, glaucoma can be treated through the use of drops or other medications to reduce the intraocular pressure and surgery to improve or replace the drainage system for the aqueous fluid. Persons in the high risk group should have their eyes checked yearly. Non at-risk individuals should have their eyes examined every 2 years starting at age 40. Early detection is the key to preventing the loss of sight from glaucoma.

Ear Injuries

Auricular Hematoma

Repeated trauma or friction to the external ear can lead to an *auricular hematoma* between the thin layer of skin that covers the ear and the cartilage which makes up the ear. As the hematoma develops, the skin will separate from the cartilage forming a palpable collection of fluid. Ice and compression can be used to limit the size of the hematoma. Prompt referral to a physician for drainage of the hematoma is recommended to prevent scarring. The development of scar tissue within the hematoma can produce a cauliflower-like appearance on the external ear known as *cauliflower ear.* To prevent rebleeding within the space, the physician will typically apply some form of compression to the area such as a button sutured to the front and back of the ear, a silicone splint or cast applied to the ear, or dental rolls applied with gauze. The compression is left in place for 7 to 14 days to insure proper healing without scarring. Athletes who participate in non-contact sports can usually return to play right away. Those individuals who participate in contact sports can return to play if protective head gear is worn. If the compression bandage is held in place with sutures, return-to-play may be delayed until the sutures are removed. Auricular hematomas are most prevalent in wrestlers; however they can be prevented by wearing protective head gear.

Ruptured Tympanic Membrane

Sudden changes in pressure within the ear or insertion of foreign objects, such as cutips, into the ear can cause the tympanic membrane to rupture. Signs and symptoms of a ruptured or perforated tympanic membrane can include sudden ear pain, sudden relief of ear pain followed by drainage from the ear, tinnitus, and a decrease in hearing.[12] The degree of hearing loss is typically related to the size of the perforation. Common causes of membrane rupture include a direct blow to the ear, increased pressure in the middle ear as a result of infection, changes in cabin pressure when flying in an airplane (such as with ascent and descent), or a sudden loud noise as might occur with an explosion or gunshot. When a tympanic membrane rupture is suspected, a thorough ear evaluation should be performed including the use of an otoscope. Inability to visualize the membrane due to wax or drainage or visual confirmation of a hole or tear in the membrane both warrant referral to a physician. Membrane ruptures will usually heal on their own within 2 to 3 weeks; however, occasionally, surgery is required to repair the opening. During the healing period, patients should wear ear plugs during shower or baths to prevent water from getting into the ear. Acetaminophen or over-the-counter NSAIDs can be taken if the patient experiences ear pain. The ability of swimmers to return to play should be determined by the treating physician.

Ear Infections

Otitis Externa

Frequent exposure to water (eg, competitive swimmers) flushes the protective cerumen (wax) from the ear and can cause infections of the external ear canal; this infection is called *otitis externa*. The constant moisture also softens the ear canal's tissue, providing further opportunity for infection by bacteria or fungi. Using cotton swabs to scour the ear can further irritate the canal and increase the risk of infection. Lakes, rivers, or improperly chlorinated pools commonly contain bacteria responsible for these infections.

Otitis externa produces ear drainage, canal swelling, and erythema that can be visualized with the otoscope. These effects decrease hearing, cause itching, and produce pain when the auricle is gently pulled or the tragus is palpated.[12] Treatment involves irrigation with sterile saline or hydrogen peroxide, inserting antibiotic or antifungal ear drops, and discontinuing swimming. Usually within 3 days, the pain and erythema decrease and swimming can be resumed. Using ear plugs while swimming, carefully drying the ears, using drying agents (eg, boric acid solution), and avoiding the use of swabs are some simple protective measures.

Otitis Media

Otitis media (interna) is an infection of the middle ear and often follows or accompanies upper respiratory infections. Signs and symptoms include ear pain without tenderness to touch, fever, a feeling of pressure in the ear, slight loss of hearing, and occasionally dizziness. Otoscopic examination will usually reveal a red tympanic membrane that may be bulging or retracted. If the membrane bulges, the light reflex may become diminished or absent; when retracted, the bony prominences of the inner ear may become more apparent. In some cases of otitis media, the membrane will appear yellowish in color with possible fluid bubbles visible behind the membrane. Otitis media requires referral and is treated with antibiotics and analgesics.[12]

Impacted Cerumen

Impacted cerumen can cause symptoms similar to otitis externa, including itching, pain, and impaired hearing. A physician may remove the cerumen by scraping with a blunt tool under direct visualization or suctioning the ear canal. Irrigation with saline or other solutions is not recommended if a history of ear infection or drainage exists. Self-application of cotton swabs or solvents to remove the cerumen may irritate the skin, creating opportunity for infection to develop, and should be avoided.

Nose Injuries

Epistaxis (Nosebleed)

Nosebleeds can result from a variety of conditions including trauma (nasal or facial fracture), infection, dry nasal passages, allergies, or hypertension. In most cases, nosebleeds can be easily controlled by instructing the patient to lean forward slightly and pinch the nostrils between the tip and the bridge of the nose. Leaning the head forward will allow the blood to drain from the nose rather than running down the back of the throat. Swallowing the blood from a nose bleed can cause nausea and vomiting in some individuals. Applying an ice bag to the nose can also help control a nosebleed. In cases that do not respond to this treatment or in cases involving a nasal fracture, the nose can be packed with rolled gauze or tampons cut into small sections to control the bleeding. Patients who experience frequent unexplained nosebleeds should be referred to a physician for follow-up. Nosebleeds accompanied by occipital headaches are classic signs and symptoms for hypertension.

Nasal Fracture

Nasal fractures are common in sports and typically involve epistaxis. Once the bleeding is controlled, the nose and surrounding facial bones should be visually inspected and palpated for deformity. Fractures involving a deviated septum can impair breathing within one nostril. Ice can be applied to the nose to reduce the pain and swelling and the patient should be referred to a physician for follow-up.

Nasal Allergies and Infections

Allergic Rhinitis

There are two types of allergic rhinitis: seasonal and perennial. Seasonal allergic rhinitis occurs most often during particular seasons, such as during the peak pollen season in the spring. As the name suggests, perennial allergic rhinitis occurs throughout the year and is often caused by animal dander, dust, cockroach droppings, or mold. Both types of rhinitis are caused by specific triggers or allergens that produce a histamine response that leads to sneezing, congestion, and itchy, watery eyes. Treatment should focus on avoiding known triggers and medication to relieve the symptoms. As discussed in Chapter Three, antihistamines are commonly used to treat the symptoms caused by rhinitis.

Sinusitis and Sinus Infections

When the mucous membranes that line the sinus cavities become irritated and inflamed, sinusitis can occur. Patients with sinusitis may complain of congestion or drainage from the sinuses, headache, and sinus pressure. When the sinus drainage thickens and accumulates within the sinuses, a bacterial or viral infection can develop, leading to a sinus infection. In addition to the symptoms associated with sinusitis, patients may experience pain in the teeth and over the sinuses. Decongestants and antibiotics are typically used to treat a sinus infection. As long as the athlete does not have a fever and the symptoms are all above the neck, he or she can still participate in his or her sport.

Throat Infections

Infective Laryngitis, Pharyngitis, and Tonsillitis

Infection or inflammation of the throat are common symptoms of other immune system pathology (eg, upper respiratory infection, sexually transmitted disease, allergies), although they can occur as isolated conditions. *Pharyngitis* and *tonsillitis* both produce throat pain, painful or difficult swallowing (and subsequent avoidance of food), and pain in the ears when swallowing. Inspection reveals a red (erythematous) throat with purulent or mucoid exudate covering the pharynx (pharyngitis) or the notably inflamed tonsils (tonsillitis). *Laryngitis* causes changes in the quality of the voice, such as hoarseness or complete inability to speak. Itching may require frequent throat clearing. Fever, difficulty or pain with swallowing, or even dyspnea may occur with severe laryngitis. A physician may observe purulent exudate on the larynx with a laryngoscope.

After a physician rules out serious pathology, treatment for throat infection is rest, analgesics, and nutrition. Contagious bacterial infections, such as streptococcal pharyngitis (*"strep throat"*), may require antibiotics and temporary isolation (24 to 36 hours) to prevent communicating the infectious organism to others. Individuals with strep throat will typically present with throat pain, fever, swollen glands, and difficulty with swallowing.

Mouth Disorders

Gingivitis

Gingivitis is a bacterial infection of the gums and typically presents with swollen, red, and bleeding gums along with bad breath. Persons with gingivitis should be treated by a dentist to prevent the progression of the infection. Maintaining good oral hygiene is essential for oral health.

Periodontitis

Periodontitis occurs when the inflammation and infection from gingivitis spreads to the ligaments and bones that support the teeth. Signs and symptoms include those of gingivitis along with infections or abcesses along the gums and partially loose teeth. Persons with periodontitis should be referred to a dentist for evaluation and treatment.

Dental Caries

Dental caries refers to general tooth decay associated with demineralization of the tooth enamel. Plaque, formed from food, saliva, bacteria, and mucous, begins to develop within 20 minutes of eating and then begins to adhere to the teeth. The plaque's acidity causes demineralization that can progress to holes in the teeth (cavities). Patients will complain of sensitivity to hot and cold beverages and may also have bad breath (halitosis). A chalky white spot on a tooth is the first sign of dental caries. Treatment options vary depending on the extent of the disease, but will generally include fillings, crowns, root canals, or tooth extraction.

Oral Candidiasis

Oral candidiasis is a fungal infection involving the mucous membranes in the mouth and is most commonly caused by the fungus *Candida alicans.* Antibiotic use and immunosuppression are the most common causes of this fungal infection. Patients will typically present with creamy white to yellow plaques on the tongue, buccal mucosa (inside of check), and palate, which later develop into raw, tender lesions. Topical or systemic antifungal medications are the standard treatment for this disorder.

Oral Cancer

Each year, over 30,000 people are diagnosed with oral cancer and 8000 individuals die from this disease. There is a direct link between tobacco use and oral cancer and the combined use of tobacco products and alcohol increases the risk for developing oral cancer by 15 times. Signs and symptoms include hoarseness that lasts for an extended period of time, pain or difficulty swallowing or chewing, and masses in the mouth or neck. The lip, tongue, and floor of the mouth are the most common sites for oral cancer. Treatment includes chemotherapy and radiation.

Summary

Although injuries or illnesses involving the eye, ear, nose, throat, and mouth are not the most common conditions encountered by the athletic trainer, they have the potential for serious complications such as loss of sight or hearing. Athletic trainers should be skilled in evaluating the eye, ear, nose, throat, and mouth including the use of an otoscope and ophthalmoscope. Early recognition and prompt referral are important aspects of the management of these conditions.

Case Study

One of your basketball athletes reports to you after having a teammate accidentally poke her in the eye during a one-on-one drill. She says that it feels like something is in her eye and the bright lights in the hallway hurt her eye.

Critical Thinking Questions

1. What steps would you take in evaluating this athlete?
2. Given the information provided at this time, what eye conditions would you include in your differential diagnosis?
3. What factors would determine whether you allow this athlete to return to play or refer her to an ophthalmologist?

References

1. National Athletic Trainers' Association. *Athletic Training Educational Competencies.* 4th ed. Dallas, TX: National Athletic Trainers' Association; 2005.
2. Ledford J, Pineda R. *The Little Eye Book: A Pupil's Guide to Understanding Ophthalmology.* Thorofare, NJ: SLACK Incorporated; 2002.
3. Le Sage N, Verreault R, Rochette L. Efficacy of eye patching for traumatic corneal abrasions: a controlled clinical trial. *Ann Emerg Med.* 2001;38:129-134.
4. Michael JG, Hug D, Dowd MD. Management of corneal abrasion in children: a randomized clinical trial. *Ann Emerg Med.* 2002;40:67-72.
5. Flynn CA, D'Amico F, Smith G, Should we patch corneal abrasions? A meta-analysis. *J Fam Pract.* 1998;47:264-270.
6. Arbour JD, Brunette I, Boisjoly HM, Shi 2H, Dumas J, Guertin C. Should we patch corneal erosions? *Arch Ophthalmol.* 1997;115:313-317.
7. Campanile TM, St Clair DA, Benaim M. The evaluation of eye patching tn the treatment of traumatic corneal epithelial defects. *J Emerg Med.* 1997;15:769-774.
8. Wilson SA, Last A. Management of corneal abrasions. *American Family Physician.* 2004;70(1):123-128.
9. Laio J, Zagelbaum BM. Eye injuries in sports. *Ath Ther Today.* 1999;4(5):36-41.
10. Robson J, Behrman AJ, Globe rupture. http://www.emedicine.com/emerg/topic218.htm. Accessed July 9, 2006. Last updated July 13, 2005.
11. Romeo SJ, Hawley CJ, Romeo MW, Romeo JP. Facial injuries in sports. *Physician Sportsmed.* 2005;33(4): 45-53, 55-56.
12. Fincher AL. Use of the otoscope in the evaluation of common injuries and illnesses of the ear. *J Athl Training.* 1994;29:52-59.

Online Resources

American Academy of Family Physicians: Family Doctor Online
familydoctor.org/online/famdocen/home.html
American Academy of Ophthalmology
www.aao.org
American Academy of Pediatrics
www.aap.org/topics.html
Eye Care America
www.eyecareamerica.org
Medline Plus
medlineplus.gov
Merck Manuals
www.merck.com/mmpe/sec08.html
National Eye Institute
www.nei.nih.gov
Prevent Blindness America
www.preventblindness.org

Lab Exercise 11-1
Use of the Ophthalmoscope in Evaluation of the Eye

Objectives

After completing this lab activity, students will be able to:

1. Identify the features of the ophthalmoscope.
2. Evaluate the eye using the ophthalmoscope.

Competencies

This lab exercise addresses the following psychomotor competencies from the NATA's *Athletic Training Educational Competencies, 4th ed*:

- Medical Conditions and Disabilities: 4e

Instructions

1. Review Table 11-3 for the proper steps in using the ophthalmoscope in evaluating the eye.
2. Using your lab partner as a model, practice the 14 steps outlined in Table 11-3.
3. Examine the eyes of four additional subjects. Practice examining both left and right eyes.
4. Draw a picture of the left and right eye of each subject you evaluate illustrating what you see with the ophthalmoscope.

Lab Exercise 11-2
Use of the Otoscope in Evaluation of the Ear

Objectives

After completing this lab activity, students will be able to:

1. Identify the key anatomical landmarks of the external ear and tympanic membrane.
2. Identify the key features of the otoscope.
3. Evaluate the ear canal and tympanic membrane for injury or illness.
4. Evaluate the nasal passageways for injury or illness.

Competencies

This lab exercise addresses the following psychomotor competencies from the NATA's *Athletic Training Educational Competencies, 4th ed*:

- Medical Conditions and Disabilities: 4e

Instructions

1. Review Table 11-4 for the proper steps in performing an otoscopic examination.
2. Using your lab partner as a model, complete Steps 1 through 5 from Table 11-4.
3. Notify your lab instructor when you have completed Steps 1 through 5. Do not make your first attempt at performing Steps 6 through 10 without your lab instructor's supervision.
4. Once the speculum is placed within the external canal, begin training your eyes to look beyond the tympanic membrane.
5. Complete the evaluation form (p. 292) while evaluating your partner's ears.
6. Perform an otoscopic evaluation of both the right and left ears of five different people.
7. Remember to clean the speculum between each examination.
8. Draw a picture of each ear that you evaluate with the otoscope illustrating what you see during your assessment.

Lab Exercise 11-2 (continued)
Use of the Otoscope in Evaluation of the Ear

Ear Evaluation

Patient's Name____

	Right Ear	Left Ear
External Ear		
Normal appearance	______	______
Tragus tender with palpation	______	______
Auricle tender with traction	______	______
Redness	______	______
Swelling	______	______
Cuts or bruises	______	______
Ear Canal		
Normal appearance	______	______
Tender with insertion of speculum	______	______
Bleeding or drainage present	______	______
Redness	______	______
Foreign body present	______	______
Excessive wax present	______	______
Membrane		
Normal appearance	______	______
Unable to view due to wax build-up	______	______
Retracted	______	______
Bulging	______	______
Red	______	______
Air bubbles present	______	______
Fluid level present	______	______
Perforation	______	______
Hearing		
Normal	______	______
Decreased	______	______

Chapter Twelve

Dermatological Conditions

Chapter Outline and Objectives

Introduction

❖ Describe the common types of lesions associated with most common skin injuries and illnesses.

Review of Anatomy and Physiology

❖ Describe the basic anatomy of the integumentary system.

Mechanical Trauma

❖ Describe the clinical presentation, differential diagnosis, treatment, prevention, and return-to-play guidelines for common skin injuries and illnesses caused by mechanical trauma.

- Blisters
- Calluses
- Acne Mechanica
- Talon Noir

Skin Infections

Bacterial Infections

❖ Describe the clinical presentation, differential diagnosis, treatment, prevention, and return-to-play guidelines for common bacterial skin infections.

- Community-Acquired Methicillin-Resistant *Staphylococcus aureus* (CA-MRSA)
- Impetigo
- Furuncles and Carbuncles
- Folliculitis

Viral Infections

❖ Describe the clinical presentation, differential diagnosis, treatment, prevention, and return-to-play guidelines for common viral skin infections.

- Herpes Simplex Virus
    - Herpes Labialis
    - Herpes Gladiatorum
- Molluscum Contagiosum
- Warts
- Plantar Warts

Fungal Infections

❖ Describe the clinical presentation, differential diagnosis, treatment, prevention, and return-to-play guidelines for common fungal skin infections.

- Tinea Pedis
- Tinea Cruris
- Tinea Unguium
- Tinea Corporis
- Tinea Versicolor

Parasitic Infections

❖ Describe the clinical presentation, differential diagnosis, treatment, prevention, and return-to-play guidelines for common parasitic skin infections.

- Scabies
- Pediculosis

Inflammatory Skin Conditions

❖ Describe the clinical presentation, differential diagnosis, treatment, prevention, and return-to-play guidelines for common inflammatory skin conditions.

- Acne Vulgaris
- Contact Dermatitis
- Chronic Eczema
- Psoriasis

Environmental Skin Conditions

❖ Describe the clinical presentation, differential diagnosis, treatment, prevention, and return-to-play guidelines for common skin conditions caused by environmental conditions.

- Sunburn
- Frostnip
- Frostbite

Miscellaneous Skin Conditions

❖ Describe the clinical presentation, differential diagnosis, treatment, prevention, and return-to-play guidelines for miscellaneous skin conditions.

- Urticaria
- Insect Stings
- Skin Cancer

This chapter addresses the following competencies from the *Athletic Training Educational Competencies, Fourth Edition*[1]:

Domain	Cognitive	Psychomotor
Acute Care of Injuries and Illnesses	4, 15, 16, 27e, 29, 30	
Medical Conditions and Disabilities	1–3, 15, 16	
Pathology of Injuries and Illnesses	4–6	

INTRODUCTION

Skin injuries or illnesses tend to occur more frequently in athletes and other active individuals than in sedentary individuals. Regardless of their patient population, athletic trainers should be familiar with the more common dermatological conditions and how to manage them. Also to prevent the spread of contagious skin infections, athletic trainers should be familiar with the guidelines for withholding infected athletes from practice and competition.

Most skin conditions will present with a specific lesion (macules, papules, plaques, nodules, pustules, bullae, vesicles, wheals, or scales) (Figures 12-1a through 12-1i). Also, some conditions are known to present with one type of lesion and then transition to a second type of lesion. Recognition of the type of lesion involved and the history of the skin condition will help the athletic trainer develop a differential diagnosis. The common types of lesions, their descriptions, and examples of actual pathology are provided in Table 12-1.

A discussion of all dermatological conditions is well beyond the scope of this textbook. This chapter will address the conditions that an athletic trainer is most likely to encounter in his or her clinical practice. These conditions are grouped into five categories: (1) those caused by mechanical trauma, (2) those associated with an infection (bacterial, viral, fungal, or parasitic), (3) those associated with localized inflammatory reactions (acne vulgaris, contact dermatitis, chronic eczema, and psoriasis), (4) those caused by environmental exposure (frostnip, frostbite, and sunburn), and (5) miscellaneous conditions. Also, urticaria, insect bites, and skin cancer are discussed. The discussion of each skin condition will include the clinical presentation, differential diagnosis, treatment, prevention, and return-to-play guidelines, when applicable.

REVIEW OF ANATOMY AND PHYSIOLOGY

The skin is the largest organ of the body and, along with its derivatives (sweat and oil glands, hair, and nails), forms the integumentary system. The skin performs many functions including protecting the body against germs, helping in the regulation of body temperature, and assisting with the elimination of wastes through sweat. It is divided into two layers: the epidermis and dermis (Figure 12-2). The epidermis is made up of keratinized, stratified, squamous epithelial tissue that consists of four distinct layers: statum corneum, stratum granulosum, stratum spinosum, and stratum basale. The dermis is made up of strong, flexible connective tissue.

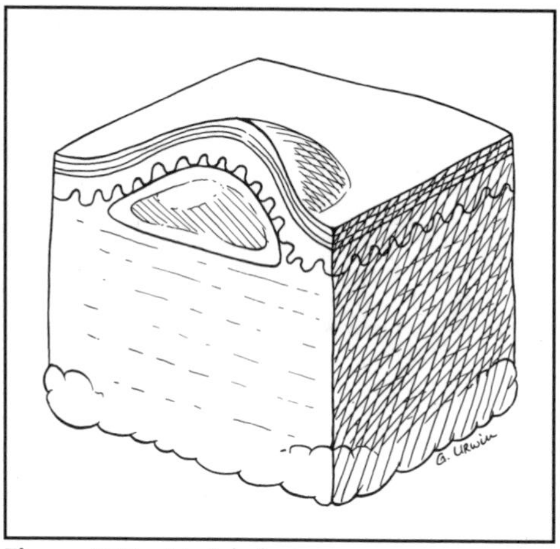
Figure 12-1a. Vesicle lesion.

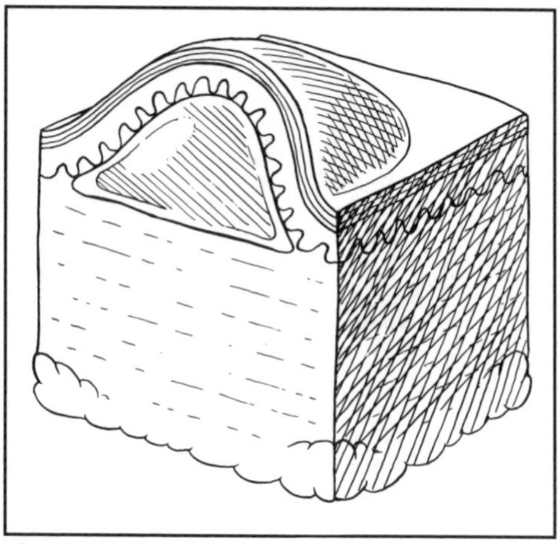
Figure 12-1b. Bulla lesion.

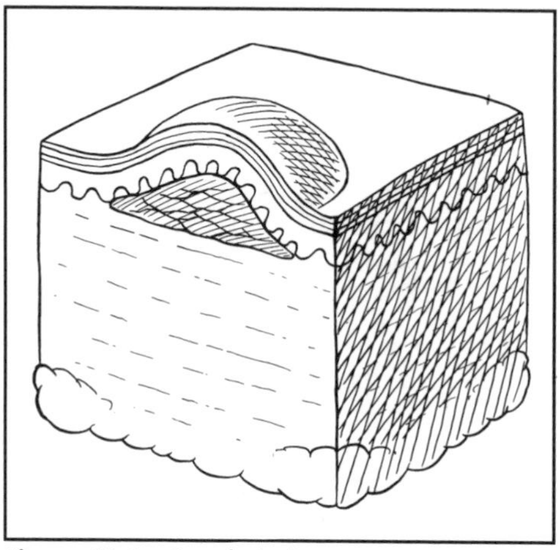
Figure 12-1c. Papule lesion.

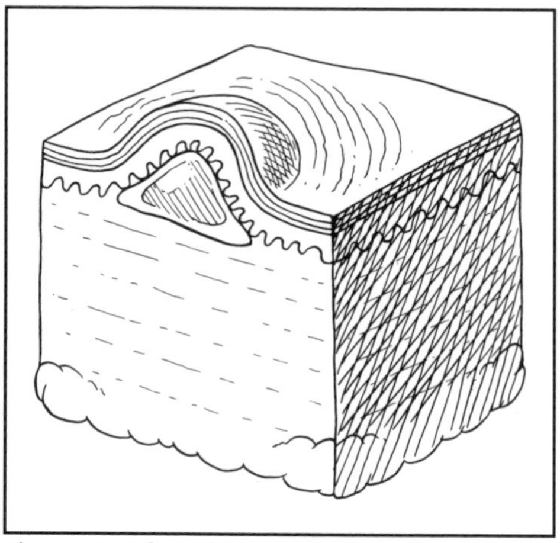
Figure 12-1d. Pustule lesion.

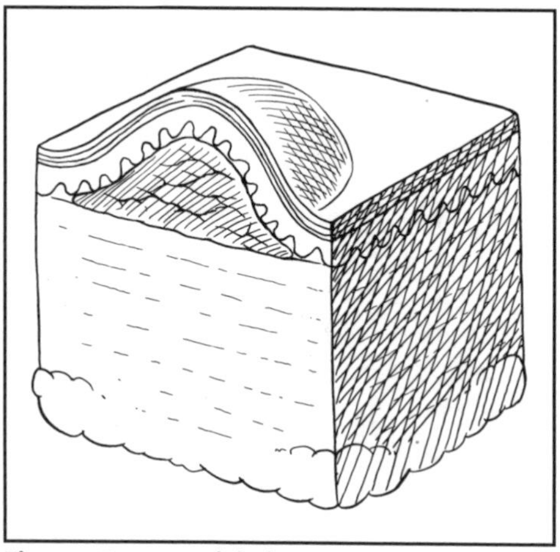
Figure 12-1e. Nodule lesion.

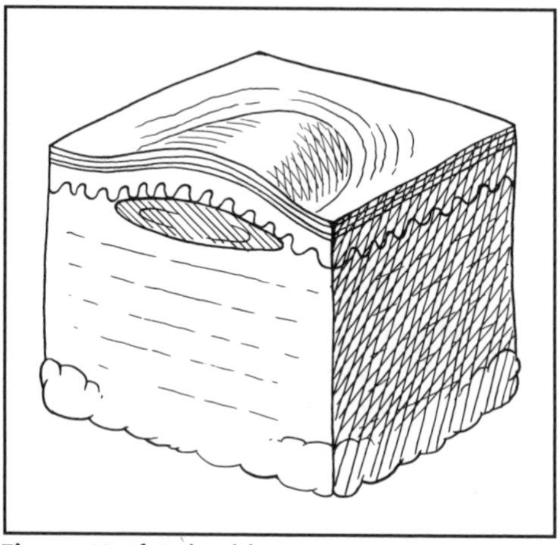
Figure 12-1f. Wheal lesion.

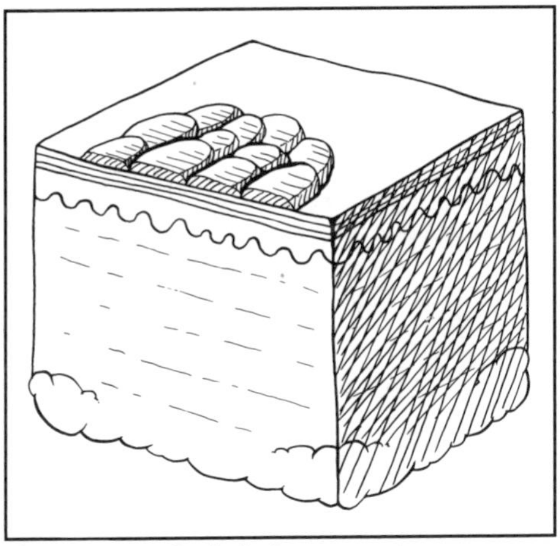

Figure 12-1g. Scale lesion.

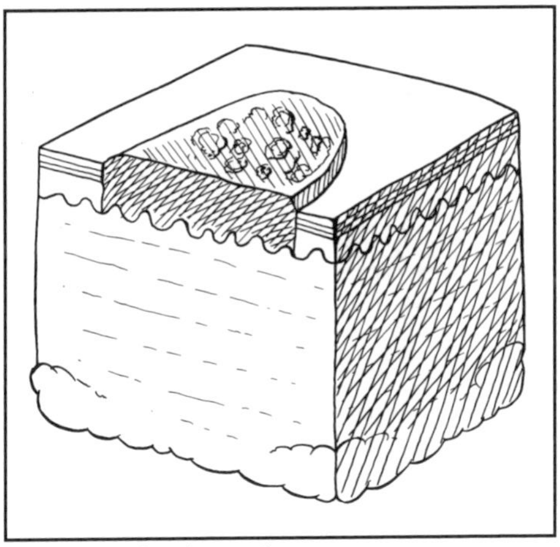

Figure 12-1h. Plaque lesion.

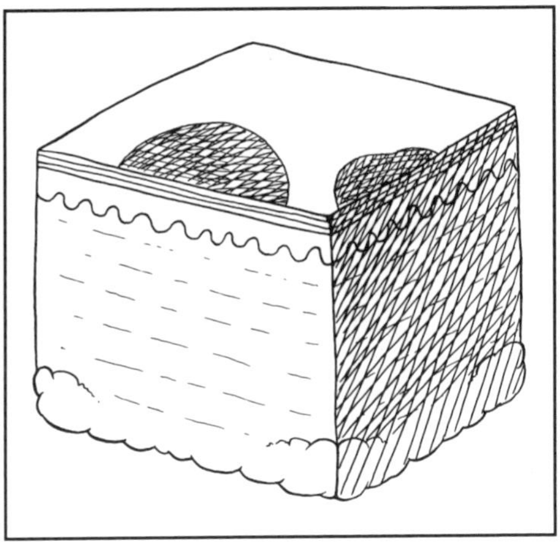

Figure 12-1i. Macule lesion.

The sweat glands are located throughout the skin and help to regulate body temperature and excrete wastes. Each coiled, tubular gland has a secretory portion that lies within the dermis and a duct that travels to the surface of the skin where it forms a funnel-shaped pore.

The sebaceous, or oil, glands are located in all areas of the skin except over the palms of the hands and feet. These glands secrete an oily substance called sebum. Blockage of a sebaceous gland duct leads to an accumulation of sebum, which causes a "whitehead" to form. Acne is caused by an inflammation of the sebaceous glands and appears as pustules (pimples) and cysts on the skin.

Hair follicles extend from the dermis up to the epidermal surface. Infection of the hair follicle can lead to folliculitis. The nails provide a protective covering for the dorsal aspect of the fingers and toes. Each fingernail and toenail consists of a free edge, body, and root. The skin surrounding the nail forms the eponychium (cuticle), and proximal and lateral nail folds (Figure 12-3).

Table 12-1
Common Skin Lesions Associated With Infections and Allergic Reactions

Lesion	Description	Example
Vesicles	Small, fluid-filled blister: <10 mm	Impetigo; herpes labialis; herpes gladiatorum
Bullae	Thin-walled sacs of fluid: >10 mm (large blisters)	Blister
Papules	Solid, round bumps: <5 mm	Warts; molluscum contagiosum
Nodules	Solid, raised bumps: >10 mm	Late stages of acne mechanica; furuncles
Pustules	Small, inflamed, pus-filled blister-like lesions	Acne mechanica; acne; furuncles
Wheals	Circumscribed lesions of inflamed skin	Urticaria
Scales	Excess epidermis forming small flakes	Eczema; tinea pedis
Plaques	Broad, raised (palpable) area on the skin	Psoriasis
Macules	Small, flat (not palpable) spots or blemishes	Tinea versicolor

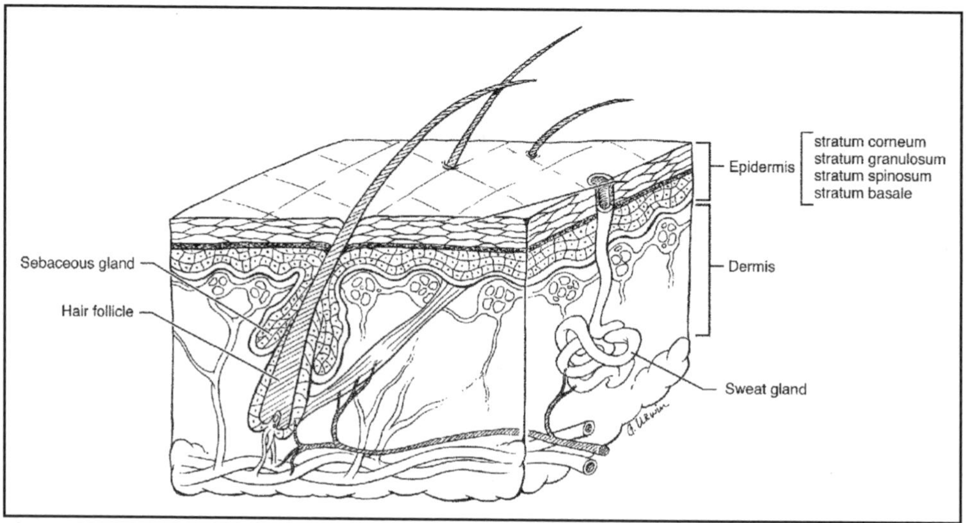

Figure 12-2. Anatomy of skin.

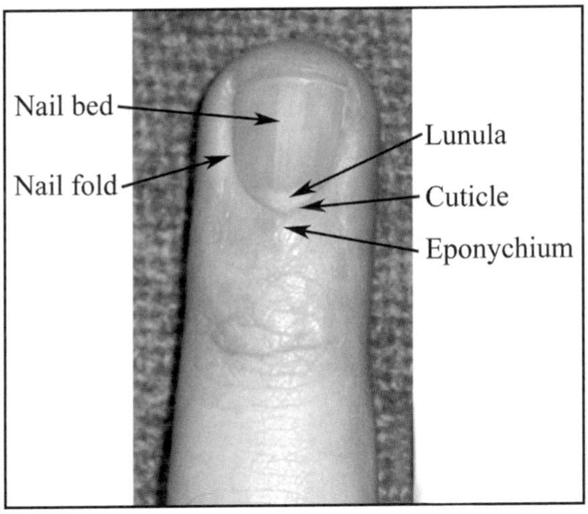

Figure 12-3. Finger anatomy.

Mechanical Trauma

Mechanical trauma accounts for a large number of skin conditions among athletes and other active individuals. These conditions are usually caused by either acute trauma, such as lacerations and abrasions, or repetitive trauma, such as blisters, calluses, acne mechanica, and talon noir. The proper treatment for lacerations and abrasions are covered in most introductory athletic training textbooks, therefore, this chapter will only address those conditions caused by repetitive trauma. It should be noted, however, that all open skin wounds, including acute lacerations and abrasions, are susceptible to bacterial infection. For this reason, athletic trainers should educate their patients that all skin conditions should be thoroughly evaluated.

Blisters

Blisters occur most frequently on the soles of the feet and the palms of the hands. Appearing as tender vesicles filled with either clear or serous fluid, blisters are typically caused by a combination of moisture and repetitive friction. Just prior to the development of a blister, individuals may complain of a "hot spot."

To prevent blisters on the feet, individuals should wear absorbent socks or two pairs of socks made up of two different materials, and properly fitted shoes. Gradually increasing the intensity of a workout or slowly breaking in new shoes can help to develop calluses rather than blisters. Lubricating the skin or applying moleskin to a friction site can also help prevent blisters.

When treating small blisters, the roof of the blister should be left intact to help protect against infection and prevent friction to the tender skin below. When treating large blisters that are prone to tearing or rupture with further friction, the fluid should be drained by puncturing the blister with a sterile needle or scalpel. The puncture should be made at the base of the blister. When punctured with a scalpel, the fluid can be milked out of the blister using a sterile gauze pad. When using a sterile needle, the fluid can be suctioned or drained into the attached syringe. Once drained, the blister should be covered with antibiotic ointment and a sterile dressing. When covering a blister prior to physical activity, possible dressings might include a donut pad with lubricating gel or antibiotic ointment, a piece of "second-skin," or moleskin. A drained blister or a blister whose roof becomes torn should be treated as an open wound. As with all open wounds, caution should be taken to prevent a bacterial infection.

Calluses

Like blisters, calluses occur most often on the plantar surface of the foot and the palms of the hands. These thickened areas of skin occur in response to repetitive friction. Ensuring that shoes are fit properly and hand grips are soft can prevent many calluses. Most calluses remain asymptomatic unless they become overly large. If calluses begin to impair an athlete's performance, or should a blister develop under the callus, the callus can be pared down using a scalpel. An alternative treatment would include soaking the area and applying salicylic acid preparations followed by abrasion of the callus using a file or pumice stone. Calluses do not prevent an athlete from participating in practice or competition.

Acne Mechanica

Acne mechanica typically presents as either papules or pustules in mild to moderate cases and may transition to cysts or nodules in more severe cases.[2] This condition is not to be confused with acne vulgaris, which is discussed later in this chapter. Acne mechanica is typically caused by the combination of pressure, friction, heat, and occlusion, which often occurs under protective equipment. Acne mechanica is sometimes referred to as sports-induced acne because of its prevalence in athletes, and "football acne" because of its specific prevalence in football athletes. This condition may occur anywhere, but occurs most often on the forehead, chin, shoulders, and upper back. Acne mechanica is generally treated with topical or systemic antibiotics such as topical retinoids or benzoyl peroxide, depending on the severity.[2,3] To prevent this condition on their shoulders and upper backs, athletes should be encouraged to wear an absorbent, cotton t-shirt under their protective equipment, as well as remove their perspiration-soaked clothing and shower immediately after activity. Differential diagnosis might include contact dermatitis and certain forms of folliculitis.[3] Acne mechanica does not exclude an athlete from participation and will usually resolve on its own once the season ends.

Talon Noir

Talon noir, or black heel, is associated with sports involving sudden stops and starts, such as tennis and basketball. The lateral shearing forces cause intra-epidermal bleeding which presents as horizontally arranged rows of small dots along the posterior or posterolateral heel. The bluish-black dots that make up talon noir will often resemble the seeds of a plantar wart. Talon noir can also be seen on the palms of the hands in racket sports or weight lifting. Paring down the superficial skin layers using a scalpel will usually remove the pigmented black heel. It should be noted that when paring down the superficial skin layers does not remove the black dots, possible melanoma should be suspected. Talon noir does not prevent participation in any sports or recreational activity.

SKIN INFECTIONS

Common skin infections affecting athletes and other active individuals can be classified as bacterial, viral, fungal, or parasitic. There are several risk factors that are common to each of these types of infections, including: (1) a warm, moist environment produced by perspiration and increased body temperature, (2) occlusive clothing and equipment, (3) close skin-to-skin contact, and (4) acute and chronic trauma to skin. Many of these infectious skin conditions require restrictions on participating in sports, particularly in sports that involve direct skin-to-skin contact such as wresting.

Bacterial Infections

Most bacterial infections can be classified into one of three categories: (1) those that are contagious, like impetigo, (2) those which continued competition can cause further tissue damage, like cellulitis, furuncles, and carbuncles, and (3) those which are neither contagious nor pose further risk to the patient, like folliculitis.[4] The common bacterial infections that an athletic trainer might encounter in his or her practice are summarized below.

Community-Acquired Methicillin-Resistant Staphylococcus aureus (CA-MRSA)

MRSA skin and soft tissue infections were once only associated with hospitals; however, they are now becoming more prevalent in the community, with the first reported case in the athletic setting occurring in 1998. CA-MRSA infections are resistant to commonly prescribed β-lactam antibiotics, which include the penicillin group and the cephalosporin group, making them a challenge to treat.

The typical presentation of a CA-MRSA infection is similar to that of a common staphylococcus ("staph") skin infection, making it difficult to distinguish without a bacterial culture. Both types of infections can present with small pimple-like lesions, pustules, or boils. In their early stage, these lesions are often mistaken for an insect bite, delaying proper treatment. Both staph and CA-MRSA infections can quickly progress to a much larger inflamed, painful, indurated lesion[5] (Figure 12-4). CA-MRSA infections can also attack existing cuts and abrasions.

The Centers for Disease Control and Prevention (CDC) describe common risk factors for CA-MRSA infections as the five Cs, which are listed in Table 12-2. Without proper precautions, these infections can easily spread to an entire sports team. The National Athletic Trainers' Association (NATA) published an official statement on the prevention of CA-MRSA infections.[6] The NATA's recommendations are summarized in Table 12-3. It is important that all open wounds be covered at all times, and any individual suspected of having a CA-MRSA infection be referred to a physician for a bacterial culture. Accurate diagnosis of CA-MRSA can help to determine the appropriate antibiotic to be used in treatment. Often times, the individual will need to be hospitalized for intravenous (IV) antibiotics.

Repeated occurrences of staph or CA-MRSA infections within the same individual or among a single team warrants the performance of nasal swab testing to identify if someone is a carrier. Individuals who carry the bacteria in their noses, but are not ill, are said to be colonized. Approximately 30% of the general population are colonized with *Staphylococcus aureus* (*S. aureus*) and 1% are colonized with CA-MRSA.[5]

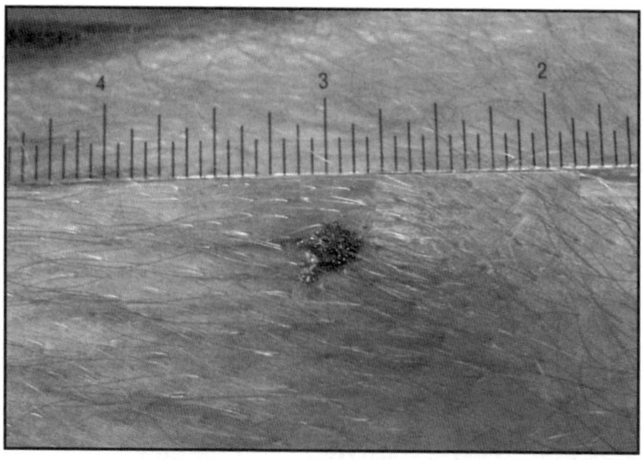

Figure 12-4. Community-acquired methicillin-resistant *Staphylococcus aureus* (CA-MRSA) infection. For a full-color version, please see page CA-I of the Color Atlas.

Table 12-2

CDC Risk Factors for MRSA Infections: The Five C's

- Close skin-to-skin contact
- Contaminated items such as towels, razors, or soap
- Crowding
- Cleanliness (poor hygiene)
- Compromised skin integrity

Table 12-3

Steps for Preventing CA-MRSA Infections

- Wash hands thoroughly with soap and water or an alcohol-based hand cleaner before and after treating a wound.
- Individuals should shower immediately after activity.
- Do not treat individuals with open wounds in a common whirlpool or tub.
- Individuals should not share towels, razors, athletic clothing, or equipment.
- Athletic clothing and towels should be properly washed after each use.
- Facilities and equipment should be kept clean.
- Refer all individuals with active skin lesions that do not respond to initial therapy.
- Proper first aid procedures should be followed when treating all wounds.
- Individuals with suspicious lesions should be referred for a bacterial culture to establish a diagnosis.
- All skin lesions should be covered before participation in sports activity.

(Adapted from NATA Position Statement on MRSA Infections [www.nata.org].)

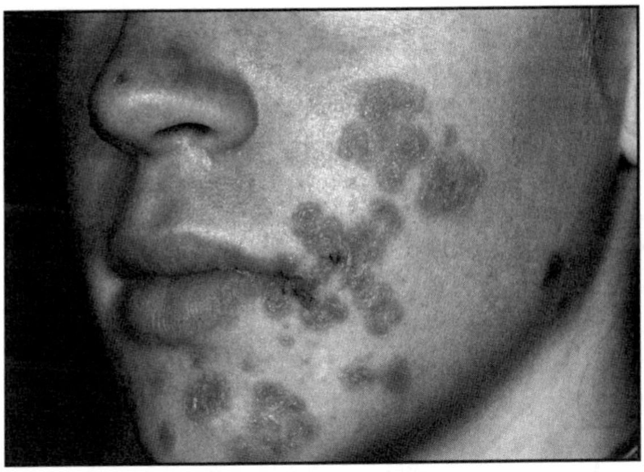

Figure 12-5. Impetigo. For a full-color version, please see page CA-I of the Color Atlas. (Published in *Clinical Dermatology: A Color Guide to Diagnosis and Therapy,* 3rd ed, Habif TP, 240, Copyright Elsevier [1996].)

There are currently no published return-to-play guidelines for the management of CA-MRSA infections in athletes. Many physicians are using the guidelines established for other bacterial infections and the National Collegiate Athletic Association's (NCAA) rules for wrestlers to guide their decisions in returning athletes to practice and competition.

Impetigo

Impetigo is most commonly caused by the *S. aureus* bacteria; however, some cases may involve the *S. pyogenes* bacteria. It typically presents with honey-colored, crusted, well-defined, erythematous vessicles and occurs most frequently on the face and other exposed areas (Figure 12-5). It is particularly common in wrestlers, swimmers, and gymnasts.[2] Football and rugby athletes are also considered at-risk for developing impetigo due to their close skin-to-skin contact.[7] In its earliest stages, impetigo may be confused with tinea corporis, herpes simplex, or acneiform papules. Treatment of impetigo typically includes debridement with hydrogen peroxide and 7 to 10 days of oral antibiotics. Topical antibiotics such as mupirocin (Bactroban, GlaxoSmithKline, Brentford, Middlesex, UK) are used for localized lesions, whereas oral medications are recommended for the treatment of extensive or bullous impetigo.[2] It is prudent to rule out MRSA in athletes with impetigo.[7] Athletes with moist, crusted lesions should be withheld from practice or competition. Athletes may return to play when the lesion crusts have dried, they have completed 5 days of antibiotic treatment, and they have had no new lesions appear within the last 48 hours.[2] Following these guidelines, active lesions should not be covered to allow participation. Inactive lesions can be covered by a nonpermeable dressing during activity.

Furuncles and Carbuncles

Furuncles, or boils, typically present as tender, red nodules that contain a core of necrotic tissue and pus. They may initially appear as a small nodule which turns into a 5- to 30-mm pustule. Open wounds pose an increased risk for the development of furuncles. Furuncles may be prevented by wearing longer clothing to cover exposed skin. All open wounds should also be covered. Single furuncles are treated with moist hot compresses to promote drainage. At times, furuncles may require lancing in order to allow the wound to drain. Furuncles are not contagious (unless they become infected with *S. aureus* or MRSA); however, returning to play too soon may cause further tissue damage. Carbuncles are formed by clusters of furuncles and are treated similarly to furuncles. Generally, it is recommended that athletes complete at least 5 days of treatment and have no draining or moist lesions, as well as have no new lesions within the last 48 hours before returning to activity.

Folliculitis

Folliculitis is a gram negative infection (*S. aureus*) of the hair follicles most often caused by friction from clothing or equipment.[2] Mild cases typically involve the superficial portion of the hair follicle, resolve on their own, and usually do not require treatment. More extensive cases involve the deeper portion of the hair follicle and are associated with redness and tenderness. Hot tub folliculitis is caused by *Pseudomonas aeruginosa* and presents with papules and pustules on skin areas that were covered by a bathing suit.[2] These lesions usually appear 2 to 3 days after exposure to the hot tub or swimming pool and typically last for 7 to 10 days. The presence of skin abrasions increase the risk for developing hot tub folliculitis as does poor maintenance of chlorine levels in pools and hot tubs.[7] Systemic signs and symptoms can be associated with hot tub folliculitis and may include fever, nausea, vomiting, headache, pharyngitis, and otitis externa. Systemic involvement warrants referral to a physician and the use of oral antibiotics.[3] Hot tub folliculitis can be prevented by maintaining chlorine and pH levels and regularly cleaning whirlpools and hot tubs. Folliculitis should not prohibit an athlete from sports participation.

Viral Infections

Most viral skin infections encountered by athletic trainers are caused by one of the following viruses: herpes simplex (HSV), *Molluscum contagiosum* (MCV), or human papilloma (HPV). Sweating, in combination with occlusive clothing and equipment, provides a perfect environment for viral skin infections. Spread of these infections requires direct skin contact with infected lesions or their secretions. Prevention of viral infections focuses on covering all abrasions and other open wounds, early detection through regular skin screenings, early treatment, and exclusion of athletes from participation when recommended by rules and guidelines.

Herpes Simplex Virus

There are two types of HSV: type 1 (HSV-1) and type 2 (HSV-2). HSV-1 is associated with herpes labialis and herpes gladiatorum, whereas HSV-2 is associated with the sexually transmitted genital herpes. Both HSV-1 and HSV-2 can produce primary and secondary infections. The primary episode is typically more severe and may produce systemic symptoms. HSV can become dormant in the neural ganglia leading to periodic recurrences. These recurrent infections usually have a shorter duration and less severe symptoms.

Herpes Labialis

Herpes labialis (cold sore or fever blister) is caused by HSV-1 and can present as a single vesicle or a cluster of vesicles on the lips (Figure 12-6). Exposure to the sun and physical or emotional stress seem to be triggers for the development of cold sores or fever blisters. Individuals will usually report prodromal symptoms of tingling or burning prior to the appearance of the lesions. Treatments are intended to reduce pain or discomfort and to promote early healing. There are a variety of over-the-counter (OTC) ointments for treating the discomfort of herpes labialis; however, prescription oral antiviral medications are more effective in reducing the duration

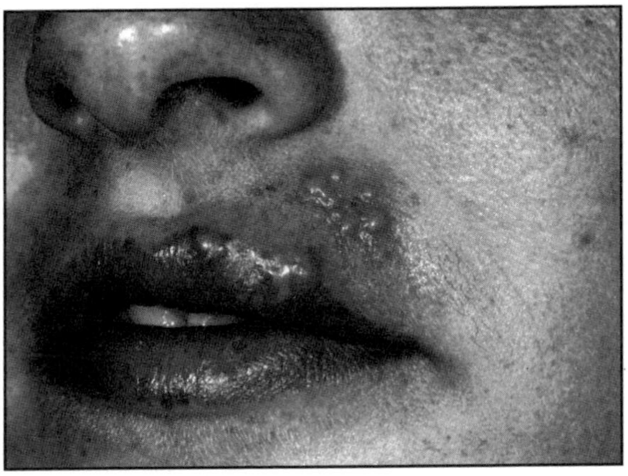

Figure 12-6. Herpes labialis. For a full-color version, please see page CA-II of the Color Atlas. (Published in *Clinical Dermatology: A Color Guide to Diagnosis and Therapy,* 3rd ed, Habif TP, 340, Copyright Elsevier [1996].)

of the infection. Acyclovir, famciclovir, and valacyclovir are three commonly prescribed oral antiviral medications.[8,9]

Athletes should be withheld from participation if they have moist lesions and their sport involves direct skin-to-skin contact with the involved area. The NCAA requires that wrestlers with a primary herpes labialis infection be withheld until they meet the following criteria: (1) the athlete is asymptomatic, (2) no new lesions have developed for 3 consecutive days, (3) all of the lesions are crusted, and (4) the athlete has been taking an appropriate dose of a systemic antiviral medication for at least 5 days.[10]

Herpes Gladiatorum

Herpes gladiatorum, also caused by HSV-1, commonly affects wrestlers, hence the name.[9,11] Open wounds such as abrasions or other cuts in the skin are necessary for HSV transmission to occur. Herpes gladiatorum typically presents with clustered vesicular lesions on an erythematous base. These lesions will usually progress to a crusty stage before resolving in 1 to 3 weeks. Many individuals will report itching or burning in the area of the lesions prior to the actual appearance of the vesicles.[11] Systemic symptoms of fever,[9,11] chills, headache, sore throat,[11] malaise, myalgia, and regional lymphadenopathy[9] have been reported with herpes gladiatorum.

A differential diagnosis might include staphylococcal furunculosis, herpes zoster, or contact dermatitis. The patient's history and location of the lesions may be helpful in identifying herpes gladiatorum. The head, face, and extremities are the most common sites affected by herpes gladiatorum; however, the trunk and eyes may also be involved.[11] Ocular HSV can be a serious complication leading to blindness; therefore, individuals with herpetic lesions close to the eyes should be referred to a physician as soon as possible. In isolated cases, it may be necessary to perform a cell culture to distinguish HSV from a bacterial infection. Although viral cultures are considered the gold standard in HSV diagnosis, it can take up to 4 to 5 days to get the results. A Tzanck test or direct fluorescent antibody test can provide a more rapid diagnosis.

As with herpes labialis, treatment with oral antiviral medications will often shorten the course of herpes gladiatorum.[9] All lesions should be kept clean and dry throughout treatment to prevent secondary bacterial infections. Prophylactic use of antiviral medications can be helpful in preventing recurrent HSV infections.[9]

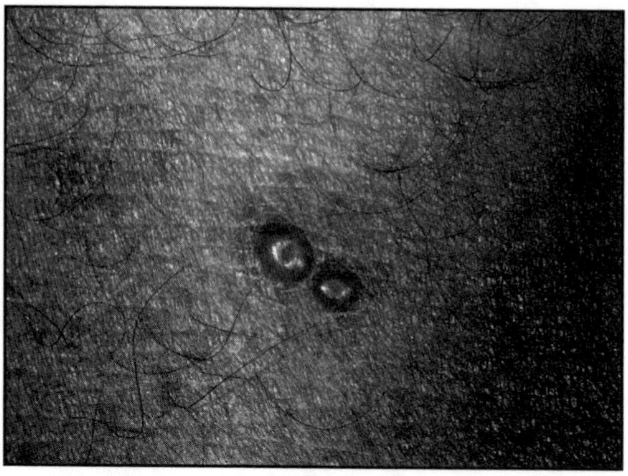

Figure 12-7. Molluscum contagiosum. For a full-color version, please see page CA-II of the Color Atlas. (Published in *Color Atlas of Dermatology,* 3rd ed, White G, 52-53, Copyright Elsevier [2004].)

The criteria for returning wrestlers with herpes gladiatorum to competition are the same as that for herpes labialis. It should be noted that the NCAA prohibits covering of an active (moist lesions without proper treatment) HSV infection to permit participation.[10]

Molluscum Contagiosum

Molluscum contagiosum is caused by the poxvirus *Molluscum contagiosum* (MCV) and is spread in the sports environment through direct skin contact. Wrestlers, rugby athletes, swimmers,[7] and gymnasts[8] are most commonly affected by this virus. MCV is also transmitted through sexual contact and is therefore considered to be a common sexually transmitted disease.[12]

MCV typically presents with a rash that includes white, pinkish, or skin-colored, dome-shaped papules with a center dimple (Figure 12-7).[12,13] The rash will usually be made up of individual or grouped lesions that range in size from as small as 3 to 5 mm to as large as 10 mm.[12,13]

Definitive diagnosis is made through histology or through a *Molluscum* preparation.[14] Treatment of MCV usually focuses on the destruction of the papules. Topical agents such as salicylic acid, thrichloroacetic acid, phenol, podophyllin, and tretinioin can be used.[14] A quicker removal can be accomplished by a physician through curettage, laser therapy, or cryotherapy.[13]

The NCAA requires that MCV lesions be curetted or removed in order for a wrestler to compete in a meet or tournament. After the lesions have been removed, the area should be covered with a gas-permeable dressing held in place with prewrap and elastic tape.[10]

Warts

Warts are caused by the human papilloma virus (HPV). There are several different types of warts which are categorized by their general appearance and location (Table 12-4). Warts are contagious and are spread by either skin-to-skin contact or contact with a contaminated surface. Warts that are located on an exposed area of skin will typically have a hard surface; those located in moist, occluded areas will typically be soft. The treatment for warts generally focuses on destroying the lesions by freezing, burning, electrocautery, or applying topical acids.[13]

Because warts are contagious, athletes should have their warts covered prior to practice or competition. Wrestlers with warts on their faces should be withheld from participation since these lesions cannot be effectively covered.[10]

Table 12-4
Types of Warts

Lesion	Description	Common Location
Common	Irregularly surfaced, domed lesions	Hands and fingers
Flat	Smooth, flat-topped lesion	Face and extremities
Periungual	Abraded or peeling appearance	Nail margins of the toes and fingers
Filiform	Finger-like projections	Face
Plantar	Broad, raised (palpable) area on the skin	Soles of the feet

Plantar Warts

Plantar warts are found on the soles of the feet and are probably the most common wart seen by the athletic trainer. They may commonly occur within calluses, where they hide the usual swirls or "fingerprints" of the callus (Figure 12-8). Due to the weight bearing forces on the feet, plantar warts grow into the foot rather than growing above the skin surface. As a result, individuals with plantar warts will commonly report a sensation of walking on a pebble. When plantar warts become painful or hinder performance, they can be pared down with a scalpel. This removal of the superficial layers of the wart will reveal tiny blood vessels which appear as a pattern of pin-sized black dots. Paring down the plantar wart will also help differentiate this lesion from corns or calluses.[13] Applying a donut pad over the plantar wart will often alleviate the individual's discomfort and allow him or her to participate without discomfort. OTC salicylic acid preparations can also be used to treat plantar warts. The effectiveness of these OTC treatments can be improved by soaking the plantar warts first and then paring down the dead skin with a pumice stone before applying the salicylic acid. More extensive treatments require referral to a physician and include cryotherapy, electrocautery, excision, and the application of chemicals. These treatments can limit the mobility of an athlete and therefore may result in time lost from workout or competition.

Keeping the feet dry and wearing shoes in locker rooms and showers can help prevent the spread of plantar warts.[7] Wrestlers with plantar warts are allowed to participate since their warts are covered by their shoes.[10]

Fungal Infections

Superficial fungal infections are the most common type of dermatological infections in athletes. These fungal infections are caused by dermatophytes and are named for the sites they attack: tinea capitis (scalp), tinea barbae (beard area), tinea pedis (feet), tinea manum (hands), tinea cruris (groin area), tinea unguium (fingernails and toenails), and tinea corporis for infection of all other skin areas.[15] A warm, moist environment serves as the primary predisposing factor for all of these infections. This chapter will discuss tinea pedis, tinea cruris, tinea unguium, tinea corporis, and tinea versicolor since they are the conditions that are most commonly encountered by athletic trainers.

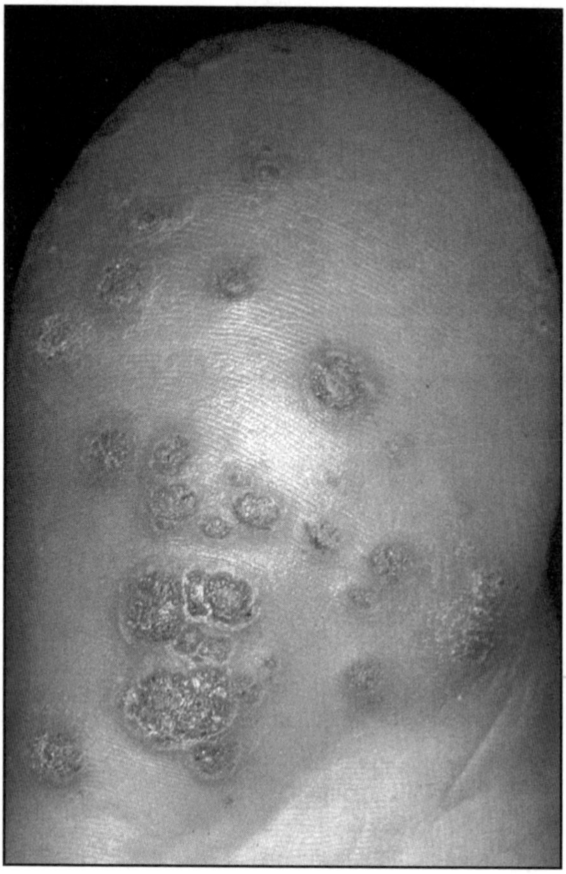

Figure 12-8. Plantar warts. For a full-color version, please see page CA-II of the Color Atlas. (Published in *Clinical Dermatology: A Color Guide to Diagnosis and Therapy,* 3rd ed, Habif TP, 330, Copyright Elsevier [1996].)

Tinea Pedis

Tinea pedis is most commonly caused by the dermatophyte *Trichophyton rubrum.* There are three forms of tinea pedis, with each one having a distinct clinical presentation. The first and most common form, interdigital tinea pedis, occurs in the web spaces of the toes and presents with a scaly, peeling area that may also be erythematous, with maceration and fissuring (Figure 12-9).[16] It is not uncommon for these lesions to spread to either the dorsal or plantar surfaces of the foot. The second form of tinea pedis presents with vesicles or bullae on the midfoot, while the third involves hyperkeratotic scale on the plantar surface of the foot. Individuals with tinea pedis, regardless of the type, will complain of itching, especially after the removal of their socks.[16]

Mild, localized fungal infections usually respond well to a topical antifungal powder such as tolnaftate (Tinactin [Schering-Plough, Kenilworth, NJ]). Moderate cases usually respond better to a topical cream such as clotrimazole (Mycelex [Bayer Healthcare Pharmaceuticals, Montville, NJ], Lotrimin [Schering-Plough]), miconazole (Monistat [Janssen Pharmaceuticals, Titusville, NJ]), econazole (Spectazole [Johnson & Johnson, New Brunswick, NJ]), sulconazole (Exelderm [Bristol Myers Squibb, New York, NY]), or terbinafine (Lamisil [Novartis, Cambridge, Mass]) twice daily for 2 to 4 weeks.[9] The athlete should be instructed to apply these topical medications at least 2 cm beyond the infected lesions onto the healthy skin around the area.[15] Extensive cases of tinea pedis may require oral antifungal medications such

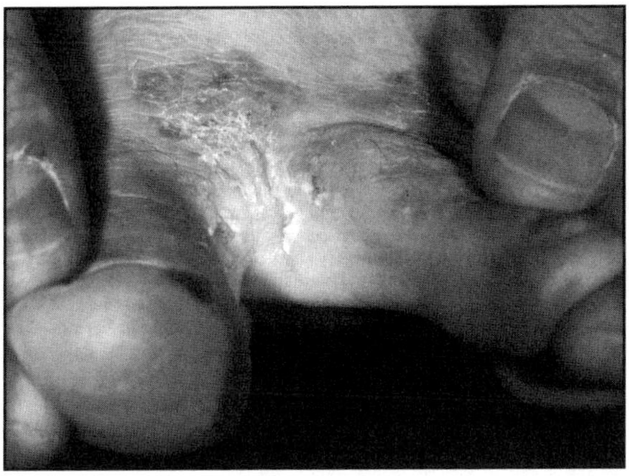

Figure 12-9. Tinea pedis. For a full-color version, please see page CA-III of the Color Atlas. (Published in *Clinical Dermatology: A Color Guide to Diagnosis and Therapy,* 3rd ed, Habif TP, 367, Copyright Elsevier [1996].)

as terbinafine (Lamisil) or itraconazole (Sporanox [Janssen Pharmaceuticals]) in addition to a topical cream.[16] If a bacterial infection occurs secondary to the fungal infection, oral antibiotics should be used in addition to the antifungal medications.

Tinea pedis can be prevented if individuals will make a habit of wearing shower shoes or other types of shoes in gym locker rooms and shower areas. Athletes should also keep their feet dry by wearing breathable, synthetic socks and using tolnaftate powder (Tinactin). Tinea pedis should not restrict an individual from participation in athletics or other activities.

Tinea Cruris

Tinea cruris (jock itch) is most commonly caused by *T. rubrum* or *T. mentagrophytes* and typically involves the proximal medial thighs, inguinal folds of the groin, and buttocks.[14] This fungal infection will usually present with large, round, scaly, plaques that have pustules and papules at the edges (Figure 12-10).[14] Tight clothing, obesity, and chronic corticosteroid use are risk factors associated with developing tinea cruris.

Clinical diagnosis can be made by the appearance and location of the lesions. Topical OTC antifungal medications are usually very effective in treating tinea cruris. Individuals who do not respond to this treatment should be referred to a physician for definitive diagnosis with a KOH stain or fungal culture and to receive systemic antifungals.

Tinea Unguium

Tinea unguium is also caused by *T. rubrum* and affects the fingernails and toenails. Distal subungual onychomycosis is the most common form of this nail fungus and appears as a white, hyperkeratotic patch under the nail (Figure 12-11). The nail will also become thickened and discolored and will eventually separate from the nail bed. Proximal subungual onychomycosis occurs closer to the cuticle, with the fungus invading the proximal nail fold.

Trauma can predispose a nail for tinea unguium. Other predisposing factors include hyperhidrosis, diabetes mellitus, age, and poor venous and lymphatic drainage.[14]

Unlike other fungal infections, tinea unguium does not respond well to topical antifungals. Systemic antifungals such as itraconazole (Sporanox), terbinafine

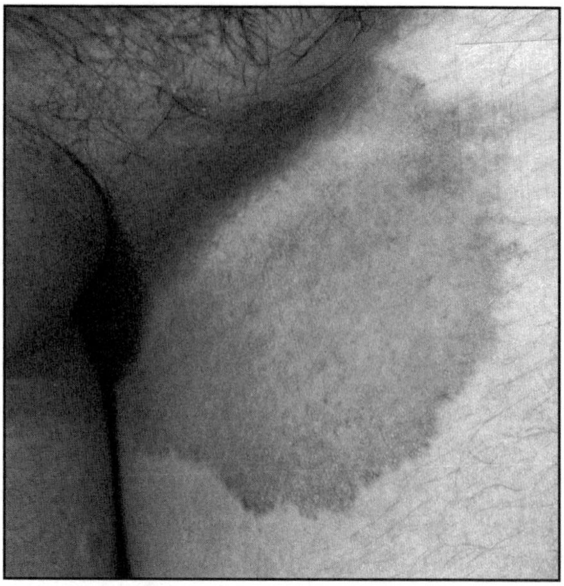

Figure 12-10. Tinea cruris. For a full-color version, please see page CA-III of the Color Atlas. (Published in *Clinical Dermatology: A Color Guide to Diagnosis and Therapy,* 3rd ed, Habif TP, 371, Copyright Elsevier [1996].)

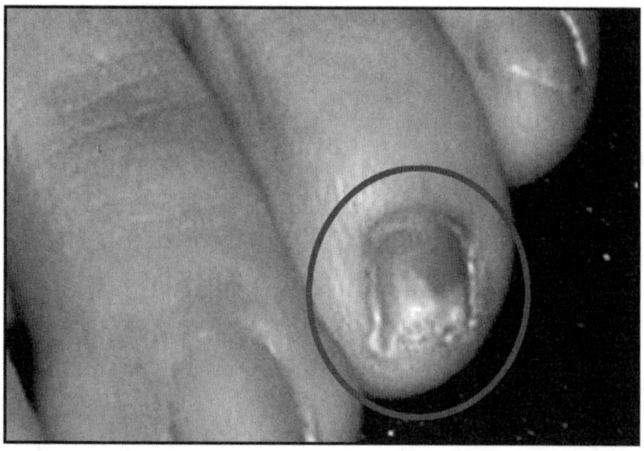

Figure 12-11. Tinea unguium. For a full-color version, please see page CA-III of the Color Atlas.

(Lamisil), and fluconazole (Diflucan [Pfizer, New York, NY]) are commonly prescribed. The presence of tinea unguium does not prevent an athlete from participating in his or her sport.

Tinea Corporis

Tinea corporis (ringworm) is most commonly caused by the *Trichophyton rubrum* dermatophyte. Because this fungal infection is highly prevalent in wrestlers, it is often referred to as tinea gladiatorum.[17,18] Tinea gladiatorum typically presents with a circular, erythematous, pruritic (itchy) plaque, with a raised edge, scaling, and central clearing (Figure 12-12).[4,17-20] Upon inspection, early lesions may have a similar appearance to dermatitis, with later lesions resembling psoriasis, or eczema. Tinea corporis can be differentiated from psoriasis by the central clearing of the tinea lesions. Some tinea corporis lesions may also be more papular and therefore resemble impetigo or early HSV lesions.[19,20] Individuals will usually complain of itching and burning.[17,18] Definitive diagnosis can be made by a physician using a KOH stain.

Color Atlas

Please refer to Chapter Twelve, pages 301–320 for the full text describing the following pictures.

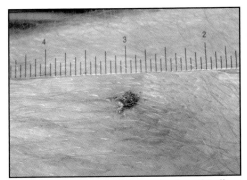

Figure 12-4. Community-acquired methicillin-resistant *Staphyloccocus aureus* (CA-MRSA) infection. Also shown on page 302.

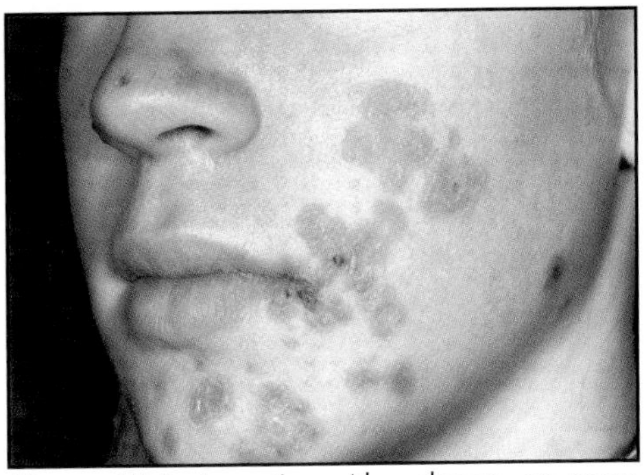

Figure 12-5. Impetigo. Also shown on page 303. (Published in *Clinical Dermatology: A Color Guide to Diagnosis and Therapy,* 3rd ed, Habif TP, 240, Copyright Elsevier [1996].)

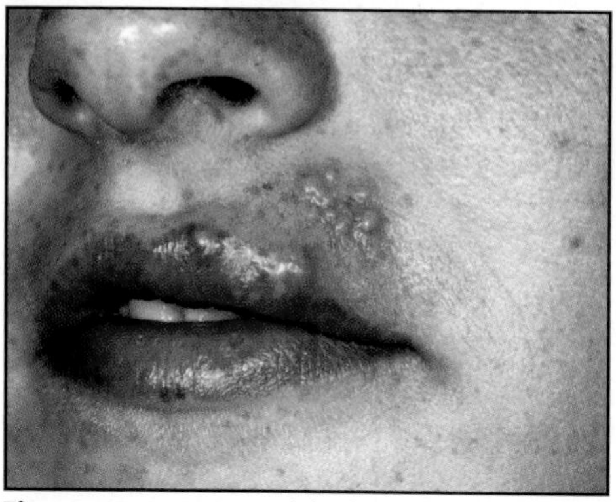

Figure 12-6. Herpes labialis. Also shown on page 305. (Published in *Clinical Dermatology: A Color Guide to Diagnosis and Therapy,* 3rd ed, Habif TP, 340, Copyright Elsevier [1996].)

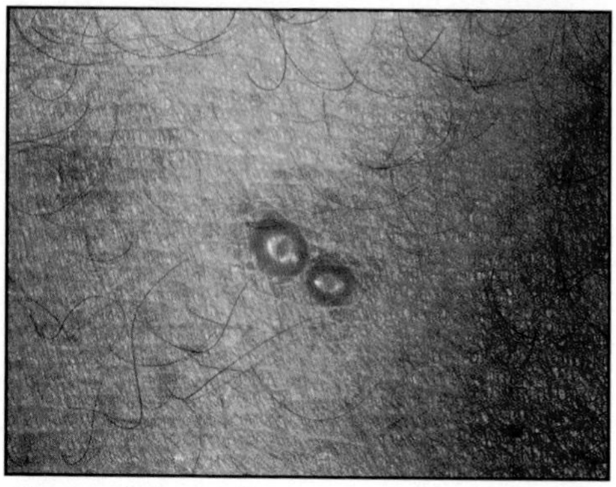

Figure 12-7. Molluscum contagiosum. Also shown on page 306. (Published in *Color Atlas of Dermatology,* 3rd ed, White G, 52-53, Copyright Elsevier [2004].)

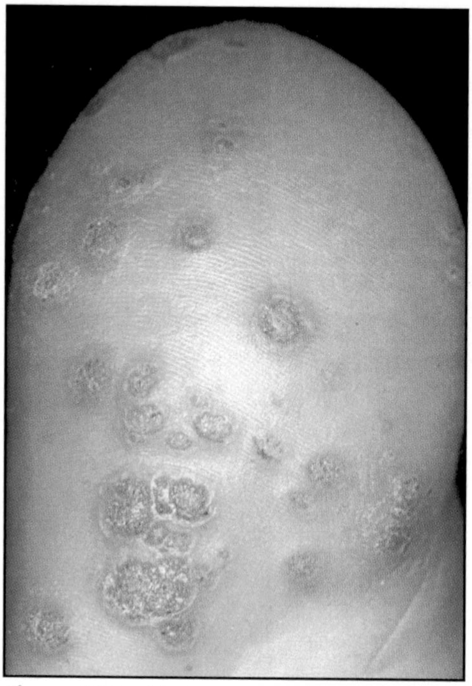

Figure 12-8. Plantar warts. Also shown on page 308. (Published in *Clinical Dermatology: A Color Guide to Diagnosis and Therapy,* 3rd ed, Habif TP, 330, Copyright Elsevier [1996].)

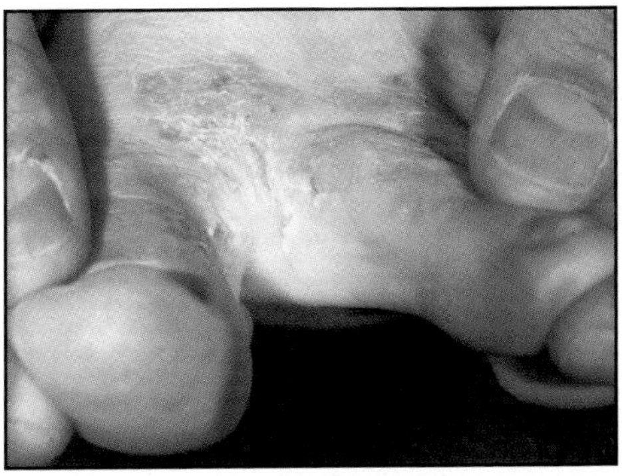

Figure 12-9. Tinea pedis. Also shown on page 309. (Published in *Clinical Dermatology: A Color Guide to Diagnosis and Therapy,* 3rd ed, Habif TP, 367, Copyright Elsevier [1996].)

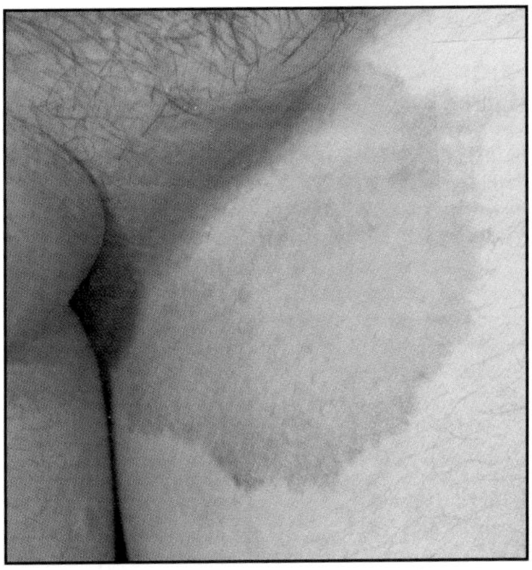

Figure 12-10. Tinea cruris. Also shown on page 310. (Published in *Clinical Dermatology: A Color Guide to Diagnosis and Therapy,* 3rd ed, Habif TP, 371, Copyright Elsevier [1996].)

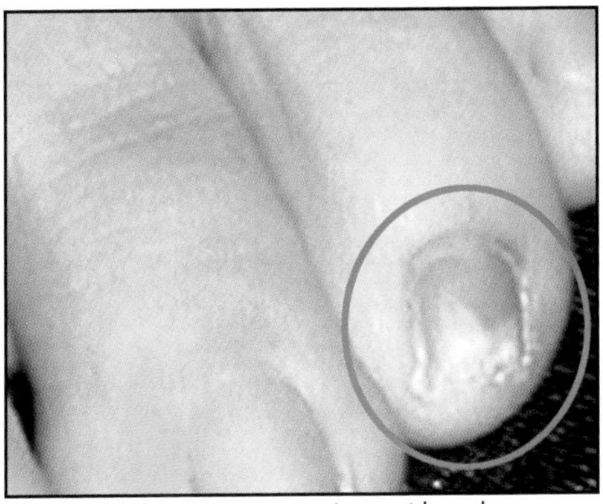

Figure 12-11. Tinea unguium. Also shown on page 310.

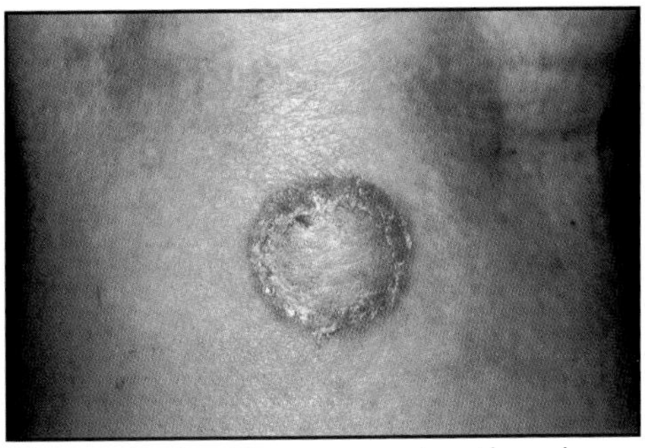

Figure 12-12. Tinea corporis. Also shown on page 311. (Published in *Color Atlas of Dermatology,* 3rd ed, White G, 167, Copyright Elsevier [2004].)

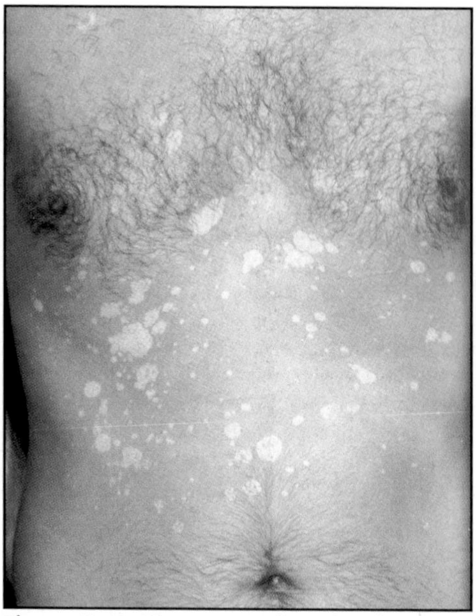

Figure 12-13. Tinea versicolor. Also shown on page 312. (Published in *Clinical Dermatology: A Color Guide to Diagnosis and Therapy,* 3rd ed, Habif TP, 402, Copyright Elsevier [1996].)

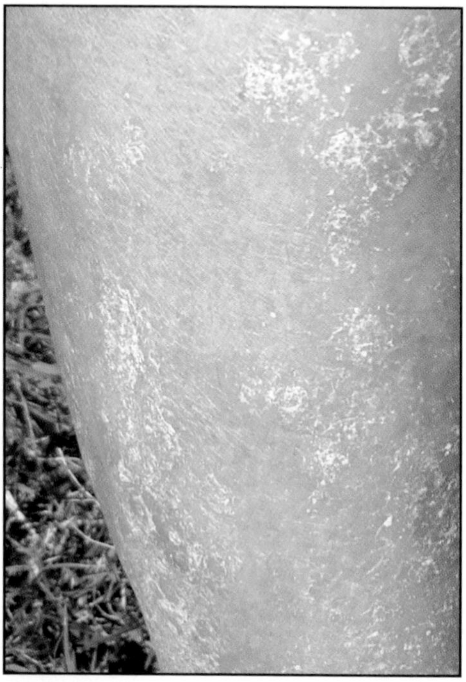

Figure 12-14. Psoriasis. Also shown on page 316.

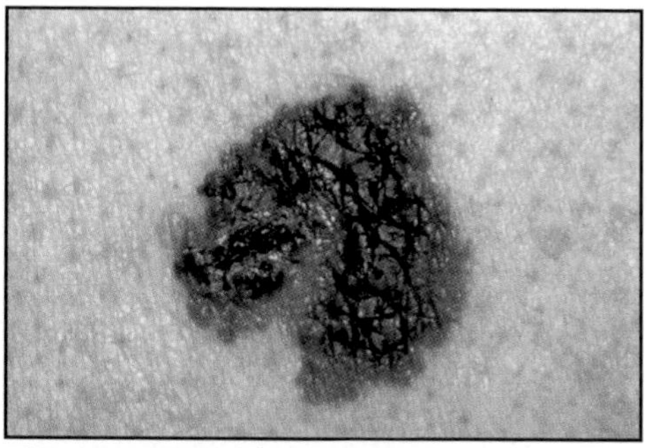

Figure 12-15. Skin cancer. Also shown on page 320. (Published in *Color Atlas of Dermatology,* 3rd ed, White G, 249, Copyright Elsevier [2004].)

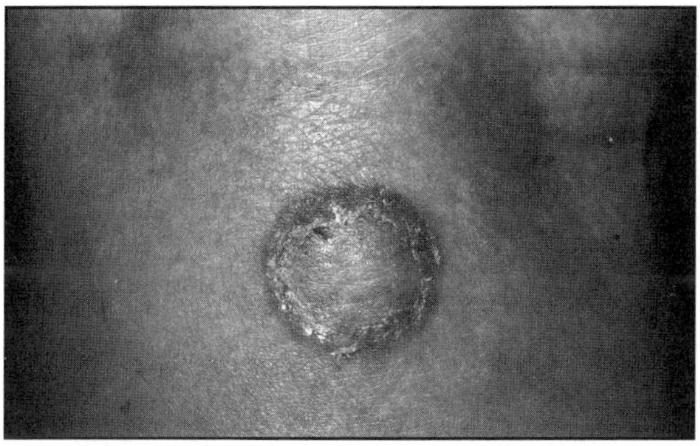

Figure 12-12. Tinea corporis. For a full-color version, please see page CA-III of the Color Atlas. (Published in *Color Atlas of Dermatology,* 3rd ed, White G, 167, Copyright Elsevier [2004].)

Tinea gladiatorum is spread through skin-to-skin contact and occurs most prevalently on the head, neck, and arms.[17,19-21] Wrestling mats or other equipment are not believed to be a factor in the spread of this skin condition.[18,21]

Athletes with tinea corporis gladiatorum should be treated with antifungal medications for at least 2 to 4 weeks, whereas the normal population may only require 1 to 2 weeks of treatment. Topical treatments such as clotrimazole (Lotrimin), miconazole nitrate (Micatin [McNeil Consumer Healthcare, Fort Washington, Pa]), and ketoconazole (Nizoral [McNeil Consumer Healthcare]) are effective for noninflammatory cases.[17] These topical treatments, however, require consistent application to all lesions. In general, single lesions can be treated with topical medications; whereas, two or more lesions should be treated with an oral medication such as griseofulvin (Grifulvin V [Johnson & Johnson], Fulvicin-U/F [Schering-Plough], Gris-Peg [Pedinol Pharmacol, Farmingdale, NY]), fluconazole (Diflucan), itraconazole (Sporanox), and terbinafine (Lamisil).[4,17,20] Oral antifungal medications are also recommended for lesions that fail to resolve with topical treatments. It is recommended that topical treatment be continued for 2 weeks after lesions have disappeared. The NCAA requires athletes with tinea corporis gladiatorum to be withheld from practice and competition until they have received a minimum of 72 hours of topical antifungal treatment.[10] Once the athlete returns to practice or competition, the lesions should be covered until the flaking stops. The lesions can be covered with a gas-permeable dressing, prewrap, and elastic tape.[4] If the lesion cannot be covered, the athlete should be withheld from practice an additional 5 days. The NCAA recommends that dressings be changed after every match and that the routine for covering tinea corporis lesions include "selenium sulfide washing of lesion or ketoconazole shampoo (Nizoral), followed by application of naftifine gel or cream (Naftin [Merz Pharmaceuticals, Greensboro, NC]) or terbinafine cream (Lamisil)."[10]

To prevent tinea corporis gladiatorum, athletes should shower immediately after practice and have their workout clothes laundered daily. Athletes should also report skin lesions as soon as they appear so that treatment can begin promptly. Athletic trainers should identify skin lesions requiring disqualification from competition or exclusion from practice.[4,17] Strict adherence to prevention protocols has been shown to reduce the number of cases of tinea corporis in wrestlers.[22] Athletes with questionable lesions should be referred to a physician for confirmation of the lesion.

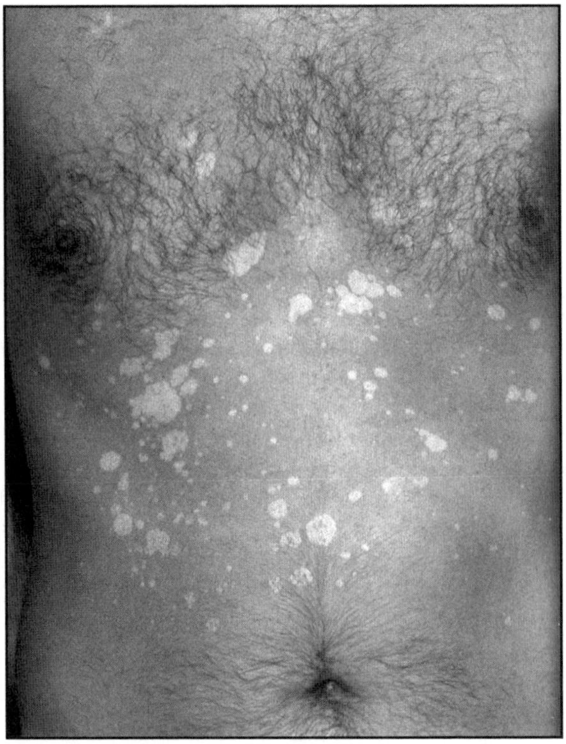

Figure 12-13. Tinea versicolor. For a full-color version, please see page CA-IV of the Color Atlas. (Published in *Clinical Dermatology: A Color Guide to Diagnosis and Therapy,* 3rd ed, Habif TP, 402, Copyright Elsevier [1996].)

Tinea Versicolor

Tinea versicolor is a superficial fungal infection caused by the *Malassezia furfur* organism. It presents with macules or patches that have either a hypopigmented or hyperpigmented appearance and may also include a dust-like scale (Figure 12-13). This change in skin pigment produces variations in skin color from white to red to brown. The back, trunk, abdomen, and arms are the areas that are most commonly affected by the *M. furfur* organism.

Tinea versicolor occurs in approximately 2% to 8% of the population and is more commonly found in regions of the country with hot, humid climates. This condition is more noticeable in the spring and summer months since the involved areas do not tan like the adjacent skin areas do. Tinea versicolor is usually recognized by its unique clinical presentation; however, if necessary, a physician can confirm the diagnosis using an ultraviolet black (Wood) light or a KOH stain.

Tinea versicolor can be treated using topical or oral antifungal medications. The topical agents usually require that the cream or lotion be left on for as little as 10 minutes or as long as overnight before being rinsed off. For this reason, many patients prefer the oral antifungals for their convenience. The changes in pigment usually resolve within one to two months after initiation of treatment. Regardless of the medication used, tinea versicolor has a high rate of recurrence, therefore, prophylactic dosing is recommended, particularly during the hot summer months. This condition is not contagious; therefore, it will not prevent participation in sports.

Parasitic Infections

Scabies

Scabies is a contagious parasitic infection caused by the *Sarcoptes scabiei*. It is spread through direct skin contact. The most commonly affected sites include the finger and toe webs, flexor surfaces of the wrists, elbows, axillae, buttocks, breasts, and male genitalia. After transfer from the host, a pregnant mite will burrow into the epidermis to lay her eggs, although symptoms may not develop for 3 to 4 weeks after exposure. Initially, a vesicle or papule may develop; however, the extreme itching of the lesions often cause these to be removed. Severe itching is the most common symptom.

Diagnosis of scabies infestation is made by scraping the lesion and placing the collected contents on a microscopic slide with mineral oil. The presence of mites, eggs, or feces represents a positive diagnosis.[16]

Scabies is treated with prescription strength lotions or creams, such as permethrin and crotamiton, that are applied from the neck down and left on for 8 to 14 hours. The treatment should be repeated 1 week later to ensure that all newly hatched mites are killed. All persons who have had contact with the infected individual (ie, teammates, family members, roommates, coaches, etc) should also be treated, and clothing and bedding should be washed.

Because scabies is very contagious, infected athletes should be withheld from contact sports during the treatment period. The NCAA guidelines require that wrestlers have a negative scabies test at the tournament in order to complete.

Pediculosis

Pediculosis refers to a parasite infestation with lice. The three most common sites affected include the head (pediculus capitis), body (pediculus corporis), and genital area (pediculus pubis). The lice are spread by direct skin contact. Once infested, it may take up to 10 days for nits (eggs) to hatch. The newly hatched lice begin biting causing 2- to 4-mm red papules and itching.

As with scabies, pediculosis can be diagnosed through microscopic examination of skin scrapings. A louse comb can also be used to identify and remove lice. Treatment requires 7 days of permethrin (Nix [Insight Pharmaceuticals, Langhorne, Pa]) lotion and lindane shampoo.[16] All persons having had contact with the infected individual should also be treated and all clothing and bedding washed and dried. NCAA guidelines require that infected individuals complete treatment and show no signs of lice in order to compete.

Inflammatory Skin Conditions

Most inflammatory skin conditions can be classified as either localized or of systemic origin. This chapter addresses four localized inflammatory conditions: acne vulgaris, eczema, dermatitis, and psoriasis. The term eczema refers to a variety of inflammatory skin conditions. In many instances, the terms eczema and dermatitis are used interchangeably. This chapter will use dermatitis to refer to the acute conditions and eczema to refer to the chronic conditions.

Acne Vulgaris

Acne vulgaris is an inflammatory condition involving the sebaceous glands and hair follicles. Clinically, this condition presents as blackheads and pimples (pustules) that may progress to erythematous macules, papules, and cysts. The face, neck, upper back, shoulders, and thighs are the most common sites affected. Acne has familial tendencies and can also occur as a side effect of steroid use.

The sebaceous glands secrete an oily substance called sebum. When the hair follicles and sebaceous glands become blocked, sebum will accumulate and become inflamed. The body's immune system responds which then leads to the development of pustules. If the wall of the pustules ruptures, the inflammation extends down into the dermis producing a deep, red, tender cyst or nodule.

Acne is graded according to severity. Mild acne is the term used to describe an outbreak with 3 to 10 lesions, while moderate acne consists of 10 to 30 lesions. Severe acne involves greater than 30 lesions. Acne is also classified as either noninflammatory, which includes cases with blackheads and pimples, or inflammatory which involves cysts and nodules.

Treatment begins with educating the patient on the importance of washing acne sites twice a day and avoiding cosmetics and lotions that might lead to blockage of the sebaceous glands or hair follicles. Medical treatment involves the use of one or more of the following types of medications: (1) topical retinoids, (2) oral retinoids, (3) topical antibiotics, or (4) oral antibiotics. Mild acne usually responds to topical treatments with retinoids (adapalene, tazarotene, tretinoin), antibiotics (erythromycin, tetracycline, clindamycin), or combinations of the two (zinc/erythromycin, benzoyl peroxide/erythromycin). Side effects of these medications include erythema, photosensitivity, pruritis, dryness, and peeling. Due to the photosensitivity, patients taking these medications should avoid excessive exposure to the sun and use liberal amounts of oil free sunblock when planning to be outdoors. Moderate to severe acne is generally treated with a combination of systemic antibiotics and topical retinoids. Common oral antibiotics used to treat acne include oxytetracycline, erythromycin, oxycycline, lymecycline, and trimethoprim. Acne vulgaris does not prevent patients from participating in competitive sports.

Contact Dermatitis

Acute allergic contact dermatitis is caused by exposure to or contact with a specific allergen. The rash produced by exposure to poison ivy is a classic example of contact dermatitis. The sap from the poison ivy leaves produces vesicles and papules that are usually very pruritic (itchy). There are a variety of allergens that can produce contact dermatitis; however, some individuals are hypersensitive to specific allergens. Table 12-5 lists several of the common allergens that are associated with allergic contact dermatitis. Changes in bath soap or laundry detergent can also cause contact dermatitis. Symptoms common to most cases of contact dermatitis include itching, erythema, clustered papulovesicles, and wet, weeping skin.[23,24] In some cases, symptoms may take up to 7 days to develop. Symptoms may develop much sooner (after 1 day) when patients have been exposed to a particular allergen before.[23]

The clinical diagnosis of contact dermatitis is often made based on the history and the location and pattern of lesions. For example, acute inflammation from the substances within a neoprene knee sleeve will produce lesions in the localized area that was in contact with the sleeve. Differential diagnosis for contact dermatitis may include skin infections (bacterial, fungal, and viral) and atopic dermatitis.

Table 12-5
Common Allergens Associated With Allergic Contact Dermatitis

- Rubber products (shoe insoles, wet suits, orthopedic appliances)
- Topical creams (analgesics, antibiotics, antiseptics)
- Athletic tape (resin, adhesive backing)
- Epoxy (face gear)
- Leather sporting equipment
- Fiberglass

The first step in treating contact dermatitis is to identify the irritant or allergen and eliminate exposure to it, although this is not always possible. Topical corticosteroid ointments are usually effective in reducing the itching caused by contact dermatitis. In severe cases, OTC antihistamines, such as diphenhydramine may also be used to relieve the discomfort of itching. When treating athletes with contact dermatitis, a second generation antihistamine like loratadine (Claritin [Schering-Plough]) should be used to avoid any sedative side effects. When individuals have a known sensitivity to specific allergens, efforts should be taken to prevent recurrent exposure. Individuals with persistent symptoms should be referred to a physician for further evaluation.

Chronic Eczema

Contact dermatitis can become chronic as a result of cumulative exposure to an allergen. Chronic dermatitis is more frequently referred to as eczema and will usually present with slightly different symptoms than acute cases. Chronic eczema is associated with dry skin, thickening of the epidermis (lichenification), and fissure or cracks in the skin. Treatment is similar to that for acute contact dermatitis; however, the additional use of lubricants or non-alcohol based skin moisturizers can help with the dry skin.

Neither acute contact dermatitis nor chronic eczema is contagious; therefore it is unnecessary to restrict athletes from participation. However, repeated scratching of these lesions can lead to secondary skin infections. Return-to-play decisions in these cases would have to be made on an individual basis.

Psoriasis

Although there are several different forms of psoriasis, this chapter will focus on the most common form, plaque psoriasis. Plaque psoriasis is a chronic inflammatory skin condition commonly found on the extensor surfaces of the body (knees, elbows, knuckles). This T cell mediated disorder activates a cascade of inflammatory processes that lead to rapid growth of epidermal and vascular cells. The characteristic lesions appear as symmetrical, round, erythematous plaques with silver-colored scales (Figure 12-14).[25]

Treatment of plaque psoriasis usually involves a variety of topical and oral drugs used separately or in combination with each other. Because psoriasis is prone to recurrence, patients have to periodically change their treatment routines to

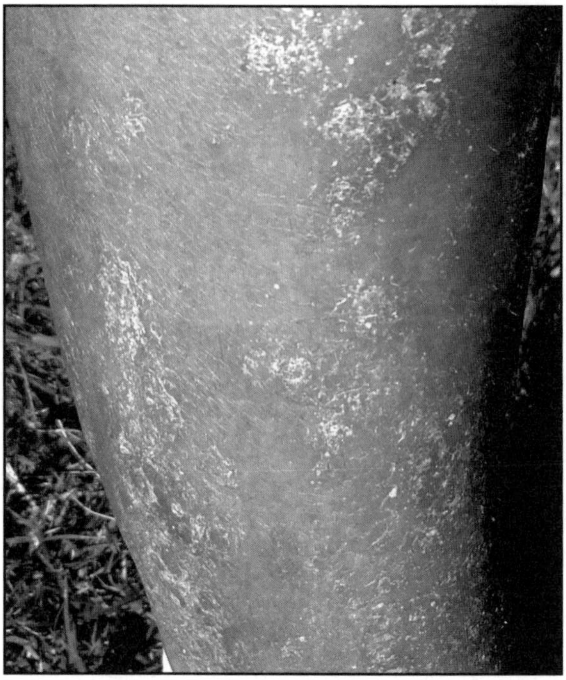

Figure 12-14. Psoriasis. For a full-color version, please see page CA-IV of the Color Atlas.

include drugs from different classes or groups. Improving the moisture content of the skin is one of the primary goals of many topical treatments. Other topical treatments include coal tars, calcipotriene ointment, and corticosteroids. Most of the oral systemic treatments are associated with significant side effects and thus require regular medical follow-ups. Sunlight or artificial UVA light is usually very effective in treating psoriasis. However, depending on the number and size of psoriasis lesions, many patients avoid sunlight due to their self-consciousness of the lesions.

The differential diagnosis for plaque psoriasis may include dermatophytosis (tinea infections) and eczema. Psoriasis is not contagious and does not prohibit an athlete from participating in sports activities.

Environmental Skin Conditions

Prolonged exposure to the environment, whether it is hot or cold, can cause adverse affects that can lead to skin damage. This chapter will address sunburn, frostnip, and frostbite.

Sunburn

Extended exposure to UV rays, particularly during the peak times of 10 am to 2 pm, can cause sunburn. The degree of skin injury can vary based on a variety of factors including total time of exposure, altitude (the intensity of the sun is greater at higher altitudes), and fairness of the skin. First-degree sunburns produce erythema, while second-degree burns will have erythema and blistering; third-degree burns will have erythema, blistering, and ulcerations.[26]

Cool compresses, lotions, and creams can be used to treat first-degree sunburns. Using nonsteroidal anti-inflammatory drugs (NSAIDs) alone or a combination of NSAIDs and topical corticosteroids can reduce the discomfort associated with mild sunburns. More serious burns may require a corticosteroid dose-pack.[26]

The best treatment for sunburn is prevention. Individuals should avoid the peak times of 10 am to 2 pm and wear protective clothing such as a wide-brim hat and long sleeves. Waterproof or water-resistant sunscreens with a sun protection factor (SPF) of 15 or greater should always be worn when exercising outdoors. It is recommended that individuals working or exercising outdoors reapply sunscreen every 2 hours.[27] As mentioned previously, individuals who are taking medication for the treatment of acne, are more susceptible to sunburn, and should therefore take extra precautions when outdoors.

Mild sunburn injuries do not require a restriction of athletic or recreational activity. However, sunburns involving blisters should be watched carefully and covered during participation to reduce the risk of secondary bacterial infections.

Frostnip

Frostnip is a superficial skin injury caused by extended exposure to cold temperatures, and most commonly affects the exposed skin areas. Frostnip generally produces numbness and a blue-white tint to the affected area. Warming the area will usually return normal sensation and color fairly quickly. Individuals can return to play when their color and sensation are normal. Frostnip can be prevented by covering exposed skin areas.

Frostbite

Frostbite involves deeper tissues and can, if not recognized and treated promptly, lead to damage of the subcutaneous tissue, muscle, and bone. The degree of tissue damage is often not known for several days after the exposure to cold. First degree frostbite will involve numbness, tingling, redness or grayish pale skin, and tissue edema. Second degree frostbite will develop clear blisters in addition to the symptoms produced by first degree frostbite. Third-degree frostbite will produce bloody blisters, whereas fourth-degree injuries are associated with deep tissue damage to muscle and bone.[26]

Treatment for frostbite focuses on rewarming the affected tissue with either body contact or warming baths (102°F to 108°F) for 13 to 15 minutes. Thawing and refreezing can lead to more extensive tissue damage; therefore, rewarming should not be performed until the threat of refreezing is gone. Dressing in layers can help maintain body heat and thus prevent frostbite. Individuals suffering from frostbite should be removed from participation in outdoor activities. When treating frostnip or frostbite, evaluation and treatment for hypothermia is also required.

Miscellaneous Skin Conditions

Urticaria

Urticaria is a common skin condition which produces hives and wheals in response to a particular stimulus. There are a variety of mechanisms for producing urticaria; however this chapter will discuss those associated with exposure to cold or in response to rapid elevation of body core temperature (cholinergic urticaria).

Cold Urticaria

Cold urticaria is caused by exposure to cold and is commonly associated with the application of therapeutic modalities such as ice massage, ice bags, or ice slush baths. Exposure to cold environmental temperatures may also cause this condition. Common symptoms include hives and itching, which usually develop shortly after contact with a cold agent or exposure to cold temperatures. Most cases involve local reactions only; however, in severe cases, individuals may develop a systemic reaction such as anaphylaxis. Patients should be screened for a history of cold urticaria before any cold modality is applied. Symptoms associated with localized reactions will usually resolve spontaneously without incidence.

Cholinergic Urticaria

Cholinergic urticaria results in a systemic reaction to a rapid rise in core temperature of 1.8°F or greater, such as may occur during physical exercise. Other causative factors may include hot showers or baths, fever, or anxiety. Although the pathophysiology is not completely understood, cholinergic urticaria is believed to be caused by a cascade of events that starts with the release of acetylcholine (ACH) which leads to mast cell degranulation and the release of histamine.

In some cases, this inflammatory reaction may present as itching on the extremities without a specific rash. Other individuals will develop either diffuse hives or distinct wheals ranging in size from small (2 to 4 mm) to large (5 to 10 mm), with itching still a common complaint. In most cases, these symptoms will resolve within 3 to 4 minutes.

In moderate to severe cases, cholinergic urticaria may produce systemic symptoms such as labored breathing or tightness of the throat. These more advanced cases are many times difficult to distinguish from exercise-induced anaphylaxis, which can be life-threatening. Active individuals with a known history of systemic symptoms associated with cholinergic urticaria should see a physician to discuss the need for a EpiPen (Meridian Medical Technology, Bristol, Tenn) prescription.

Implementing a more gradual warm-up program may help to prevent cholinergic urticaria reactions. Taking a non-sedating antihistamine, such as loratadine (Claritin [Schering-Plough]), 1 hour before exercise can also be helpful in preventing cholinergic urticaria during exercise.[23,28]

Insect Stings

Insect stings have the potential to cause serious systemic allergic reactions. Approximately 1% of children and 3% of adults are allergic to some type of insect sting or bite. Bees, wasps, hornets, yellow-jackets, and fire ants are the insects most commonly linked to allergic reactions Allergic reactions to insect stings in children tend to be localized and subcutaneous, whereas reactions in adults tend to be more systemic in nature. These systemic symptoms may range from generalized urticaria, dizziness, throat tightness, and shortness of breath, to anaphylactic shock. Adults who have experienced a previous localized reaction have a 10% to 15% chance of experiencing a systemic reaction in the future. Also, adults who have had at least one systemic reaction to an insect sting have up to a 70% chance of experiencing future systemic reactions. Therefore, athletic trainers should be aware of those patients who have a history of an allergy to insect stings, particularly those who work or exercise outdoors.

Local reactions to insect stings can be treated with antihistamines to reduce the itching and oral corticosteroids to reduce the inflammation and swelling. Anaphylactic reactions, however, require immediate emergency care. It is essential to have an EpiPen on hand for the treatment of these individuals. Although guidelines state that the standard adult dose of epinephrine (0.3 mL) can be administered a second or third time (waiting 10 to 15 minutes between doses) for individuals who do not respond to the first dose,[29] EpiPens are single-dose devices. Individuals with

Table 12-6
Risk Factors for Skin Cancer

- Sun exposure without the use of sunscreen
- Presence of numerous moles or large moles
- Fair skin, freckling, red or blond hair
- Family history of skin cancer
- Immune suppression
- History of severe sunburns during childhood or adolescence

a history of severe anaphylactic reactions should have multiple EpiPens on hand. If multiple doses of epinephrine are required, the individual must be closely monitored, as the epinephrine may cause cardiac arryhthmias. Anaphylactic reactions can be recurrent, therefore, all individuals suffering from anaphylaxis, regardless of the dose of epinephrine administered, should be monitored closely for 3 to 6 hours following an attack.[29]

At least 50 deaths are attributed to allergic reactions from insect stings each year.[29] Individuals with a known allergy to insect stings should avoid contact with these insects whenever possible. Individuals who are stung or bitten by an insect during athletic or recreational participation should be monitored closely. Return-to-play decisions should be made on a case-by-case basis; however, anyone demonstrating a systemic allergic reaction should be removed from activity.

Skin Cancer

Skin cancer is the most common form of all cancers. There are two types of skin cancer: nonmelanomas and melanomas. Nonmelanoma skin cancer occurs most often and involves the basal and squamous cells of the epidermis. Nonmelanoma is generally less serious as it rarely spreads to other parts of the body. Melanoma skin cancer occurs in the lower epidermis and is formed from melanocytes. Melanoma is much more serious since it commonly spreads to other parts of the body. In fact, malignant melanoma accounts for more than 80% of skin cancer deaths.[27]

Society's quest for the perfect tan has led many individuals to have an increased risk for developing skin cancer. Table 12-6 outlines the common risk factors associated with skin cancer. The American Cancer Institute has also reported that men have a higher incidence of developing skin cancer than women.

The American Cancer Society promotes the acronym ABCD for recognizing changes in the skin that might be associated with skin cancer (Table 12-7). When inspecting a mole, you should look for asymmetry, border irregularity, nonuniformity in color, and diameter greater than that of a pencil eraser. The presence of any of these features suggests a risk of skin cancer and requires referral to a physician (Figure 12-15). Moles that appear suddenly, or existing moles that change in appearance, should also be evaluated by a physician.

A physician's diagnosis of skin cancer requires a thorough history, physical examination, and skin biopsy (incisional, excisional, shave, or punch). Once a diagnosis is made, the entire mole is removed and the lymph nodes are checked for cancer cells. Additional tests are then conducted to determine whether the cancer has spread to any other part of the body (see Chapter Five).

Table 12-7
ABCD Rule for Detecting Skin Cancer

A	Asymmetry	One side of the mole does not match the other side.
B	Border irregularity	Mole has irregular or notched edges.
C	Color	Nonuniformity of color. Mole has shades of multiple colors: tan, brown, black, red, blue, or white.
D	Diameter	Mole is larger than the size of a pencil eraser (1/4 inch).

Table 12-8
Steps for Preventing Skin Cancer

- Avoid being outside during the middle of the day when the UV light is at its peak intensity.
- Wear protective clothing (long-sleeved shirt and wide-brim hat).
- Apply sunscreen (SPF 15 or greater) and lip balm.
- Wear sunglasses.
- Avoid tanning beds and sun lamps.
- Perform regular skin checks.

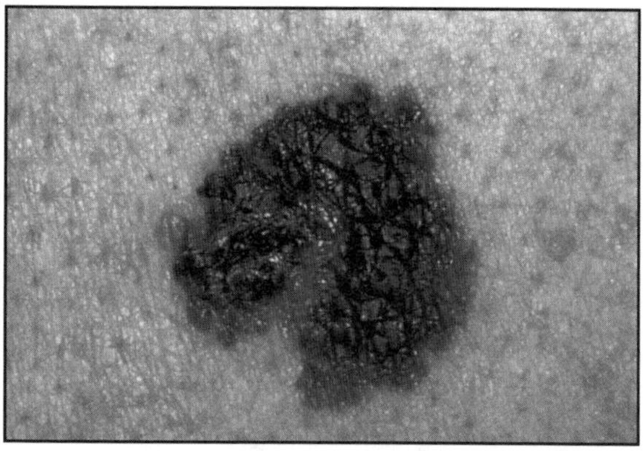

Figure 12-15. Skin cancer. For a full-color version, please see page CA-IV of the Color Atlas. (Published in *Color Atlas of Dermatology,* 3rd ed, White G, 249, Copyright Elsevier [2004].)

The treatment regimen chosen for patients with malignant melanoma depends on the size of the tumor and the stage of the cancer. Localized cases may be treated with surgical excision only. Skin cancer that has metastasized or spread to other parts of the body is usually treated with chemotherapy. Five-year survival rates for patients with melanoma vary depending on the stage of the cancer; however, in general, the lower the stage the higher the survival rate (stage 0: 97%; stage I: 90% to 95%; stage II: 45% to 78%; stage III: 28% to 70%; stage IV: 10%).

There are a variety of steps that can be taken to prevent skin cancer as outlined in Table 12-8. The use of sunscreen is a very important part of any skin cancer prevention plan; however, most people do not use it correctly. As mentioned for the prevention of sunburn, a sunscreen with SPF of 15 or greater should always be used. Sunscreen should be applied 20 to 30 minutes before going outdoors and reapplied often.

Summary

Common dermatological conditions encountered by the athletic trainer can range from minor rashes to infections to even cancer. Some of these conditions are contagious, such as impetigo, CA-MRSA infections, herpes gladiatorum, and molluscum contagiosum and, therefore, require early detection, proper treatment, and restrictions on sports participation in order to prevent spread from one individual to another. Although most skin conditions are relatively minor, others can be life-threatening, such as insect stings and skin cancer. All dermatological conditions should be taken seriously; therefore, athletic trainers should educate their patients to report all skin lesions when they are first noticed.

Case Study

Last week, four football players at the high school where you work developed painful, draining boils. They have continued to participate in football practice with the areas covered. You have been treating them with twice-daily cleaning and antibiotic dressings, but the wounds seem to be getting worse rather than better. They have enlarged in size, increased in drainage, and become more painful. Today, another two players have come to you with similar-appearing lesions.

Critical Thinking Questions

1. What are some of the possible conditions that may be affecting these athletes? What is a likely explanation for the lesions worsening despite treatment?
2. What are the next reasonable steps in management of these six athletes? Include their participation status as well as any referrals, treatments, precautions, and instructions to the athletes and their parents.
3. What are some reasonable steps you may take to prevent other football players from developing the same problem?

References

1. National Athletic Trainers' Association. *Athletic Training Educational Competencies.* 4th ed. Dallas, TX: National Athletic Trainers' Association; 2005.
2. Rogachefsky AS, Bergfeld WF, Taylor JS. Dermatology. In: Fu FH, Stone DA, eds. *Sports Injuries: Mechanisms, Prevention, Treatment.* 2nd ed. Philadelphia, PA: Lippincott Williams & Wilkins; 2001:889-906.
3. Freiman A, Barankin B, Elpern DJ. Sports dermatology part 1: common dermatoses. *CMAJ.* 2004;171(8):851-853.
4. Dienst WL, Dightman L, Dworkin MS, Thompson RK. Pinning down skin infections: diagnosis, treatment, and prevention in wrestlers. *Physician Sportsmed.* 1997;25(12):45-56.
5. Schnirring L. MRSA infections. *Physician Sportsmed.* 2004;32(10):12-17.
6. National Athletic Trainers' Association. Official statement on community-acquired MRSA infections (CA-MRSA). Dallas, TX: National Athletic Trainers' Association. www.nata.org/statements/official/MRSA_Statement.pdf. Accessed 2005.
7. Adams BB. Sports dermatology. *Dermatol Nurs.* 2001;13(5):347-348, 351-348, 363.
8. Cyr PR, Dexter W. Viral skin infections: preventing outbreaks in sports settings. *Physician Sportsmed.* 2004;23(7):33-38.

9. Stacey A, Atkins B. Infectious diseases in rugby players: incidence, treatment and prevention. *Sports Med.* 2000;29(3):211-220.
10. National Collegiate Athletic Association (NCAA). Skin infections (Appendix D). *NCAA Wrestling Rules and Interpretations.* Indianapolis, IN: National Collegiate Athletic Association; 2005:WA12-WA16.
11. Becker TM. Herpes gladiatorum: a growing problem in sports medicine. *Cutis.* 1992;50(2):150-152.
12- Velasquez BJ. When is a skin rash more than just a rash? Sexually transmitted diseases: a dermatological perspective. *Athl Ther Today.* 2002;7(3):16-23.
13. Stulberg DL, Hutchinson AG. Molluscum contagiosum and warts. *Am Family Phys.* 2003;67:1233-1240.
14. Trent JT, Federman D, Kirsner RS. Common viral and fungal skin infections. *Ostomy Wound Manage.* 2001;47(6):28-34.
15. Erbagci Z. Topical therapy for dermatophytoses: should corticosteroids be included? *Am J Clin Dermatol.* 2004;5(6):375-384.
16. Winokur RC, Dexter WW. Fungal infections and parasitic infestations in sports. *Physician Sportsmed.* 2004;32(10):23-33.
17. Kohl TD, Lisney M. Tinea gladiatorum: wrestling's emerging foe. *Sports Med.* 2000;29(6):439-447.
18. Kohl TD, Martin DC, Nemeth R, Evans DL, Berks County Scholastic Athletic Trainers' Association. Wrestling mats: are they a source of ringworm infection? *J Athletic Training.* 2000;25:427-430.
19. Landry G. Treating and avoiding herpes and tinea infections in contact sports. *Physician Sportsmed.* 2004;32(10):43-44.
20. Landry G, Chang C. Herpes and tinea in wrestling. *Physician Sportsmed.* 2004;32(10):34-42.
21. Adams BB. Tinea corporis gladiatorum: a cross-sectional study. *J Am Acad Dermatol.* 2000;43(6):1039-1041.
22. Hand JW, Wroble RR. Prevention of tinea corporis in collegiate wrestlers. *J Athletic Training.* 1999;34:350-352.
23. Fisher AA. Sports-related cutaneous reactions: part II. Allergic contact dermatitis to sports equipment. *Cutis.* 1999;63(4):202-204.
24. Smith A. Contact dermatitis: diagnosis and management. *Br J Community Nurs.* 2004;9(9):365-371.
25. Schnenberger DW. Curbing the psoriasis cascade. *Postgrad Med.* 2005;117(5):9-16.
26. Snowise M, Dexter WW. Cold, wind, and sun exposure. *Physician Sportsmed.* 2004;32(12):26-32.
27. Dewald L. The ABCDs of skin cancer: a primer for athletic trainers and therapists. *Athl Ther Today.* 2002;7(3):29-32.
28. Sweeney TM, Dexter WW. Cholinergic urticaria in a jogger. *Physician Sportsmed.* 2003;31(6):32-36.
29. Golden DB. Stinging insect allergy. *Am Fam Physician.* 2003;67(12):2541-2546.

Chapter Thirteen

Neurological System

CHAPTER OUTLINE AND OBJECTIVES

Introduction

Review of Anatomy, Physiology, and Pathogenesis

- ❖ Describe the basic structures of the neurological system and their functions.
- ❖ Review pathophysiological mechanisms of the neurological system.

Signs and Symptoms

- ❖ Discuss the general signs and symptoms of neurological pathology.

Pain Patterns

- ❖ Identify the referred pain patterns associated with pathology of the central and peripheral nervous systems.

Medical History and Physical Examination

- ❖ Discuss medical history findings relevant to neurological pathology.
- ❖ Perform physical examination tasks relevant to the neurological system.
    - Sensation
    - Motor
    - Reflexes
    - Meningeal Irritation
    - Balance and Coordination
    - Cranial Nerves
    - Cognitive Function

Pathology and Pathogenesis

Central Nervous System Disorders

- Discuss the signs, symptoms, management, and medical referral guidelines for pathology involving the central nervous system.
  - Cerebrovascular Events
  - Headaches
  - Brain Trauma
  - Epidural or Subdural Hematoma
  - Post-Concussion Syndrome
  - Second-Impact Syndrome
  - Neurological Infections
  - Cerebral Palsy and Anoxic Brain Injury
  - Epilepsy, Seizure, and Convulsion Disorders

Spinal Cord Disorders

- Discuss the signs, symptoms, management, and medical referral guidelines for pathology involving the spinal cord.
  - Spinal Cord Trauma
  - Spinal Bifida
  - Multiple Sclerosis

Peripheral Nervous System (and Combined Central-Peripheral) Disorders

- Discuss the signs, symptoms, management, and medical referral guidelines for pathology involving both the central and peripheral nervous systems simultaneously.
  - Reflex Sympathetic Dystrophy
- Discuss the signs, symptoms, management and medical referral guidelines for pathology involving the peripheral nervous system.
  - Motor Unit and Neuromuscular Disorders
    - Motor Neuron
      Amyotropic Lateral Sclerosis
      Poliomyelitis
      Post-Polio Syndrome
    - Axon
      Peripheral Neuropathy
      Guillain-Barré Syndrome
    - Neuromuscular Junction
      Myasthenia Gravis
    - Muscle
      Muscular Dystrophy
  - Management of Neuromotor Diseases

This chapter addresses the following competencies from the *Athletic Training Educational Competencies, Fourth Edition*[1]:

Domain	Cognitive	Psychomotor
Acute Care of Injuries and Illnesses	4, 8, 16, 19–21, 27c, 30	4i
Medical Conditions and Disabilities	1–3, 16, 17	4c
Orthopedic Clinical Examination and Diagnosis	1, 6–9, 16	9
Pathology of Injuries and Illnesses	4–6	

Introduction

Injury or illness can affect any portion of the neurological system (brain, brainstem, spinal nerves, or peripheral nerves). Many of these conditions are very serious and can result in permanent nerve damage, disability, or even death if not detected early. Although athletic trainers most commonly encounter sport-related injuries to the brain (concussions), spinal nerve roots, or peripheral nerves, they may also treat patients who suffer from progressive or degenerative neurological diseases. Recognition of the common signs and symptoms, as well as the indications for medical referral, is essential for the proper management of neurological pathology.

Review of Anatomy, Physiology, and Pathogenesis

The nervous system can be conceptually divided into two main functional components: the central nervous system (CNS), which includes the brain and spinal cord, and the peripheral nervous system (PNF), which includes the spinal nerve roots and peripheral nerves.[2] The brain is made up of four distinct regions including the cerebrum (cerebral cortex, corpus collosum, and basal ganglia), diencephalon (thalamus, pineal body, and hypothalamus), cerebellum, and the brainstem (midbrain, pons, and medulla oblongata) (Figure 13-1). The cerebrum, which controls cognitive function and memory, is divided into two paired (left and right) hemispheres separated by the longitudinal fissure. The left hemisphere receives input from and controls movements of the right side of the body. Likewise, the right hemisphere receives sensory input from and regulates movement of the left side of the body. The outer layer of the cerebrum is made up of the cerebral cortex (gray matter). The hypothalamus links the nervous system to the endocrine system and assists with homeostasis through the regulation of thirst, temperature, fluid balance, and blood pressure. The thalamus serves as the relay point for afferent sensory information, routing these signals to the appropriate segment of the brain. The cerebellum is located inferior to the cerebrum and functions to regulate fine motor coordination, balance, and posture. The pons serves as a bridge to connect the cerebellum to the brain stem. The medulla oblongata connects the brain to the spinal cord and serves to regulate heart rate, blood pressure, respiration, digestion, coughing, and vomiting. The spinal cord carries neural impulses back and forth between the brain and the body. Table 13-1 summarizes the functions of each section of the CNS.

Neurons are the cells in the nervous system. Figure 13-2 shows a typical neuron, including a cell body, dendrites to receive electrochemical input, and one or more axons to carry electrochemical impulses to other neurons. Neuron structure varies slightly according to its location and function in the nervous system.

Other types of cells serve different functions within the nervous system. Astroglia, for instance, adhere to blood vessels to form the *blood-brain barrier.* In addition, astroglia assist in regulation of the electrochemical environment needed for proper neuron function. Microglia cells enter the nervous system from the blood to remove particles and microbes from the system. Oligodendrogliocytes bind the neuronal structures together and provide the myelin that surround and insulate axons. The astroglia, microglia, and oligodendrogliocytes are collectively known as "glial" cells.

Figure 13-1. Components of the central nervous system.

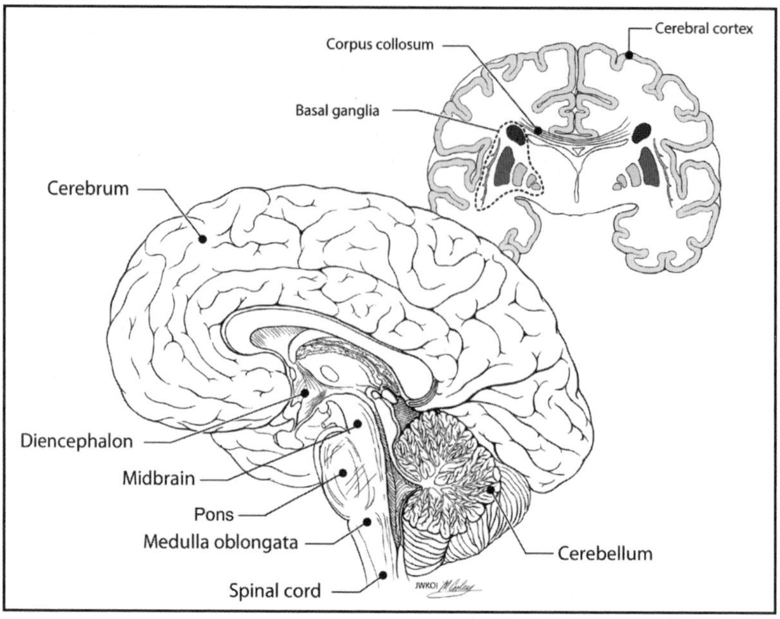

Figure 13-2. General neuron and its structures.

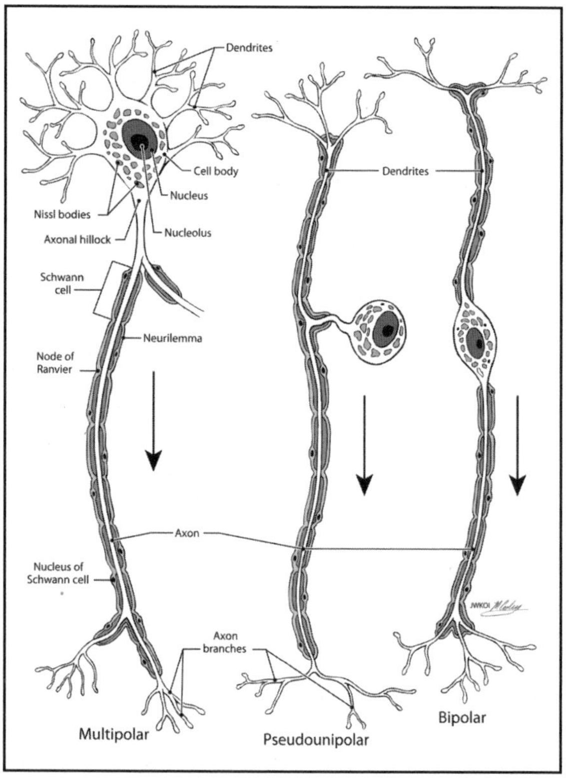

Table 13-1
Functions of the Key Components of the Central Nervous System

Structure	Motor Function
Cerebrum (cerebral cortex, basal ganglia)	Motor function Cognition Memory Sensory perception (touch, pressure, pain, temperature) Special senses (sight, hearing, smell, taste)
Diencephalon (hypothalamus, thalamus, pineal body)	Sensory relay and connection with the endocrine system Control of emotions (fear, anger) Regulation of body temperature and fluid balance
Cerebellum	Regulate control of posture and movement Balance and coordination Fine motor movements
Brainstem (pons, medulla oblongata)	Regulate the involuntary functions (HR, BP, respiration, digestion) Coughing, vomiting
Spinal cord	Reflexes including stretch (myotatic), withdrawal, crossed extension, grasp

Ependymal cells form connective tissues that line the cerebral ventricles and central spinal cord canal. These structures contain the *cerebrospinal fluid*, which bathes the CNS and transports nutrients, chemical messengers, and waste products. The cerebrospinal fluid also supports and protects the brain by permitting it to float in the fluid rather than rest on the cranium. At various points, the cerebrospinal fluid circulates into the subarachnoid space.

The entire CNS is covered with three connective tissue layers called the *meninges*. The innermost layer, the *pia mater*, lies directly on the brain and spinal cord and supports the blood vessels that supply the nerve cells and tissues. The *arachnoid mater* lies above the pia mater. Cerebral spinal fluid circulates in between the arachnoid mater and pia mater (the subarachnoid space), suspending the entire CNS in fluid. The outermost layer is the *dura mater*, a relatively tough membrane that isolates the CNS from the internal and external environments.

Blood vessels perfuse the brain, which is one of the most vascular organs of the body. Under normal circumstances, only certain compounds can pass from the blood into the brain. This blood-brain barrier is one of the most important protective mechanisms of the body. In general, lipid-soluble compounds can pass through the blood-brain barrier with greater ease than water-soluble compounds. As discussed in Chapter Three, pharmacologic agents that are designed to exert an influence on the CNS (pain relievers, anti-seizure medications, etc) must be engineered to pass through the blood-brain barrier. Some pathological conditions affect this barrier, subsequently letting toxic substances move into the CNS. In addition, the vessels within the barrier themselves are vulnerable to injury. Damage to these or other vessels within the brain can cause hemorrhage within the confined space of the cranium, resulting in compression of the brain.

The PNS begins where nerve roots exit the spinal cord at each vertebral level. Individual peripheral nerves branch out to every organ and system of the body. Much like the vascular system, virtually every cell of the body is connected to the nervous system.

The PNS is subdivided into the somatic nervous system and the autonomic nervous system. The *somatic nervous system* is responsible for voluntary control of the body, primarily through skeletal muscle contractions. This system receives input from the afferent (ascending) nerve pathways and then sends this input to the brain via afferent pathways within the spinal cord. Once this input is processed, the brain sends signals back to the spinal cord via efferent (descending) pathways where they are then sent to the corresponding muscles through other efferent pathways.

The *autonomic nervous system*, which regulates various body functions and behavior, is made up of two components: the sympathetic and parasympathetic systems. The *sympathetic nervous system* increases heart rate, respiratory rate, and neuromotor reaction, usually in response to physical stress, including exercise. The sympathetic system inhibits the gastrointestinal system to avoid diverting blood from working muscles. By contrast, the *parasympathetic nervous system* functions at rest to regulate basic metabolic processes, such as digestion. It assists recovery from sympathetic stimulation by slowing heart and respiration rates. The opposing, but balanced, output of these systems plays a major role in homeostasis. The sympathetic system responds to internal and external stresses, and the parasympathetic system restores and maintains basal function once the stress is removed.

The PNS includes 12 cranial nerves and 31 spinal nerves. The cranial nerves originate from the base of the brain or brainstem and exit from the base of the skull. These nerves are numbered as Cranial Nerve (CN) I through XII. Table 13-2 provides a listing of the cranial nerves and their functions. Cranial nerve function can be impaired by a head injury or disease state that damages these nerves.

The peripheral nerves originate from the spinal nerves which are formed by dorsal and ventral nerve roots branching off from the spinal cord. The dorsal nerve roots carry sensory fibers, while the ventral nerve roots carry motor fibers. Most peripheral nerves contain sensory and motor fibers from more than one spinal nerve. The spinal nerves are identified by their exit point from the spinal vertebrae and are grouped into four regions: cervical, thoracic, lumbar, and sacral. There are eight cervical nerves (C1 to C8) which all exit the spinal column above their adjacent vertebrae. For example, C1 exits just above the first cervical vertebra and C8 exits just above the first thoracic vertebra. The thoracic (T1 to T12) and lumbar (L1 to L5) spinal nerves exit the spinal column just below their adjacent vertebrae (T3 exits just below the third thoracic vertebrae; L2 exits just below the second lumbar vertebra). Each spinal nerve is associated with a skin sensory pattern (dermatome) and muscle or muscle group (myotome). The sensory distribution of peripheral and spinal nerves is illustrated in Figures 13-3 and 13-4, respectively. Table 13-3 provides a summary of the spinal nerve roots with their corresponding dermatomes and myotomes as well deep tendon reflexes. Testing sensory, motor, and reflex function forms the foundation for assessing neurological disorders.

Each nerve is covered with a sheath of myelin. Myelin is a protein-lipid structure that is created by Schwann cells, which reside along the length of the nerve.

Table 13-2
Assessment of Cranial Nerves

CN	Name	Function	Assessment Procedure
I	Olfactory	Smell	Instruct the patient to close his or her eyes Place a familiar and non-irritating odor (menthol, peppermint, isopropyl alcohol, coffee, etc) under the patient's nose Ask the patient, "Do you smell anything? If so, what do you smell?"
II	Optic	Vision acuity and peripheral vision	In clinical setting: use Snellen eye charts to test visual acuity; on sideline: anything that requires the athlete to focus on and identify letters, numbers, or read a section of text Wiggle fingers in periphery until seen
III	Oculomotor	Pupillary light reflex, eye movement (in toward nose, up and in, up and out, and down and out	Instruct the patient to follow your finger visually without moving his or her head Test the limits of eye motion Move finger toward nose Move finger diagonally up and out (away from nose) Move finger diagonally down and out Move finger diagonally up and in (toward nose)
IV	Trochlear	Eye movement (down and in toward nose)	This test is assessed in conjunction with CN III and VI Move finger diagonally down and in
V	Trigeminal	Face sensation, clenching of teeth, side-to-side jaw movement	Using one or two fingers, check touch sensation on the forehead, cheeks, and lateral chin
VI	Abducens	Eye movement (lateral)	This test is assessed in conjunction with CN III and IV Move finger laterally away from nose
VII	Facial	Face movement	Motor: Ask the patient perform the following tasks while you look for gross asymmetry: Smile Frown Raise both eyebrows (wrinkle forehead) Puff out cheeks Show both upper and lower teeth Tightly close both eyes

continued

Table 13-2 (continued)

Assessment of Cranial Nerves

CN	Name	Function	Assessment Procedure
VIII	Vestibulocochlear (acoustic)	Hearing, balance	Snap fingers or crumple paper near the ear Ask the patient if he or she hears anything? What does he or she hear? Perform the Rhomberg test
IX	Glossopharyngeal	Taste, gag reflex	Using a tongue blade, touch the back of the throat to initiate the gag reflex Assess the patient's ability to distinguish tastes (salty, sweet, bitter)
X	Vagus	Swallowing, gag reflex, voice quality	Ask the patient to speak
XI	Spinal accessory	Shoulder elevation	Instruct the patient to shrug his or her shoulders against your resistance (can also be assessed with break test) and note any weakness
XII	Hypoglossal	Tongue movement	Instruct the patient to stick out his or her tongue; observe for deviation to one side

CN=cranial nerve.

Myelin creates an insulating layer, similar to the covering on a wire, which keeps the electrical impulse from spreading outside of the nerve fiber. Loss of myelin results in delayed or blocked transmission of nervous impulses. Peripheral nerves may incur several types of injury. *Neurapraxia* is the disruption of nerve conduction without loss of axonal continuity. *Axonotmesis* is the disruption of nerve conduction with loss of axonal continuity, but preservation of the myelin sheath and other connective tissues. *Neurotmesis* is the loss of nerve conduction with loss of axonal continuity and damage to the connective tissues.

Table 13-3

Spinal Nerve Roots and Their Sensory, Motor, and Reflex Distributions

Nerve	Sensory	Motor	Deep Tendon Reflex
C1	None	Neck flexion	None
C2	Top of head	Neck extension	None
C3	Anterior and posterior neck	Lateral neck flexion	None
C4	Superior shoulders	Shoulder shrug	None
C5	Lateral upper arm	Shoulder abductors	Biceps
C6	Lateral forearm, thumb, and second finger	Elbow flexors or wrist extensors	Brachioradialis
C7	Middle finger	Elbow extensors or wrist flexors	Triceps
C8	Medial forearm, fourth and fifth fingers	Finger flexors	None
T1	Medial upper arm and elbow	Finger abductors	None
L1	Inguinal area; posterolateral hip	Hip flexion	None
L2	Proximal anterior thigh	Hip flexion	None
L3	Distal, anterior thigh; medial thigh	Knee extension	Patellar
L4	Medial lower leg	Dorsiflexors	Patellar
L5	Lateral lower leg, anterior lower leg and dorsum of the foot (second to fourth toes)	Great toe extension	Patellar
S1	Lateral foot	Plantar flexion	Achilles
S2	Proximal, posterior lower leg	Knee flexion	Achilles

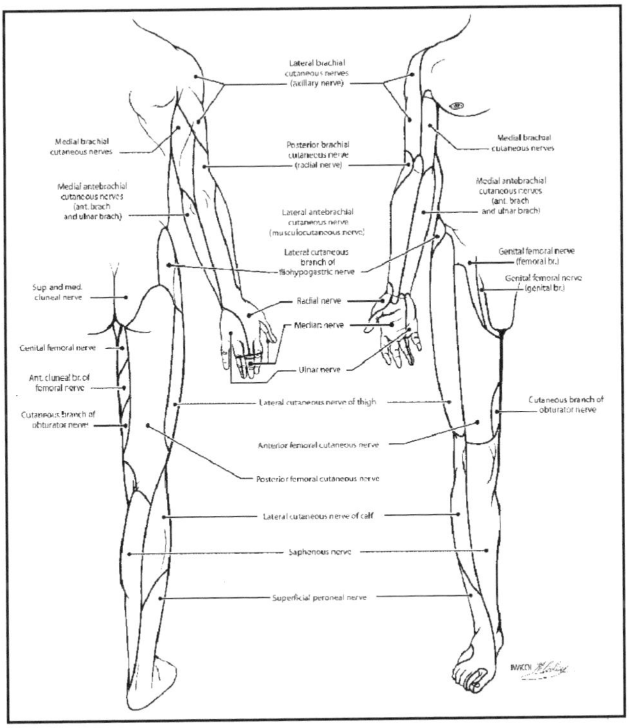

Figure 13-3. Sensory distribution of peripheral nerves.

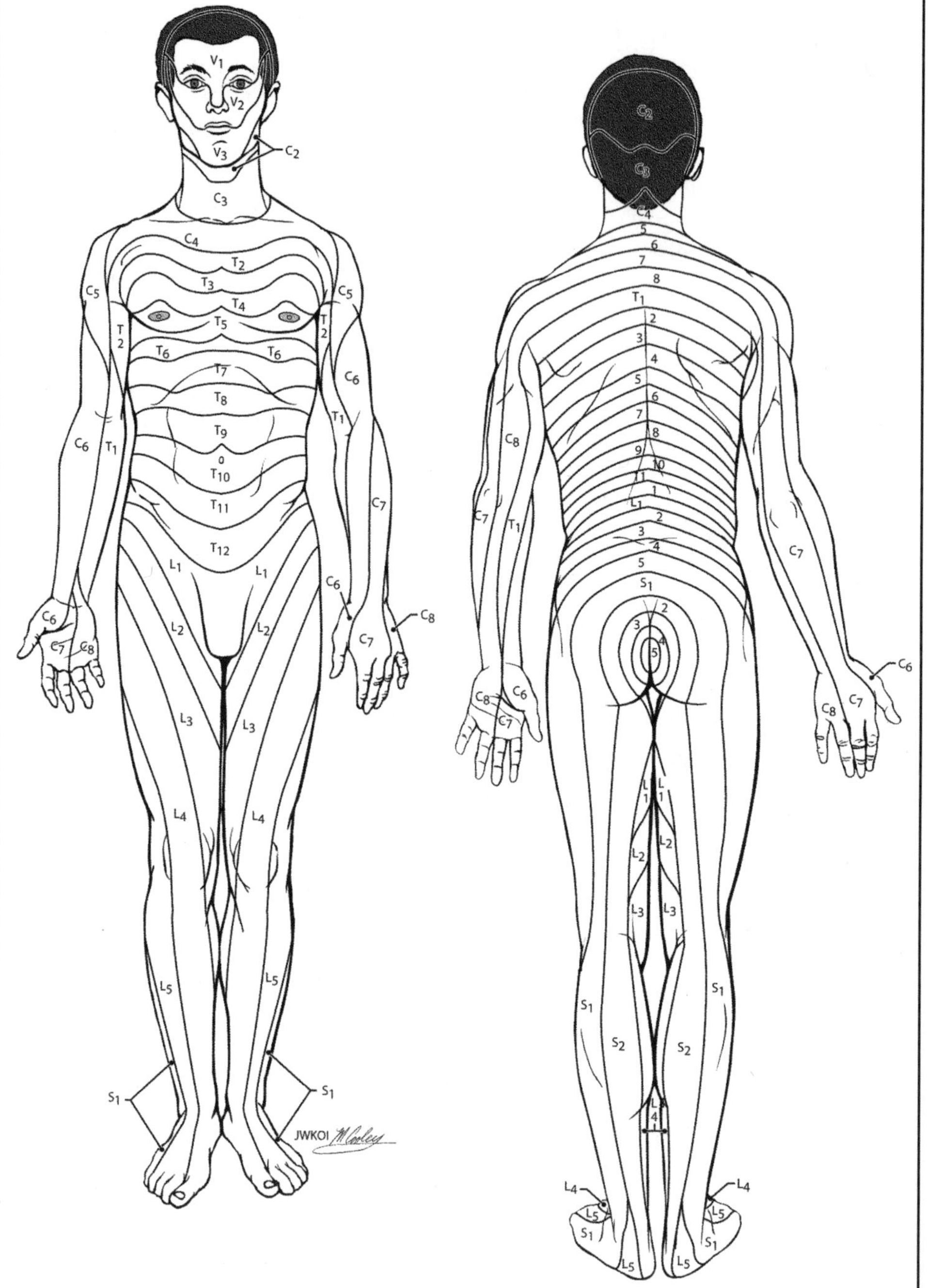

Figure 13-4. Sensory distribution of spinal roots.

Signs and Symptoms

Syncope and Coma

Syncope (see Chapter Six), a brief loss of consciousness, occurs from a sudden compromise of the brain's vascular supply. *Coma*, however, is a relatively longer state of deep unconsciousness, lasting hours or days, during which the person cannot be aroused to a normal level of consciousness. Syncope can be the first sign of impending coma, as may occur following head injury and intracranial bleeding.

Paresthesia

Pathology in the nervous system can cause a complete loss of sensation or alter the perception of tactile sensation, called *paresthesia*. Paresthesia may present as numbness, *hypoesthesia* (*decreased sensation*), *hyperesthesia* (*increased sensation*), tingling, or burning. The only body regions affected are those directly associated with the injured or diseased nerve or neurons.

Abnormal Motor Control, Coordination, or Tone

Decreased deep tendon reflexes (DTR), paralysis, weakness, tremors, ataxia, and psychomotor agitation (a loss of coordination associated with changes in mood) can be signs of significant neurological system impairment.

Headache

Pain perceived in or around the head is an extremely common symptom associated with many pathological states. Musculoskeletal stress, vascular pathology, or common toxins such as alcohol and nicotine can cause benign headaches. An acute headache that persists for several hours is very common following head trauma. Chronic, recurrent, or severe headaches that are not associated with trauma or stress, particularly if increasing in intensity, frequency, or duration, can be a symptom of serious neurological pathology.

Changes in Vision, Hearing, or Other Senses

The senses of smell, sight, hearing, taste, and facial sensation are all controlled by the cranial nerves. Injury or illness involving any of the 12 cranial nerves or brainstem can affect the normal functioning of these senses.

Changes in Mental Status

Cognitive changes occur with pathology of the cerebrum, which controls mental function, memory, and personality. Trauma, infection, degenerative or destructive neurological diseases, or biochemical toxicity may induce these changes.

Pain Patterns

Dorsal Spinal Columns

Light touch and proprioception neural impulses travel from the peripheral nerve receptors and nerves to ascend to the brain in the dorsal columns of the spinal cord. These pathways cross over to the opposite side (decussate) in the midbrain to the contralateral cerebrum.

Ventral Spinal Columns

Pain and temperature impulses travel from the peripheral receptors to pathways in the anterolateral (ventral) columns and decussate immediately upon entering the spinal cord.

Peripheral Nerves

Specific peripheral nerves transmit sensation, autonomic function, and motor control to specific regions and structures. Figure 13-3 shows sensory distributions of selected peripheral nerves; testing these regions may indicate injury to a sensory peripheral nerve.

Many neurological diseases affect a specific structure within the nervous system, but some produce lesions in several structures. The distribution of symptoms often aids physicians in preliminary diagnosis, which is confirmed by further clinical, laboratory, and imaging tests.

Medical History and Physical Examination

Family and Personal History

Genetic factors contribute to the development of certain neurological conditions, such as epilepsy, muscular dystrophy, and some degenerative CNS disorders. A personal history of neurological pathology may affect the physical examination. For example, persons with cerebral palsy or a history of stroke would not be expected to have "normal" reflexes or coordination in an affected limb. In addition, medications for such conditions should be noted since they often have many neuromotor side effects.

Inspection

Selective atrophy of certain muscles suggests peripheral nerve pathology. Certain CNS disorders can also cause tremors or affect gait and other gross movements. *Decorticate posturing,* in which the arms are rigidly flexed and the legs are fixed in extension (Figure 13-5), indicates interruption of neurological signals from the cerebral cortex. *Decerebrate posturing,* in which the arms and legs are both rigidly extended (Figure 13-6), indicates an interruption of neural signals from the cerebellum. The presence of blood or cerebral spinal fluid draining from the nose or ear indicates a possible skull fracture. Other visual signs of a skull fracture include discoloration over the mastoid process (*Battle's sign*) or the eyelids and periorbital region (*Raccoon sign*). Dilated and fixed pupils, unequal papillary response (*anisocoria*), or involuntary rapid movement of the eyes (*nystagmus*) are all also associated with a head injury.

Physical Examination

Sensation

Testing sensation on the entire body is usually unnecessary, so the physical examination concentrates around the symptomatic region. Touch sensation travels

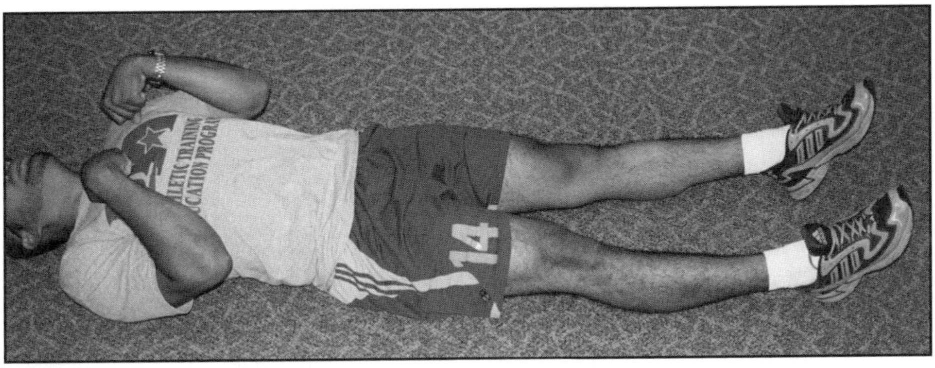

Figure 13-5. Decorticate posturing.

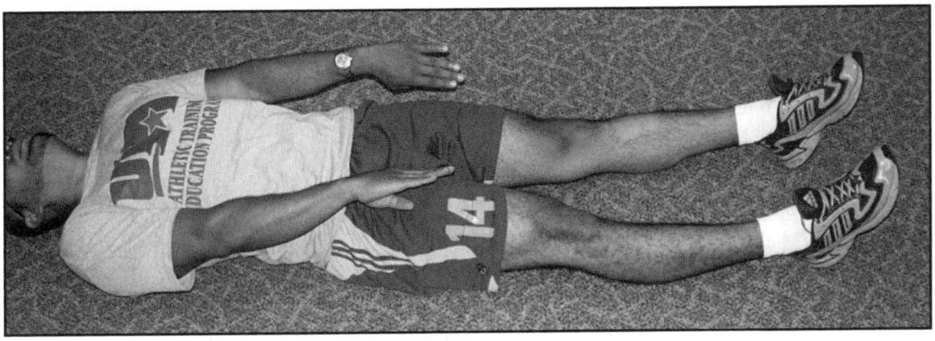

Figure 13-6. Decerebrate posturing.

in bilateral spinal pathways to the brain and is a good quick test of peripheral and spinal nerve integrity. In general, athletic trainers use the dermatome patterns to assess sensory function (see Figure 13-3) Several levels of sensation (touch, pain, vibration, discrimination) can be tested depending on the symptoms and the assessment findings. *Light touch* sensation can be assessed using a cotton ball or a finger. With all of the sensory testing, assessment should be performed bilaterally for comparison. When comparing from side to side, the examiner can ask "Can you feel this," "Tell me when you feel something," or "Does this feel the same as this?" The ability to perceive *pain* can be tested using a straight or safety pin. Occasionally substitute the dull end of the pin for the sharp end in the assessment. Ask the patient, "Does this feel dull or sharp?" The pin stick should be enough to feel sharp but not enough to draw blood. To avoid the possibility of drawing blood, a wooden cotton-tipped stick can be broken in half, with the broken end used to test pain and the cotton-tipped end used to test touch and pressure. *Vibration sense* may be the first sensation lost with a peripheral neuropathy. This sensation can be assessed using a tuning fork and is usually tested over the interphalangeal joint of the great toe or a distal interphalangeal joint in a finger. To assess vibration sense, the forked end of the tuning fork should be struck on the heel of the examiner's hand and then the stem end placed over the toe or finger to be tested (Figure 13-7). One or two fingers from the examiner's other hand can be placed under the joint so that he or she can also feel the vibration. Ask the patient if he or she can feel the vibration or instruct him or her to tell you when he or she can no longer feel the vibration. (Lab Exercise 13-1 provides an opportunity to practice the skill of sensory evaluation for both

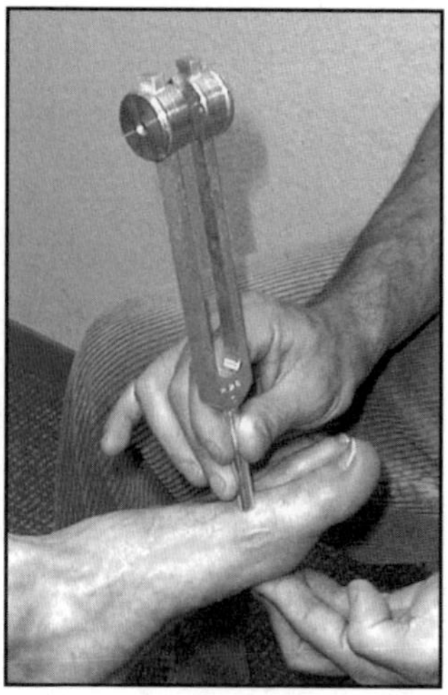

Figure 13-7. Vibration testing.

the upper and lower extremity.) Loss of *discriminatory sensation* suggests pathology involving the cerebral cortex. Two-point discrimination can be assessed using an open paperclip with the two ends placed approximately 5 mm apart. The two ends are touched simultaneously to one of the patient's finger pads. Ask the patient if he or she feels one stick or two. Alternate the use of one end with the use of two ends. Pathology of the cerebral cortex will cause a widening of the space within which the patient can detect sensation at two different points.

Motor

Similar to the sensory examination, the motor examination is usually limited to the region of injury or symptoms. For non-emergency conditions involving the neck or back, test the upper extremities with suspected cervical problems and the lower extremities with suspected lumbar problems. The motor exam primarily involves testing for myotomal weakness (see Table 13-3). The motor system is tested by asking the patient to contract specific muscle groups as the examiner provides resistance. Muscle strength can be tested through the entire range of motion or by using a break test. Weakness is noted by comparing to the same muscle on the contralateral, unaffected side. (Lab Exercise 13-2 provides an opportunity to practice a neurological assessment of the motor nerves.)

Reflexes

An increase, decrease, or absence of deep tendon reflexes (Achilles, patellar, biceps, brachioradialis, triceps) is associated with both injury and illness to the neurological system. These reflexes can be easily tested using a reflex hammer (Figures 13-8a through 13-8e). Table 13-4 outlines the steps to follow when testing the upper and lower extremity deep tendon reflexes and the normal response expected. If reflex testing fails to elicit a response bilaterally, instruct the patient to clench his or her teeth. Alternatively, when testing lower extremity reflexes, instruct the patient to clasp his or her hands in front of him or her and to try and pull them apart isometrically. Likewise, when testing upper extremity exercises, instruct the patient to cross his or her legs and perform isometric abduction. These procedures will enhance the reflex response. (Lab Exercise 13-3 provides the opportunity to

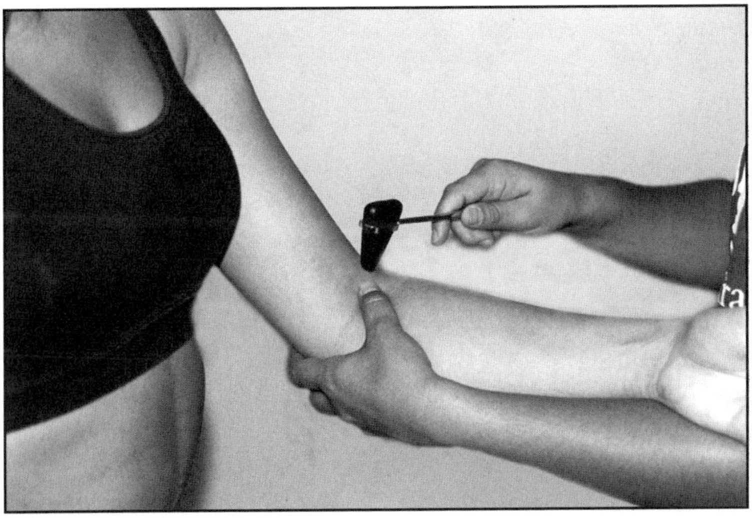

Figure 13-8a. Biceps (C5) reflex testing.

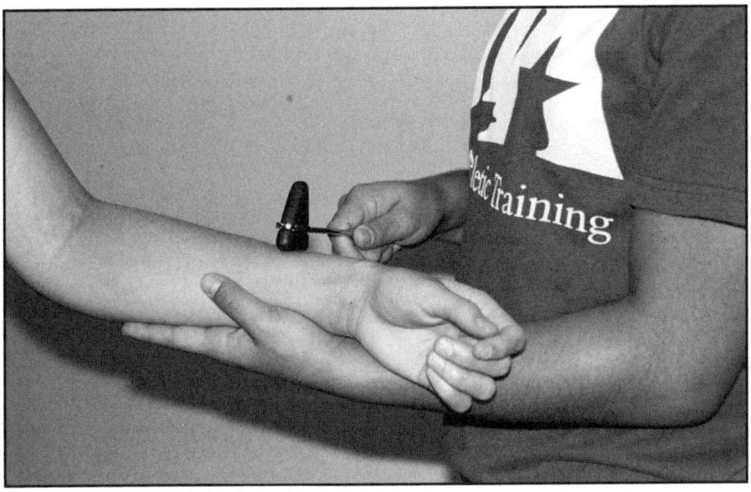

Figure 13-8b. Brachioradialis (C6) reflex testing.

practice assessing deep tendon reflexes.) Asymmetries of reflex response, in either amplitude or delay, are important. Athletic trainers document reflexes as normal, "increased," or "decreased" in comparison to the contralateral limb. In acute spinal cord injury, a symmetric loss of reflexes distal to the injury is commonly present. Unilateral changes in these reflexes can occur with injury or illness to a nerve root or peripheral nerve. Increased reflexes are associated with CNS pathology, while decreased or absent reflexes suggest pathology involving the spinal nerve roots or peripheral nerves.

Table 13-4

Assessment of Deep Tendon Reflexes

Reflex (Spinal Level)	Instructions for Assessment	Normal Response
Biceps (C5)	Position the patient seated or standing. Use one hand to support the patient's elbow in a position of 90 degrees of flexion, with the patient's forearm resting on your forearm (see Figure 13-8a). Place the thumb of the hand supporting the patient's elbow over the biceps tendon near its insertion on the radius. Using the pointed side of the reflex hammer's head, strike his or her thumb. Perform the test bilaterally for comparison.	Normally, the biceps contracts slightly, which can be observed and palpated.
Brachioradialis (C6)	Position the patient seated or standing. Use one hand to support the patient's elbow in a position of 90 degrees of flexion, with the patient's forearm resting in a neutral position over your forearm (see Figure 13-8b). Using the wide side of the reflex hammer's head, strike the brachioradialis tendon approximately 3 inches above the wrist. Perform the test bilaterally for comparison.	Striking the brachioradialis tendon normally produces supination of the forearm.
Triceps (C7)	Position the patient seated or standing. Support the patient's arm in approximately 30 degrees of shoulder extension with the elbow flexed approximately 90 degrees (see Figure 13-8c). Using the wide side of the reflex hammer's head, strike the triceps tendon just proximal to its insertion on the olecranon process. Perform the test bilaterally for comparison.	Normally, the triceps should contract or twitch slightly.

continued

Table 13-4 (continued)

Assessment of Deep Tendon Reflexes

Reflex (Spinal Level)	Instructions for Assessment	Normal Response
Patellar (L2-4)	Position the patient seated on the edge of the table with the legs hanging off the edge. Palpate the patellar tendon just distal to the inferior pole of the patella. Using the wide side of the reflex hammer's head, strike the patellar tendon distal to the inferior pole of the patella (see Figure 13-8d). Perform the test bilaterally for comparison.	The knee should move slightly into extension.
Achilles (S1)	Position the patient seated on the edge of the table with the legs hanging off the edge. Palpate the Achilles tendon in the posterior ankle. Lift the patient's foot into a neutral or slightly dorsiflexed position. Using the wide side of the reflex hammer's head, strike the Achilles tendon just proximal to its insertion onto the calcaneus (see Figure 13-8e). Perform the test bilaterally for comparison.	Normally, the foot should plantarflex slightly when the Achilles tendon is struck. The examiner should be able to palpate this response.

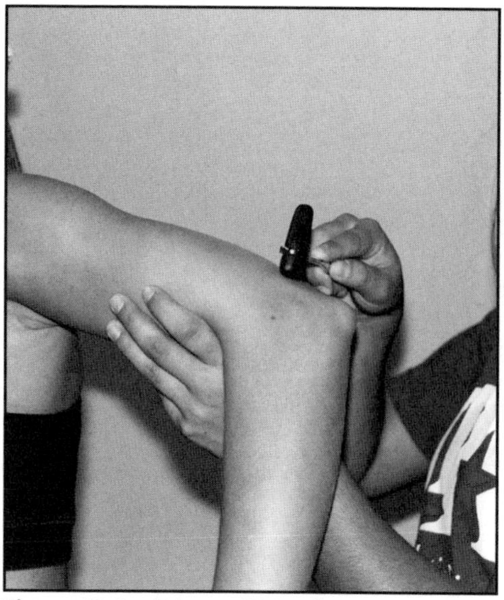

Figure 13-8c. Triceps (C7) reflex testing.

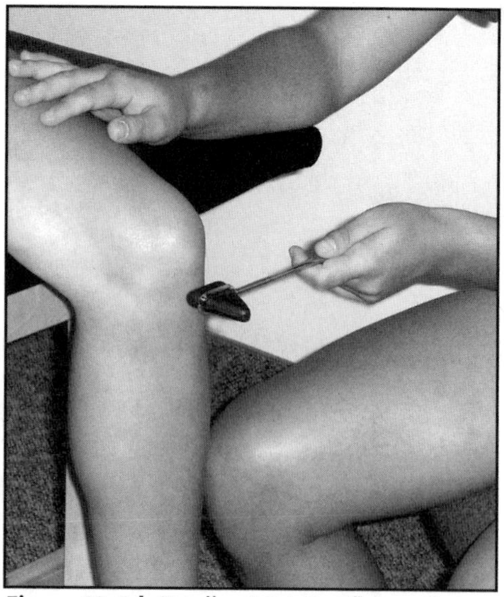

Figure 13-8d. Patellar (L2-L4) reflex testing.

Figure 13-8e. Achilles (S1) reflex testing.

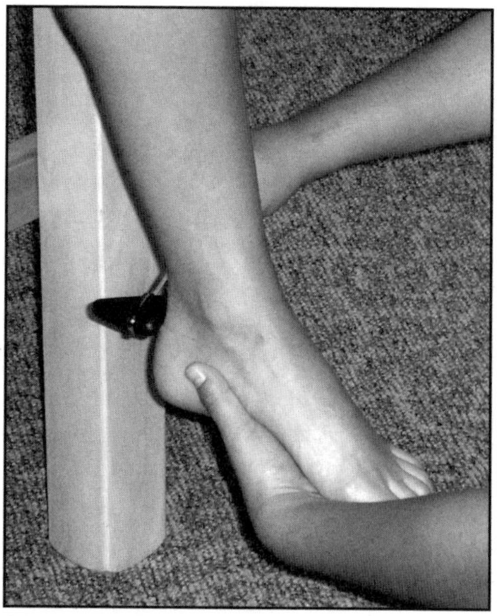

Disruption of the long motor tracts, the cerebral cortex motor neuron pathways, may be evaluated with the *Babinski test* (Figures 13-9a and 13-9b). This test is performed with the patient laying supine. Using a blunt object, such as a pen or the end of reflex hammer, the bottom of the foot is stroked from the heel to the lateral border of the foot over the ball of the foot to the great toe. Normally, this test will cause the toes to flex. A positive Babinski sign (extension of the great toe with flex-

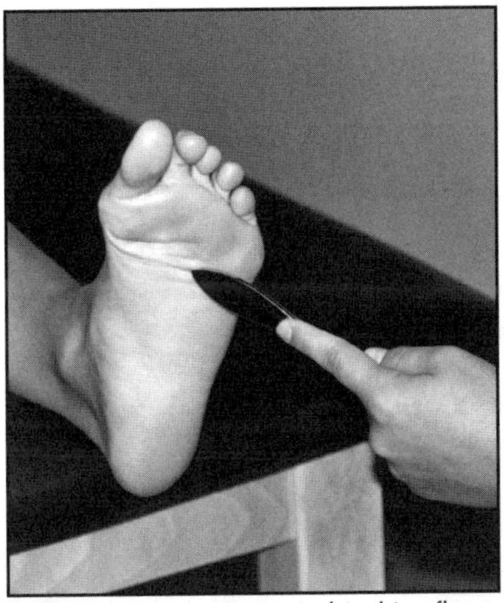

Figure 13-9a. Negative Babinski reflex.

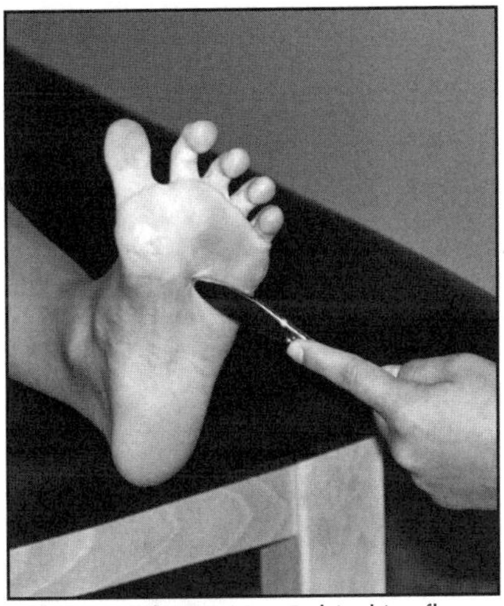

Figure 13-9b. Positive Babinski reflex.

ion and abduction of the other toes) indicates an upper motor neuron lesion (injury involving the brain or spinal cord). *Clonus*, another abnormal reflex, may be found at the ankle and occasionally the wrist. The test is conducted by quickly moving and maintaining the foot (or hand) into end-range dorsiflexion (or extension). A low-amplitude, involuntary oscillation of the foot or hand is abnormal and suggests an upper motor neuron disorder.

Meningeal Irritation

The meninges can become inflamed with certain pathologies including meningitis, vertebral disc pathology, or other conditions causing inflammation in the spinal canal. The *Kernig* and *Brudzinski* tests can be used to assess for inflammation. Both tests begin with the subject in supine. For the Kernig test, the head is raised, either actively or passively (Figure 13-10). Burning or shooting pains in the spine is a positive sign. The Brudzinski (or "straight leg raise") test involves passively raising one leg at a time, keeping the knee fully extended (Figure 13-11). At the first sign of pain in the leg or back, the knee is slightly flexed until the symptoms are relieved. The ankle is then passively dorsiflexed, which should reproduce the symptoms if meningeal irritation is present. Alternately, the head can be raised after knee flexion, which will again reproduce symptoms. If dorsiflexion and head flexion do not reproduce the symptoms, the pain is more likely from leg or back muscles. Both tests slightly stretch the lower extremity peripheral nerves and nerve roots, which creates tension on the meninges.

Balance and Coordination

Balance and coordination tests are usually conducted following head trauma to assess the extent of injury or recovery. An athletic trainer may also document status of a known neuromotor disorder by using such tests.

The *Romberg test* is used to assess vestibular and postural control. The subject stands relaxed with feet together and eyes closed, with the examiner nearby for

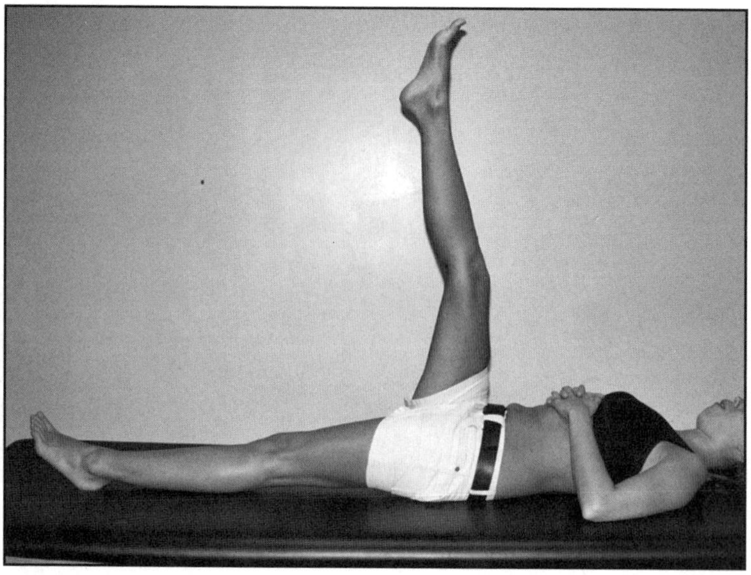

Figure 13-10. Kernig test.

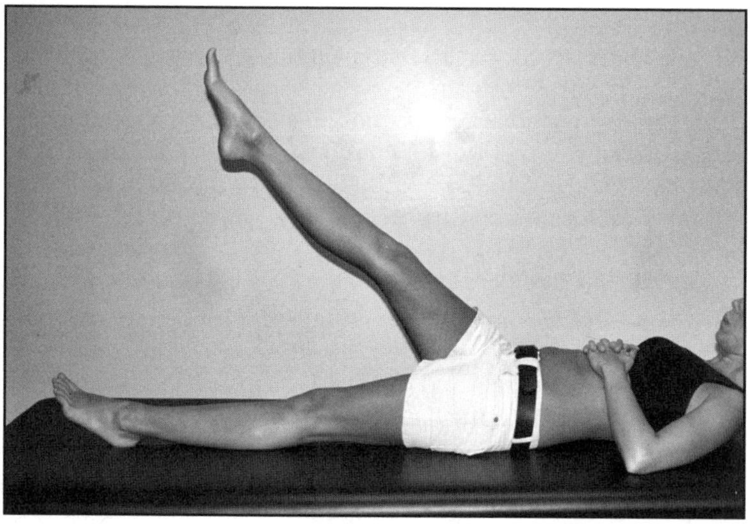

Figure 13-11. Brudzinski test.

safety. Loss of balance or significant swaying suggests neurological impairment. A variation of this test can be performed with the arms positioned in 90 degrees of abduction.

Voluntary movement coordination is assessed with two tests. The first involves the person rapidly moving their finger back and forth from their nose to a target, such as the examiner's finger. This can be done with the eyes open, then repeated with the eyes closed. Inability to contact the target consistently (after a few practice trials) indicates possible cerebellum or basal ganglia disorders. A second test is rapid pronation and supination of both hands, first "in phase" (both pronating and supinating together) and then "out of phase" (one hand pronating while the other supinates). Inability to perform and maintain either task for several seconds indicates a possible cerebellum disorder. If these balance or coordination tests are positive, further testing by a physician is indicated.

Cranial Nerves

Cranial nerve function indicates the status of the medulla oblongata and can be easily and quickly tested both in the athletic training facility and on a sports sideline. Table 13-2 provides a listing of the 12 cranial nerves, their normal function, and the steps to follow when assessing for injury or illness. (Lab Exercise 13-4 provides an opportunity to practice cranial nerve assessment.) Any sign of cranial nerve impairment suggests injury or disease and requires urgent medical referral. If any cranial nerve functions are rapidly declining, the situation is a medical emergency.

Cognitive Function

Cognitive function (memory and attention) can be quickly assessed through several screening exams. To assess the patient's orientation to person, place, and time, the athletic trainer can ask simple questions like, "What month is it?", "What is your name?", "What city do you live in?" A patient's ability to focus attention can be assessed with a simple serial test, such as counting down from 100 by 7 (*Serial 7s*) or 3 (*Serial 3s*). Memory can be assessed by asking the patients about events that occurred just prior to the head injury. Inability to remember these events indicates *retrograde amnesia*. Inability to recall events after the head injury suggests *anterograde amnesia* and can be assessed using tests such as the *3 or 5 Object Recall*. To perform this test, the athletic trainer gives the patient a list of three to five unrelated words (eg, dog, cat, blue, summer, football). To test immediate recall, the athletic trainer immediately asks the patient to repeat the words. To test delayed recall, the athletic trainer should wait 2 to 3 minutes and then ask the patient to once again repeat the words. Inability to correctly list the given words represents a positive test and warrants medical referral.

More and more athletic trainers are also beginning to use standardized, objective screening instruments to establish a cognitive baseline measure, providing a benchmark for comparison after injury.[3] The Standardized Assessment of Concussion (SAC) is one example of a standardized, cognitive test. This screening tool is easy to administer in the athletic training facility or on the sideline and has been shown to be accurate in identifying head injured athletes.

Pathology and Pathogenesis

The cerebrum, midbrain, cerebellum, medulla (brainstem), spinal cord, and associated structures (thalamus, hypothalamus, basal ganglia, pons, etc) may be damaged in a number of ways, including trauma, vascular compromise, anoxia, toxicity, and disease (degeneration, cancer, etc). Table 13-5 lists possible etiology and associated signs and symptoms by location for the CNS. Common neurological pathology is discussed below and is categorized as those conditions affecting the CNS, those affecting the PNS, and those that affect both systems simultaneously.

Central Nervous System Disorders

Cerebrovascular Events

Vascular injury (eg, stroke, aneurysm, trauma) in the CNS affects the structures supplied by the respective vessels. Signs and symptoms associated with these events appear from the neural region or structures that the vessels supply.

Table 13-5

Central Nervous System Structure, Potential Pathogenesis, and Signs and Symptoms

Structure	Potential Pathogenesis	Signs and Symptoms
Cerebrum	Cerebral palsy/anoxia, vascular, cancer, trauma, degenerative	Altered cognition, disorientation, behavioral changes, difficulty initiating movements
Basal ganglia	Vascular, degenerative, cancer	Resting tremor or movements, rigidity, wild unintentional movements
Midbrain and medulla	Vascular, trauma, multiple sclerosis	Altered breathing and cranial nerve signs
Cerebellum	Vascular, degenerative, trauma	Ataxia, intention tremor, inability to move to target, inability to rapidly alternate movement, lack of coordination or balance
Spinal cord	Trauma, vascular, cancer, lateral sclerosis, multiple sclerosis, infection	Weakness/flaccidity, atrophy, hypertonia or hypotonia or both

Strokes are the leading cause of brain injury in adults, with approximately 500,000 cases reported annually.[4] Strokes occur when blood vessels within the brain become blocked or burst. Bleeding from these injuries can accumulate in the cranium and compress the brain. The blood also stimulates an inflammatory response, causing secondary hypoxia in surrounding neural tissue, which leads to tissue necrosis.

General signs and symptoms of a stroke include severe headache, facial weakness or drooping, slurred speech, incoordination or weakness on one side of the body, poor balance, double vision, unilateral hearing loss, photophobia, nausea, vomiting, or loss of or altered consciousness.

Early detection is the key to optimum treatment of strokes; therefore, anyone suspected of having a stroke should be immediately transported to the nearest emergency room. New fibrinolytic drugs are being used successfully with some stroke victims to decrease the disability from a stroke and improve the quality of life. However, these drugs must be administered within 3 to 6 hours of the onset of symptoms.

Cerebral aneurysms are weak or thin spots within a blood vessel in the brain. Pressure within the vessel can cause bulging of a vessel wall, which can put pressure on the nerves within the brain. Aneurysms can also burst causing bleeding within the brain. Unfortunately, in most cases, aneurysms do not present with neurological symptoms until they become very large or burst. If symptoms are present, they will include severe headache, pain above or behind the eye, vision changes, numbness or weakness of one side of the face, and dilation of pupils.[5]

As with stroke, persons suspected of having a cerebral aneurysm should be referred immediately to the nearest hospital. Prognosis is much better when aneurysms can be detected before they burst. Accurate detection will require medical imaging such as MRI, CT scan, or angiography (a dye test used to visualize arteries and veins).

Headaches

Headaches can be caused by several neurovascular problems. A *migraine headache* causes intense throbbing pain, usually unilaterally, with associated symptoms of nausea, vomiting, photophobia (aversion to light), and phonophobia (aversion to sound).[6] For many patients, migraine headaches are precipitated by an aura which will typically present with flashes of light or bright colored or white spots. Many who suffer migraines have a positive family history. The causes and mechanisms of migraine headaches are poorly understood, but may be related to alterations in the neurotransmitter serotonin, inflammatory effects on the trigeminal nerve complex, or hormonal variations. Other triggers can include stress, lack of sleep, smoking, and the use of alcohol, particularly red wine. If the underlying mechanism of a patient's migraine headaches can be identified, avoidance of these triggers can help prevent future attacks. Medications are commonly used to treat migraine headaches. Many patients also find it beneficial to withdraw to a dark room and sleep.

A *cluster headache* is an intense, gnawing pain that is deep and non-throbbing in nature, occurring unilaterally around one eye. Lacrimation (tearing), rhinorrhea ("runny nose") or nasal congestion, diaphoresis, unilateral pupillary constriction (miosis), ptosis (drooping eyelid), and psychomotor agitation may also be present as a result of trigeminal nerve and parasympathetic involvement.[7] A cluster headache episode lasts up to 45 minutes and may recur on a daily basis; the defining characteristic is the recurrence of the headache across several days followed by a long period with no headache.[6] Common exacerbating factors include psychoemotional stress and alcohol or tobacco use. Similar to migraines, the etiology and pathophysiology of cluster headaches are not well understood, but may be related to neurovascular, hormonal, or autonomic nervous system abnormalities. Cluster headaches are most commonly treated with two types of medication: one to reduce the number of headaches and the second to reduce the severity of a headache when it occurs. Because cluster headaches come on very quickly, the pain-relieving medication may be administered via inhaler or injection to ensure quick action.

A *toxic vascular headache* presents diffuse, throbbing, severe pain over the entire crown of the head; this type of headache is never unilateral.[6] Etiology includes infection (usually accompanied by fever), caffeine abuse or withdrawal, alcohol abuse or withdrawal (hangover), hypoxia, hypoglycemia (low blood sugar), and metabolic disorders.[6]

Persons with vascular headaches are awake and alert, have no fever, and demonstrate a negative neurological examination.[6] Treatment consists of rest in a quiet, dark room and prescription medication if the headaches are recurrent and disabling. If other systemic signs occur simultaneously with a severe headache, emergency medical attention is required.

Brain Trauma

A *concussion* occurs when the brain collides with the cranium, either at the site of head impact or opposite the site of impact when the brain, suspended in cerebral spinal fluid, shifts within the cranium (contrecoup injury). Trauma can temporarily disrupt neural function, alter consciousness or orientation, cause a hematoma with-

Table 13-6

General Signs and Symptoms of a Concussion

- Headache
- Confusion or disorientation
- Dizziness or lack of balance
- Loss of memory (retrograde amnesia: memory of events prior to head injury; anterograde amnesia: memory of events after a head injury)
- Change in pupil reaction to light
- Unequal pupils
- Nausea and/or vomiting
- Ringing in the ears
- Loss of consciousness (depending on the degree of injury)

in the brain tissue, or cause structural damage to neurons. It is important to assess neurological function (cranial nerve assessment) not only at the time of injury, but also at regular intervals for several days. Reevaluation every few minutes for several hours may be necessary in cases of complete loss of consciousness. Reevaluation at least every 15 to 30 minutes for two hours and every 4 to 6 hours for 2 days is prudent following a head injury of any severity.

There are several grading scales in the literature that have been commonly used to grade concussion injuries. Currently, there are three main approaches to grading concussions: (1) grading the concussion during the initial evaluation, (2) grading the concussion after the resolution of all symptoms, and (3) not grading the injury, but rather focusing instead on the patient's recovery as determined by symptoms, cognitive testing, and postural-stability testing. The athletic trainer and team physician should decide on the approach to be followed and then be consistent in its use.

Epidural or Subdural Hematoma

Rupture of cranial or brain blood vessels can cause epidural and subdural hematomas. Bleeding from a damaged vessel occurs either outside of the dura mater (epidural) or between the dura mater and arachnoid mater (subdural). As the hematoma expands in the limited space of the cranium, the brain tissue is compressed and begins to fail.

Epidural hematomas are formed by arterial bleeding and therefore may occur within hours of the head injury. Although individuals with a developing epidural hematoma may initially have been knocked unconscious or show signs and symptoms of concussion (Table 13-6), they will usually also have had a short period of very lucid (mentally clear) consciousness. This period of lucidness can be misleading and remove suspicion of a serious head injury. As mentioned previously, all individuals who suffer a head injury should be monitored closely. As the pressure of the hematoma builds within the cranium, the individual may report a headache with increasing intensity, common concussion signs and symptoms (see Table 13-6), and signs of cranial nerve impairment. Epidural hematomas represent life-threatening emergencies; therefore, individuals should be referred immediately.

Subdural hematomas involve venous bleeding and therefore may take several days before signs of deterioration begin. In patients who experienced loss of consciousness, prolonged amnesia, or who continued to have symptoms at bedtime, parents, family members, or roommates should be instructed to check the person's orientation and level of consciousness throughout the night. The athletic trainer or physician should reassess the patient the following morning. Any individual who has lost consciousness should be withheld from strenuous activity until neurological testing by a physician has been performed.

Post-Concussion Syndrome

Post-concussion syndrome is a spectrum of signs and symptoms that appear or persist for several days or weeks following brain injury. The etiology of post-concussion syndrome is highly debated, with some researchers attributing it to microdamage in the CNS while others believe the origin is primarily psychological. Symptoms include headache, dizziness, attention deficits, and changes in mood. Neurological testing should be conducted to document residual deficits in cranial nerve function, reflexes, balance, coordination, and mental function, and this information should be passed to the treating physician. Vigorous physical activity should be avoided until the symptoms resolve completely. Chronic symptoms without relief in severity, frequency, or duration should be referred to a physician for medical testing.

In rare instances, acute brain trauma causes an immediate seizure that lasts several minutes. This situation is managed as any other type of seizure with emergency referral upon recovery of consciousness.

Second-Impact Syndrome

Although rare, *second-impact syndrome* can occur when an individual receives a second blow to the head while he or she is still symptomatic from his or her initial concussion.[8] This second blow may be very minimal in force or even involve a minor contrecoup injury, such as might occur from a tackle or fall. The second blow is thought to disturb the brain's normal autoregulation of blood flow causing vasodilation and increasing intracranial pressure.[8] Individuals suffering from second-impact syndrome will deteriorate very quickly (within 2 to 5 minutes) following the second blow, demonstrating both general concussion signs and symptoms and progressing signs of cranial nerve impairment. Loss of consciousness may occur very quickly. Second-impact syndrome is associated with a 50% rate of mortality; therefore, prevention is the key. Individuals should not be returned to activity when they still show any signs or symptoms of a concussion.

Recent research has shed new light on the effect of concussions on cognitive function and the concern that many individuals are returned to play too quickly. As a result, the NATA has issued a position statement regarding the management of sports-related concussion. This document includes discussion on the recognition of concussion injuries, evaluation strategies, assessment tools, return-to-play decisions, home care, disqualification criteria, and equipment issues. The key points from this statement are summarized in Table 13-7.[3] Athletic trainers should be familiar with this position statement document and discuss it with their team physician.

The external forces responsible for causing a head injury can also cause a cervical spine injury. Therefore, patients with a trauma-related head injury should also be assessed for a possible cervical spine injury. Most orthopedic assessment textbooks provide extensive information on head and neck injuries. Athletic trainers should consult an evaluation textbook for more detailed assessment of these injuries.

Table 13-7
Summary of Recommendations from the NATA's Position Statement Regarding the Management of Sports-Related Concussion

- A head injury should not be described as a "ding" under any circumstances.
- Athletic trainers should recognize the signs and symptoms of head injury.
- Athletic trainers should educate athletes, parents, and coaches about concussions.
- For every concussion, athletic trainers should document details about the mechanism of injury, initial signs and symptoms, findings of serial testing, instructions given to patients and parents, recommendations of physicians, and date and time of return to participation.
- Athletic trainers and team physicians should establish a plan for management of concussion.
- Vital signs should be checked for every 5 minutes following concussion and be monitored for several days.
- Clinical examination, cognitive testing, and postural-stability testing should all be used when making a determination regarding return to sports participation following concussion; ideally, these findings are compared to baseline (pre-injury) values.
- Athletic trainers should use only tests that have been validated and in which they have appropriate training to administer.
- A loss of consciousness or amnesia lasting more than 15 minutes requires a same-day examination by a physician and disqualification from returning to participation that day.
- Athletes who are symptomatic at rest or during exertion 20 minutes after injury should be disqualified from returning to participation that day.
- A more conservative judgment regarding return to participation is warranted for athletes with a history of concussion.
- Younger athletes (<18 years) recover more slowly and have greater risk of long-term sequelae, and therefore require a more conservative judgment regarding return to participation than do adults.
- After concussion, medications should be avoided unless prescribed by a physician, including over-the-counter anti-inflammatories. Patients may be instructed to rest, but encouraged to participate in whatever activities of daily living that do not cause symptoms. Patients need not be awakened unless there had been a loss of consciousness or prolonged amnesia or symptoms are still present at bedtime.
- Oral and written instructions should be provided to the adult responsible for the athlete overnight following a concussion.
- Athletic trainers should enforce the standard use of helmets in appropriate sports and ensure that all equipment meets safety standards.

(Adapted from Guskiewicz KM, et al. National Athletic Trainers' Association Position Statement: Management of Sports-Related Concussion. J Athl Train. *2004;39:280-297.)*

Neurological Infections

Bacteria and viruses can cause inflammation of the meninges, called *meningitis*. These organisms may enter the CNS through the bloodstream, the cranial sinuses, or after surgical or traumatic wounds that expose the meninges. The CNS has relatively few immune defenses, so bacteria replicates rapidly. As the concentration of bacteria increases, fluid is drawn into the cranium and cranial blood vessels. Intracranial pressure increases rapidly, causing compression and ischemia of the brain. In addition, the inflammatory response increases the permeability of the blood-brain barrier, allowing inappropriate substances into the brain and further increasing pressure. In response to the increasing cranial pressure, the blood pressure drops rapidly and death may occur from either shock or cerebral ischemia.

Acute bacterial meningitis, caused by *Streptococci*, *Haemphili*, or *Meningococci* species, can be fatal within hours of infection. An intolerable headache, very stiff or rigid neck, violent vomiting, and a rapidly rising fever occur and worsen in only a few hours. Altered cognition, syncope, seizures, and coma may also occur. Clinical signs include a rash on the head and an inability to flex the neck passively without also causing flexion of the hips and knees (Brudzinski's sign). Emergency transport for hospitalization and aggressive antibiotic and corticosteroid therapy is the course of treatment. Bacterial meningitis is highly contagious and can become epidemic in schools, the military, athletics, and other environments in which people spend extended time in close physical contact. Exposure to a person who has bacterial meningitis requires a course of prophylactic antibiotics and medical monitoring. Vaccines that are effective against the more common of the *Meningococi* species are available and may be useful in preventing the disease in at-risk populations.

Viral meningitis is most commonly caused by mumps, coxsackievirus, Epstein-Barr, and herpes simplex type II viruses. Viral meningitis causes the same signs and symptoms as bacterial meningitis, but less severe. It is less threatening than bacterial meningitis and typically requires only supportive and symptomatic treatment. Viral meningitis is also less contagious than the bacterial form.

Other organisms, including drugs, lead poisoning, and parasites, cause less severe forms of meningitis. Differentiating the type of meningitis requires medical procedures and laboratory tests performed by a physician. When presented with history, signs, and symptoms consistent with meningitis, the athletic trainer should document the person's vital signs, particularly body temperature, and make an emergency medical referral.

Return-to-play decisions for athletes with meningitis will depend on the type of meningitis, the degree of complications, and the time frame necessary for symptom resolution.

Cerebral Palsy and Anoxic Brain Injury

Cerebral palsy (CP) is an anoxic, metabolic, or ischemic brain injury acquired at birth.[2,9] The resulting neurological deficits are not progressive, not communicable, and cannot be transmitted genetically. The most evident and common consequences involve posture and voluntary movement, although sensory, perceptual, or mental disturbances may also occur.

Impairment in CP depends on the cerebral regions that are damaged. Motor disorders can involve one limb (monoplegia), the unilateral upper and lower extremities (hemiplegia), only the lower extremities (diplegia), or the entire body (tetraplegia).[2,9] The major type of CP is spastic and presents with hypertonicity (constant spasm). Other types, comprising less than 25% of all cases, include flaccid (hypotonia), ataxic, and dyskinetic (athetoid).[2,9]

Athletic trainers may encounter persons with mild or moderate CP in athletics or participating in other physical activities. Adults with CP may have a history of multiple corrective surgeries, or sustain overuse injuries, weakness, and impairment of range of motion at affected joints. Rehabilitation to address CP specifically is usually provided by physical, occupational, and speech therapists.

Epilepsy, Seizure, and Convulsion Disorders

Seizures result from a sudden electrochemical discharge in the brain and can cause a wide range of signs and symptoms.[10,11] They can be partial, affecting only a portion of the brain, or generalized, affecting the majority of the brain.[11] The first of the two major types of seizures is the *petit mal* or "absence" seizure, during which the person briefly loses cognitive awareness and may lose postural control. These seizures often last only seconds and the affected person may not realize a seizure has occurred. During conversation, observers may notice the person taking a long pause in between words or sentences or having a "blank" stare.

The second major type of seizure, the *grand mal* or "tonic-clonic" seizure, causes a sudden, complete loss of consciousness and postural control. The person usually falls to the ground and exhibits extreme postural rigidity (*tonic phase*) followed by convulsive-type contractions (*clonic phase*) involving the entire body.[11] In the period immediately following the seizure, called the *postictal phase*, the person may regain consciousness immediately or remain unconscious for some time after the seizure stops.[11] Seizures are most often associated with epilepsy, but may also be caused by chemical toxicity, hypoxia, head injury, and other pathological disorders. In either type of seizure, the person may experience an aura, such as a hallicinatory smell, sound, or vision, which precedes the onset of the seizure. Not all people with epilepsy experience an aura, and auras may also occur with conditions such as migraine headache.

Many people experience a seizure at some time during their life, but most do not develop a seizure disorder.[12] Recurrent seizures are called *epilepsy*, which has a prevalence of 3% across the population.[10] Most people with epilepsy experience seizures before 30 years of age.[10] If an athlete reports a history of epilepsy, the athletic trainer should note the medications used and their side effects, the frequency of seizures, and the nature of the seizures (petit mal, grand mal, does the athlete typically experience auras). Most epilepsy medications are tranquilizers and sedatives, which cause drowsiness or incoordination. Epilepsy very rarely causes death, although frequent seizures increase the risk of accidents.

Although many persons with epilepsy do not participate in competitive sports, there is no medical reason they could not do so. People with epilepsy are, in general, not at higher risk for injury than their peers. Exercise may actually inhibit seizures, since most seizures occur at rest rather than during activity.[10] Persons with a seizure disorder who choose to swim or scuba dive require close supervision to avoid accidental drowning. Motor sports are contraindicated for persons who experience one or more seizures per year.[10] Collision and contact sports, however, pose no particular increased risk.[10,12]

Participation in sports or regular group physical activity may provide psychological benefits. Persons with epilepsy often feel excluded because of their condition and are at increased risk for emotional disturbances and suicide. Being accepted as part of a team or peer exercise group may help allay feelings of exclusion.[10] The athletic trainer should educate coaches and peers as necessary, including the nature of seizures, how to respond to a seizure, and reasonable precautions during activity.

Management of a seizure is first concerned with protecting the person from harm.[12] Removing furniture and bystanders from the immediate vicinity to avoid head or limb injury may be necessary. Towels or pillows can protect the person's head. Nothing should be inserted into the mouth, nor should the mouth be forced open. The person may bite his or her tongue, become incontinent, or produce copious saliva ("foam at the mouth"). Turning the person to their side may prevent blocking the airway by these fluids. Once the clonic stage of the seizure ceases, assess airway, respiration, and other vital signs. If clear, begin a secondary evaluation of face, tongue, head, and joints to identify injuries. Upon recovery of consciousness, the person will be confused and fatigued, and should therefore be moved to a quiet area to rest and be reassured.

A first seizure or a seizure lasting more than 5 minutes requires a physician referral. If a seizure does not fit into the person's pattern of previous seizures, a medical referral is appropriate. Any injury incurred during a seizure should be appropriately stabilized and referred to a physician as usual. In adolescents, discontinuing epilepsy medication often is the precipitating factor for a seizure.

Spinal Cord Disorders

Spinal Cord Trauma

Traumatic spinal cord injury can be complete, which disrupts all ascending and descending tracts, or incomplete, disrupting only some of the spinal tracts. With complete lesions, all voluntary and autonomic neural functions controlled by spinal neurons distal to the injury are immediately and permanently lost. Function is partially preserved with incomplete lesions depending on the exact site and extent of damage. In addition to the initial structural damage, secondary tissue damage from contusion, inflammation, neurapraxia, and compression within the spinal cord follows the acute injury. After the acute injury and cessation of neural function distal to the injury (spinal shock), deep tendon reflexes return and spasticity develops. Clonus develops and most autonomic reflexes return, including bowel and bladder function, although sensation and voluntary movement do not.

The assessment, management, and prevention of spinal cord injury are covered extensively in most orthopedic assessment texts, and thus are not addressed in this chapter. We encourage athletic trainers to consult an orthopedic assessment text and review this information regularly.

Spina Bifida

Spina bifida describes the incomplete formation of the neural tube (vertebral arch and meninges). This condition occurs in various degrees. *Meningocele* indicates the herniation of the meninges through the defect. *Myelomeningocele* includes herniation of the spinal cord as well as meninges. Both of these conditions result in impairment distal to the defect and varying degrees of disability. They are both usually diagnosed at birth and require surgical intervention. Other medical complications, such as ventricular swelling and severe scoliosis, can occur with these conditions.

Spina bifida occulta, a condition more likely to be encountered by athletic trainers, is the incomplete formation of the posterior vertebral arch but without herniation of meninges or the spinal cord.[13] This condition is often discovered when the person has an x-ray for complaints of back pain. Occasionally, skin abnormalities, such as a skin discoloration called a "port wine mark" because of its color or a patch of hair called a "faun's beard," are present over the site of the defect. One or more spinous processes are absent upon palpation. Neurological function (sensation, reflex, motor) is usually preserved. Treatment for symptomatic cases may require trunk strengthening or, in rare cases, surgical stabilization.

Multiple Sclerosis

Most commonly appearing in early adulthood, *multiple sclerosis* (MS) is a degenerative, autoimmune disease that forms regions of intermittent inflammation ("plaques") in the CNS. These plaques cause demyelination of surrounding neurons and usually affects several regions within the CNS simultaneously (cerebral cortex, cerebellum, motor and sensory tracts), following no standard pattern.[13,14] The plaques lapse and recur, with each recurrence affecting new regions of the CNS. Eventually, demyelination causes irreversible neuronal degeneration.[13]

Signs and symptoms vary depending on where plaques occur in the CNS, but commonly include visual disturbances (diplopia—double vision—or a spot in the visual field, difficulty speaking (dysarthria), peripheral paresthesia, incoordination, weakness, and unusual fatigue.[13,14] Reflexes may increase and clonus or the Babinski reflex may appear.[14]

The etiology of MS is unknown, although immunologic factors may have a role and it occurs twice as often in women than men. Diagnosing MS is difficult and no specific test provides a definitive diagnosis. When MS is suspected, physicians will typically order an MRI which might reveal lesions within the brain. Other diagnostic tests include a spinal tap to examine cerebral spinal fluid, an electroencephalogram (EEG) and electromyogram (EMG). No cure for MS currently exists. Most cases of MS are classified as relapsing-remitting, with acute attacks being followed by complete or partial recovery. Treatment is focused on reducing the frequency of attacks and managing symptoms. Self-injections of Interferon are one example of a drug therapy used to reduce the frequency of acute episodes in cases of relapsing-remitting MS. Another form of this disease, progressive MS, is associated with more significant disability. Counseling, activity modification to avoid fatigue, exercise to preserve function, and speech therapy when needed are also essential elements in any treatment plan for MS.[13] Heat seems to exacerbate the symptoms of MS and should therefore be avoided (eg, hydrocollator packs, heated aquatic therapy, outdoor exercise on hot days, etc). Life span is not usually affected, except in the severely progressive forms of MS, but impairment and disability may become profound.[14] An athlete's ability to participate in competitive sports will depend on the type of MS and the degree of disability.

Peripheral Nervous System (and Combined Central-Peripheral) Disorders

Reflex Sympathetic Dystrophy

Reflex sympathetic dystrophy (RSD) usually occurs in the distal extremities when the CNS produces continuous sympathetic stimulation of that limb.[15] Recall that the sympathetic nervous system is the response to stress. The activity of small-fiber pain receptors from a chronic injury may contribute enough physical stress to cause RSD. Joint injury, limb trauma, lengthy immobilization, disorders affecting nerve roots, and peripheral neuropathy increase the risk of developing RSD.[15,16] In an athletic setting, RSD most commonly occurs after a severe injury or fracture is followed by immobilization and non-weight bearing.

RSD causes symptoms across several peripheral nerve distributions.[15] Symptoms include pain that is disproportional to the injury, skin hypersensitivity (even to clothes or bed sheets), and extreme reluctance to move the joint or bear weight.[15] Clinical signs include swelling, decreased range of motion, increased skin temperature, and atrophic skin, hair, and nail changes of the affected limb.[15,16] As the syndrome progresses over several weeks, atrophy and poor peripheral vascular control, as indicated by cyanosis, intolerance to cold, and pallor, develops.[15] After several months, sympathetic activity decreases and the entire limb (skin, muscle, and bone) becomes atrophic, cool, pale, and so hypersensitive it is no longer functional.[15,16]

Recognition and treatment of RSD may be very difficult.[15] RSD may be prevented by encouraging movement, particularly at uninjured joints, and weight bearing (if not contraindicated) after an injury. Rehabilitation for RSD consists of rhythmic weight-bearing, gentle joint distraction, active range of motion, desensitization techniques, and joint mobilization.[15] Transcutaneous nerve stimulation (TENS) units may be prescribed for pain relief. Analgesic medications and anesthetic injections to block the sympathetic impulses may also be used in resistant cases.[15] Persistent and aggressive treatment increase the probability of a successful outcome.

Motor Unit and Neuromuscular Disorders

The motor unit is comprised of a single motor neuron, its axon and axon branches (the peripheral nerve), and the muscles fibers controlled by the motor neuron. Motor units operate on the "all or none" principle: either the motor neuron discharges and all of the associated muscle fibers contract, or the neuron fails to discharge and no contraction occurs. Motor unit diseases can affect the motor neuron body, the axons, the neuromuscular junction where the axon joins the muscle fiber, or the muscle directly.[17] Table 13-8 outlines the neurological pathology that affects the various parts of the motor unit.

Motor Neuron

Amyotropic Lateral Sclerosis

The etiology of *amyotropic lateral sclerosis* (ALS or "Lou Gehrig's disease") is unknown. Toxic and autoimmune responses have been suggested. The disease degenerates nerve fibers and neurons and progresses from distal to proximal. Gradual, progressive weakness appears, often noticed first in the hands and arms. Spasticity, hyperactive reflexes, and tics develop as the disease progresses, followed by dysarthria and difficulty swallowing (*dysphagia*). Cognition is unaffected.

ALS occurs in adulthood, most commonly in middle age. Treatment is supportive to maintain function as long as possible, including mobility, speech, feeding, and breathing. ALS currently has no cure and half of persons with ALS die within 3 years of onset; up to 10% will live 10 years. Complications of respiratory failure usually cause death.

Poliomyelitis

The poliovirus destroys motor neurons in the anterior spinal cord, producing the disease called polio. Development of effective vaccines and immunization programs have virtually eliminated polio in America, although it still occurs in developing countries. The athletic trainer may occasionally encounter someone who recovered from childhood polio. Recovery depends on the amount of motor neuron destruction and strengthening of unaffected motor units.

Table 13-8
Neuromuscular Disorders

Structure	Potential Pathology
Motor neuron	Amyotropic lateral sclerosis (ALS; Lou Gehrig's disease) Poliomyelitis and postpolio syndrome
Axon	Peripheral neuropathy Guillain-Barré syndrome
Neuromuscular junction	Myasthenia gravis
Muscle	Muscular dystrophy (MD) Myopathy, polymyositis, dermatomyositis

Post-Polio Syndrome

Post-polio syndrome is common among polio survivors who contracted the disease before widespread vaccination. This syndrome is characterized by the appearance of symptoms two to three decades after the initial infection.[18] Arthralgia, myalgia, weakness, atrophy, and unusual muscle fatigue (and, of course, a history of poliovirus infection) define postpolio syndrome.[18] The syndrome progresses slowly and is treated symptomatically, with assistive devices and activity modification as necessary.

Axon

Peripheral Neuropathy

Peripheral neuropathy is a "catch-all" term describing many disorders of the nerve fiber. Motor and sensory changes can occur, as well as loss of vasomotor control. Sensory changes can range from numbness or mild tingling to painful hypersensitivity. Many different conditions can produce peripheral neuropathy, including diabetes mellitus, trauma, toxicity, infection, or demyelinating disease. Treatment and prognosis for recovery depend on the underlying disorder. Hence, identification of the underlying disorder is paramount.

Guillain-Barré Syndrome

An autoimmune response to viral infection is thought to cause *Guillain-Barré syndrome*, an acquired demyelinating polyneuropathy—meaning that it affects many nerves. In this disease, a sudden, disabling symmetric weakness of both legs occurs, progresses to the arms, and is accompanied by loss of the deep tendon reflexes. Cognitive function is maintained, although the ability to speak may be affected. Guillain-Barré progresses rapidly and may lead to loss of respiratory control. Anyone presenting with bilateral weakness or numbness in the legs should be referred immediately to avoid respiratory failure. Weakness peaks about three weeks after onset, but a full recovery may take months. In some persons, residual weakness may persist for years and neuropathies may recur.

Neuromuscular Junction

Myasthenia Gravis

Myasthenia gravis (MG) is an autoimmune disorder of the neuromuscular junction, where the motor neuron connects to muscle fibers. The autoimmune response destroys postsynaptic acetylcholine receptors at the neuromuscular junction. When acetylcholine is released, the decrease in receptors results in a lower than normal change in electrical potential. The decreased potential translates into inefficient muscle contraction, clinically manifested as weakness and fatigability.

Extreme muscle fatigue, double vision (*diplopia*), and *ptosis* (sagging eyelids) develop suddenly and progressively worsen over several hours or days. Respiratory muscles may be affected, and dysarthria, dysphagia, and dyspnea may occur. Deep tendon reflexes are not affected. Medical treatment consists of corticosteroids and drugs that act at the neuromuscular junction. No cure exists, although most functional ability can be restored and maintained with careful medical management.

Muscle

Muscular Dystrophy

Muscular dystrophy (MD) describes a class of genetic disorders that affect muscle fiber structure. In the most common type, Duchenne muscular dystrophy, muscle fibers progressively degenerate and are replaced by non-contractile connective tissue. The proximal, limb-girdle muscles of the shoulder and pelvis are affected first, producing a wide-base gait, difficulty with stairs, frequent falls, and difficulty rising from the floor. The disease appears in early childhood and wheelchair use is necessary by about 10 years of age. Eventually the respiratory muscles are affected, causing death usually before the age of 20.

Other forms of MD are less disabling and allow a normal life span. No cure for MD exists, although gene therapy has shown promise. Corticosteroids may counter the inflammation accompanying muscle fiber destruction. Moderate exercise to maintain function and nutritional counseling to avoid obesity (which increases demand on muscles) are recommended. Intense activity damages muscle tissue and should be avoided.

Management of Neuromotor Diseases

Virtually all diseases of the motor unit adversely affect strength, endurance, and flexibility.[19] Incoordination of posture and voluntary movements may also occur and reflex responses may increase or decrease. Many neuromotor diseases cause progressive weakness and paralysis. Weakness produces limited movement and often leads to secondary problems such as obesity, joint stiffness or contracture, and skin lesions, all of which further inhibit motion and compound the effects of the underlying disease.[19] As a result, metabolic demands of movement and activity increase significantly and may cause fatigue. Aerobic capacity or strength may not increase with rehabilitation exercises, but functional tasks may become easier or more effective after conditioning.[19]

For a person with a neuromotor disease, the qualification for participation in sports is made on a case-by-case basis, depending on the nature and stage of the disease, the desired activity and level of competition, the approval of the attending physician, and the person's (or parents') goals. Adaptive sports or activities may be appropriate to protect the participant from injury and allow a rewarding experience. Many of these neuromotor conditions prevent participation in competitive athletics, but may occur among physically active individuals.

Summary

Neurological disorders can be obvious or subtle, but nearly always affect physical performance. Pathology can occur in any region of the nervous system, including the brain, brainstem, spinal cord, and peripheral nerves. Signs and symptoms depend on the location and extent of the disorder, but often include paresthesia, weakness, change in reflexes, incoordination, dysarthria, dysphagia, or dyspnea. Head trauma (eg, concussion, post-concussion syndrome, and second-impact syndrome), spinal trauma, and seizure disorders (eg, epilepsy) are the neurological disorders most likely to be encountered among athletes. Many persons with neurological disorders participate in regular physical activity. Athletic trainers should therefore be aware of the basic types of neuromotor disorders and their effects.

Case Study

Barry is a 15-year-old male who has epilepsy. His physician has cleared him for participation in soccer. Barry had his first seizure when he was 12 years old, and he has been prescribed medication that he takes on a daily basis.

Critical Thinking Questions

1. What further information would be useful to know about Barry's seizure history, type of seizure, and postictal phase?
2. What education might you provide to Barry's coaches and teammates?
3. What is your plan for seizure management if Barry should have a seizure during practice or a game? What other individuals need to be informed of the management plan?

References

1. National Athletic Trainers' Association. *Athletic Training Educational Competencies.* 4th ed. Dallas, TX: National Athletic Trainers' Association; 2005.
2. Gould BE. Neurologic disorders. *Pathophysiology for the Health-Related Professions.* Philadelphia, PA: WB Saunders Co; 1997:320-376.
3. Guskiewicz KM, Bruce SL, Cantu RC, et al. National Athletic Trainers' Association Position Statement: Management of Sport-Related Concussion. *J Athl Train.* 2004;39(3):280-297.
4. American Heart Association. *Basic Life Support for Healthcare Providers.* Dallas, TX; 2004.
5. National Institute of Neurological Disorders and Stroke (NINDS). Cerebral aneurysm fact sheet. Web page] www.ninds.nih.gov/disorders/cerebral_aneurysm/detail_cerebral_aneurysm.htm. Accessed October 21, 2005.
6. Dimeff RJ. Headaches in athletes. *Clin Sports Med.* 1992;11(2):339-349.
7. Garten CE. Headaches and athletes. *Athl Ther Today.* 2005;10(3):28-29.
8. Starkey C, Ryan JL. *Evaluation of Orthopedic and Athletic Injuries.* 2nd ed. Philadelphia, PA: FA Davis; 2002.
9. Perin B. Physical therapy for the child with cerebral palsy. In: Tecklin JS, ed. *Pediatric Physical Therapy.* Philadelphia, PA: JB Lippincott Co; 1989:68-105.
10. Cantu RC. Epilepsy and athletics. *Clin Sports Med.* 1998;17(1):61-69.
11. Fuller KS. Epilepsy. In: Goodman CC, Boissonnault WG, eds. *Pathology: Implications for the Physical Therapist.* Philadelphia, PA: WB Saunders Co; 1998:785-790.

12. Dimberg EL, Burns TM. Management of common neurological conditions in sports. *Clin Sports Med.* 2005;24(3):637-662.
13. Gould BE. Congenital and genetic disorders. *Pathophysiology for the Health-Related Professions.* Philadelphia, PA: WB Saunders Co; 1997:97-107.
14. Apatoff BR. Demyelinating diseases. In: Beers MH, Berkow R, eds. *The Merck Manual of Diagnosis and Therapy.* 17th ed. Whitehouse Station, NJ: Merck Research Laboratories; 1999:1473-1476.
15. Kasdan ML, Johnson AL. Reflex sympathetic dystrophy. *Occup Med.* 1998;13(3):521-531.
16. Rosenthal AK, Wortmann RL. Diagnosis, pathogenesis, and management of reflex sympathetic dystrophy syndrome. *Compr Ther.* 1991;17(6):46-50.
17. Homnick DN, Marks JH. Exercise and sports in the adolescent with chronic pulmonary disease. *Adolesc Med.* 1998;9(3):467-481.
18. Smith MB. The peripheral nervous system. In: Goodman CC, Boissonnault WG, eds. *Pathology: Implications for the Physical Therapist.* Philadelphia, PA: WB Saunders Co; 1998:811-837.
19. Small E, Bar-Or O. The young athlete with chronic disease. *Clin Sports Med.* 1995;14(3):709-726.

Online Resources

National Institutes of Neurological Disorders and Stroke

www.ninds.nih.gov

Lab Exercise 13-1
Assessment of Sensory Function

Objectives

After completing this lab exercise, students will be able to:

1. Perform a sensory assessment for the lower extremity.
2. Perform a sensory assessment for the upper extremity.

Competencies

This lab exercise addresses the following psychomotor competencies from the NATA's *Athletic Training Educational Competencies, 4th ed*:

- Orthopedic Clinical Examination and Diagnosis: 9

Equipment Needed

- Cotton ball or cotton-tipped applicator
- Safety pin (can also use straight pin)
- Neurological hammer with brush and pin (can be used in place of the items listed above)
- Paper clip or two-point discriminator calipers
- Tuning fork

Introduction

Injury or illness involving the spinal nerve roots or peripheral nerves can result in a loss of neurological function (ie, sensory, motor, or reflex function). This lab exercise provides the opportunity to practice upper and lower extremity sensory evaluation techniques including the assessment of light touch, pain, two-point discrimation, and vibration sense.

Part 1: Light Touch

Light touch sensation can be evaluated using a cotton ball, the soft end of a cotton-tipped applicator, the brush from a neurological hammer, or a finger. Sensory assessment should follow the dermatomal patterns produced by the spinal and peripheral nerves. It is recommended that you review these sensory distributions (see Figures 13-3 and 13-4) before you begin this lab.

All light touch sensory assessment should be performed bilaterally and include each nerve distribution area. When assessing light touch, instruct the patient to close his or her eyes so that he or she cannot see where you are touching. As you touch within each nerve distribution area, ask the patient if he or she can feel you touching him or her. To validate the patient's responses, you may want to occasionally ask the patient if he or she feels anything when you have not touched him or her. Starting proximally, test each sensation area moving in a distal direction. Test results should be recorded as normal (N), reduced (R), or absent (A).

You should become comfortable with performing a complete sensory assessment following a set sequence from proximal to distal; however, you should also be able to distinguish individual nerve distribution sites should you identify an area of sensory loss.

Lab Exercise 13-1 (continued)
Assessment of Sensory Function

1. Practice with your lab partner until you can easily and accurately perform a complete sensory assessment of the upper extremity following a set sequence from proximal to distal.
   C5
   C6
   C7
   C8
   T1

2. Practice with your lab partner until you can easily and accurately perform a complete sensory assessment of the lower extremity following a set sequence from proximal to distal.
   L1
   L2
   L3
   L4
   L5
   S1

3. Once comfortable with the location and sequence of the nerve root distribution patterns, have your lab partner test you on your knowledge of the individual nerve root distributions. Following the random order below, perform a light sensory assessment at each nerve distribution site. Your partner should provide feedback as to your performance (ie, correct or incorrect).

Nerve	**Correct (Y/N)**
C8	_____
L2	_____
L5	_____
C5	_____
S1	_____
T1	_____
C7	_____
L4	_____
C6	_____
L1	_____
L3	_____

____
Lab Partner's Signature

Lab Exercise 13-1 (continued)
Assessment of Sensory Function

Part 2: Pain Sensation

The relative sharpness or dullness of pain can be evaluated using a safety pin or the pin from a neurological hammer. Lightly touch each nerve distribution area with the pin comparing bilaterally at each site. You should ask "Does this feel the same as this?" You should be consistent in the degree of pressure applied with the pen from side to side. Then ask the patient to turn his or her palms upward and to close his or her eyes. Lightly touch the distal pad of the index finger with the pin, randomly alternating between the sharp and dull end of the pin. Ask the patient "Tell me what you feel, dull or sharp."

1. Using the pin, practice the bilateral comparison within each nerve distribution site of the upper extremity with your lab partner.
   C5
   C6
   C7
   C8
   T1

2. Using the pin, practice the bilateral comparison within each nerve distribution site of the lower extremity with your lab partner.
   L1
   L2
   L3
   L4
   L5
   S1

3. Practice the assessment of dull and sharp pain sensation with your lab partner. Have him or her close his or her eyes.
   a. While lightly touching the distal pad of the index finger, alternate the use of the sharp and dull end of the pin. Perform this assessment bilaterally.
   b. While lightly touching the distal pad of the great toe, alternate the use of the sharp and dull end of the pin. Perform this assessment bilaterally.

Lab Exercise 13-1 (continued)
Assessment of Sensory Function

Part 3: Vibration Sensation

Vibration sense is evaluated using a tuning fork. In the upper extremity, vibration sense is evaluated over the distal pad of the index finger. The distal pad of the great toe is used to assess vibration sense in the lower extremity. The tuning fork should always be placed over soft tissue rather than bone. Bone transmits the vibration more proximally rather than isolating the distal segment. First, strike the double end of the tuning fork on the heel of your hand, then touch the single end of the fork on the soft tissue area to be tested. When performing the test, the patient's eyes should again be closed. Ask the patient "Do you feel this? How about this?" Randomly stop the vibration of the fork with your other hand and then touch the test area.

1. Practice the assessment of vibration sense in the upper extremity with your lab partner.
2. Practice the assessment of vibration sense in the lower extremity with your lab partner.

Part 4: Two-Point Discrimination

Two-point discrimination can be evaluated using special two-point calipers or a bent paper clip. Like the vibration test, this test is typically performed at the distal segment over the distal pad of the index finger and the great toe. Once again, the patient's eyes should be closed. While randomly alternating the use of one point or two, ask the patient to tell you how many points he or she feels. The shortest distance at which the patient can distinguish two points should be measured in millimeters and compared to the contralateral side.

1. Practice the upper extremity two-point discrimination test with your lab partner. Compare bilaterally.
2. Practice the lower extremity two-point discrimination test with your lab partner. Compare bilaterally.

Lab Exercise 13-2
Assessment of Motor Function

Objectives

After completing this lab exercise, students will be able to:

1. Perform a neurological motor assessment of the upper extremity.
2. Perform a neurological motor assessment of the lower extremity.

Competencies

This lab exercise addresses the following psychomotor competencies from the NATA's *Athletic Training Educational Competencies, 4th ed*:

- Orthopedic Clinical Examination and Diagnosis: 9

Equipment Needed

- Examination table

Introduction

Injury or illness involving the spinal nerve roots or peripheral nerves can result in a loss of neurological function (ie, sensory, motor, or reflex function). As discussed in the chapter, neurological signs and symptoms include numbness, tingling, burning, or unexplained muscle weakness and can indicate nerve root impingement associated with disc pathology, peripheral nerve damage, cervical or lumbar spine injury, or disease involving the central nervous system. The motor exam primarily involves testing for myotomal weakness (see Table 13-3). The function of motor nerves is tested by asking the patient to contract specific muscle groups as the examiner provides resistance. Muscle strength can be tested through the entire range of motion or by using a break test. Weakness is noted by comparing to the same muscle on the contralateral side. This lab exercise provides the opportunity to practice both upper and lower extremity motor evaluation techniques.

Part 1: Upper Extremity

Upper extremity motor function is evaluated by testing the following nerve roots or peripheral nerves.

Nerve Root	Peripheral Nerve	Motor Function
C5	Axillary nerve	Shoulder abductors
C6	Musculocutaneous nerve	Elbow flexors or wrist extensors
C7	Radial	Elbow extensors or wrist flexors
C8	Median and palmar interosseous nerve	Finger flexors
T1	Ulnar	Finger abductors

Again, you should become comfortable with performing a complete upper extremity motor assessment following a set sequence from proximal to distal; however, you should also be able to distinguish individual nerve distribution sites. You should be consistent in your technique (resistance applied through range of motion or break test) throughout the motor exam.

Lab Exercise 13-2 (continued)
Assessment of Motor Function

1. Practice with your lab partner until you can easily and accurately perform a complete motor assessment of the upper extremity following a set sequence from proximal to distal.
   C5 (axillary)
   C6 (musculocutaneous)
   C7 (radial)
   C8 (median, palmar interosseous)
   T1 (ulnar)

2. Once comfortable with the location and sequence of the upper extremity nerve root distribution patterns, have your lab partner test your knowledge of the individual nerve root and peripheral nerve distributions. Following the random order below, perform a motor assessment at each nerve distribution site. Your partner should provide feedback as to your performance (ie, correct or incorrect).

Motor Nerve	**Correct (Y/N)**
Radial	_____
C8	_____
C6	_____
Median	_____
C5	_____
T1	_____
Palmar interosseous	_____
C7	_____
Axillary	_____
Musculocutaneous	_____
Ulnar	_____

____
Lab Partner's Signature

3. Perform an upper extremity motor evaluation on three additional individuals. Using Table 13-3 as a guide, have a peer evaluate your technique with three of these individuals and your lab instructor or ACI evaluate your fourth assessment.

Subject #1________________________________ Date_______________

Motor Nerve	**Peer Initials**
C5	____________
C6	____________
C7	____________
C8	____________
T1	____________

Lab Exercise 13-2 (continued)
Assessment of Motor Function

Subject #2________________________________ Date________________

Motor Nerve	**Peer Initials**
C5	____________
C6	____________
C7	____________
C8	____________
T1	____________

Subject #3________________________________ Date________________

Motor Nerve	**Peer Initials**
C5	____________
C6	____________
C7	____________
C8	____________
T1	____________

Subject #4________________________________ Date________________

Motor Nerve	**ACI or Lab Instructor Initials**
C5	____________
C6	____________
C7	____________
C8	____________
T1	____________

Part 2: Lower Extremity

Lower extremity motor function is evaluated by testing the following nerve roots or peripheral nerves.

Nerve Root	**Peripheral Nerve**	**Motor Function**
L1-L2	Lumbar plexus	Hip flexion (in seated or supine position)
L3	Femoral nerve	Knee extension
L4	Deep peroneal nerve	Ankle dorsiflexion
L5	Deep peroneal nerve	Great toe extension
S1	Tibial nerve	Plantar flexion
S2	Lateral plantar nerve	Knee flexion

You should become comfortable with performing a complete lower extremity motor assessment following a set sequence from proximal to distal; however, you should also be able to distinguish individual nerve distribution sites. You should be consistent in your technique (resistance applied through range of motion or break test) throughout the motor exam.

Lab Exercise 13-2 (continued)
Assessment of Motor Function

1. Practice with your lab partner until you can easily and accurately perform a complete motor assessment of the lower extremity following a set sequence from proximal to distal.
   L1–L2 (lumbar plexus)
   L3 (femoral nerve)
   L4 (deep peroneal nerve)
   L5 (deep peroneal nerve)
   S1 (tibial nerve)
   S2 (lateral plantar nerve)

2. Once comfortable with the location and sequence of the nerve root distribution patterns, have your lab partner test your knowledge of the individual nerve root and peripheral nerve distributions. Following the random order below, perform a motor assessment at each nerve distribution site. Using Table 13-3 as a guide, your partner should provide feedback to you regarding your performance (ie, correct or incorrect).

Motor Nerve	**Correct (Y/N)**
L5	_____
L2	_____
Femoral nerve	_____
S1	_____
Deep peroneal nerve	_____
Lumbar plexus	_____
Lateral plantar nerve	_____
L4	_____
L1	_____
Tibial nerve	_____
L3	_____
S2	_____

____
Lab Partner's Signature

3. Perform a lower extremity motor evaluation on three additional individuals. Using Table 13-3 as a guide, have a peer evaluate your technique with three of these individuals and your lab instructor or ACI evaluate your fourth assessment.

Lab Exercise 13-2 (continued)
Assessment of Motor Function

Subject #1__________________________________ Date________________

Motor Nerve	Peer Initials
L1-L2	____________
L3	____________
L4	____________
L5	____________
S1	____________
S2	____________

Subject #2__________________________________ Date________________

Motor Nerve	Peer Initials
L4	____________
S1	____________
L1-L2	____________
L5	____________
L3	____________
S2	____________

Subject #3__________________________________ Date________________

Motor Nerve	Peer Initials
S2	____________
L3	____________
L5	____________
L4	____________
S1	____________
L1-L2	____________

Subject #4__________________________________ Date________________

Motor Nerve	ACI or Lab Instructor Initials
L1-L2	____________
L3	____________
L4	____________
L5	____________
S1	____________
S2	____________

Lab Exercise 13-3
Assessment of Deep Tendon Reflexes

Objectives

After completing this lab exercise, students will be able to:

1. Assess the deep tendon reflexes of the upper extremity.
2. Assess the deep tendon reflexes of the lower extremity.

Competencies

This lab exercise addresses the following psychomotor competencies from the NATA's *Athletic Training Educational Competencies, 4th ed:*

- Orthopedic Clinical Examination and Diagnosis: 9

Equipment Needed

- Reflex hammer

Introduction

Deep tendon reflexes are tested using a reflex hammer whose head is triangular, providing both a flat end and a pointed end. The flat end is typically used to strike large surfaces while the pointed end is used to strike smaller areas. The hammer should be held between the thumb and index finger and the tendon strike should be performed with a rapid wrist movement. Placing the tendon on slight stretch before striking it should elicit a contraction response. Reflexes are recorded as absent, diminished, or normal. If the reflexes are bilaterally diminished or absent, you can use a reinforcement technique to enhance the reflex response. When testing an upper extremity reflex, instruct your patient to clench his or her teeth just before you strike the tendon. When testing a lower extremity reflex, instruct your patient to clasp both hands together and pull one hand away from the other.

Instructions

Part 1: Upper Extremity

There are three deep tendon reflexes used to assess neurological function in the upper extremity: the biceps, brachioradialis, and triceps. A detailed, step-by-step description of each reflex test is provided in Table 13-4. Figures 13-8a through 13-8c provide a visual example of each test.

1. Practice each of the upper extremity deep tendon reflexes with your lab partner. Remember that it is important to compare bilaterally after each individual reflex test. In other words, when testing the biceps reflex, you should test the uninvolved arm and then immediately test the involved arm before testing the next reflex.
   Biceps (C5)
   Brachioradialis (C6)
   Triceps (C7)

Lab Exercise 13-3 (continued)
Assessment of Deep Tendon Reflexes

2. Practice each of these reflexes on at least four additional individuals. Have a peer evaluate your technique on three of the examinations. Your lab instructor or ACI should evaluate your technique on the fourth examination.

Subject #1______________________________________ Date__________________

Reflex	**Peer Initials**
Biceps (C5)	______________
Brachioradialis (C6)	______________
Triceps (C7)	______________

Subject #2______________________________________ Date__________________

Reflex	**Peer Initials**
Biceps (C5)	______________
Brachioradialis (C6)	______________
Triceps (C7)	______________

Subject #3______________________________________ Date__________________

Reflex	**Peer Initials**
Biceps (C5)	______________
Brachioradialis (C6)	______________
Triceps (C7)	______________

Subject #4______________________________________ Date__________________

Reflex	**ACI or Lab Instructor Initials**
Biceps (C5)	______________
Brachioradialis (C6)	______________
Triceps (C7)	______________

Part 2: Lower Extremity

There are two deep tendon reflexes used to assess neurological function in the lower extremity: the patella and the Achilles. A detailed, step-by-step description of each reflex test is provided in Table 13-4. Figures 13-8d and 13-8e provide a visual example of each test.

1. Practice each of the lower extremity deep tendon reflexes with your lab partner.
   Patella (L2-L4)
   Achilles (S1)

2. Practice each of these reflexes on at least four additional individuals. Have a peer evaluate your technique on three of the examinations. Your lab instructor or ACI should evaluate your technique on the fourth examination.

Lab Exercise 13-3 (continued)
Assessment of Deep Tendon Reflexes

Subject #1_________________________________ Date_______________

Reflex	**Peer Initials**
Patella (L2-L4)	____________
Achilles (S1)	____________

Subject #2_________________________________ Date_______________

Reflex	**Peer Initials**
Patella (L2-L4)	____________
Achilles (S1)	____________

Subject #3_________________________________ Date_______________

Reflex	**Peer Initials**
Patella (L2-L4)	____________
Achilles (S1)	____________

Subject #4_________________________________ Date_______________

Reflex	**ACI or Lab Instructor Initials**
Patella (L2-L4)	____________
Achilles (S1)	____________

Lab Exercise 13-4
Assessment of Cranial Nerves

Objectives

After completing this lab exercise, students will be able to:

1. Assess the function of the cranial nerves.

Competencies

This lab exercise addresses the following psychomotor competencies from the NATA's *Athletic Training Educational Competencies, 4th ed*:

- Orthopedic Clinical Examination and Diagnosis: 9

Equipment Needed

- Penlight
- Peppermint candy (or other item to taste)
- Isopropyl alcohol prep pad (or other item to smell)
- Snellen eye chart (or other text item to read)
- Tongue depressor

Introduction

There are 12 pairs of cranial nerves which originate in the brain and innervate the head and neck. A common mnemonic used to remember these nerves is: On Old Olympus Towering Tops, A Finn And German Viewed Some Hops.

C1	Olfactory
C2	Optic
C3	Oculomotor
C4	Trochlear
C5	Trigeminal
C6	Abducens
C7	Facial
C8	Auditory
C9	Glossopharyngeal
C10	Vagus
C11	Spinal root accessory
C12	Hypoglossal

Instructions

1. Using your lab partner as a model, practice assessing the cranial nerves in a set sequence. Your lab partner should use Table 13-2 as a guide to check your accuracy and provide you with feedback.
2. Once you are comfortable performing a cranial nerve assessment in a set sequence, have your lab partner randomly select cranial nerves for you to test. Again, your lab partner should use Table 13-2 to check your accuracy.

Lab Exercise 13-4 (continued)
Assessment of Cranial Nerves

3. Perform a cranial nerve assessment on at least four additional individuals. Have a peer evaluate your technique on three of the examinations. Your lab instructor or ACI should evaluate your technique on the fourth examination.

Subject #1________________________________ Date_______________

Reflex		**Correct (Y/N)**
C1	Olfactory	__________
C2	Optic	__________
C3	Oculomotor	__________
C4	Trochlear	__________
C5	Trigeminal	__________
C6	Abducens	__________
C7	Facial	__________
C8	Auditory	__________
C9	Glossopharyngeal	__________
C10	Vagus	__________
C11	Spinal root accessory	__________
C12	Hypoglossal	__________
		__________ Peer Initials

Subject #2________________________________ Date_______________

Reflex		**Correct (Y/N)**
C1	Olfactory	__________
C2	Optic	__________
C6	Abducens	__________
C7	Facial	__________
C4	Trochlear	__________
C5	Trigeminal	__________
C3	Oculomotor	__________
C8	Auditory	__________
C12	Hypoglossal	__________
C10	Vagus	__________
C9	Glossopharyngeal	__________
C11	Spinal root accessory	__________
		__________ Peer Initials

Lab Exercise 13-4 (continued)
Assessment of Cranial Nerves

Subject #3________________________________ Date______________

Reflex		**Correct (Y/N)**
C1	Olfactory	____________
C11	Spinal root accessory	____________
C8	Auditory	____________
C7	Facial	____________
C4	Trochlear	____________
C5	Trigeminal	____________
C2	Optic	____________
C6	Abducens	____________
C12	Hypoglossal	____________
C10	Vagus	____________
C9	Glossopharyngeal	____________
C3	Oculomotor	____________

____
Peer Initials

Subject #4________________________________ Date______________

Reflex		**Correct (Y/N)**
C1	Olfactory	____________
C2	Optic	____________
C3	Oculomotor	____________
C4	Trochlear	____________
C5	Trigeminal	____________
C6	Abducens	____________
C7	Facial	____________
C8	Auditory	____________
C9	Glossopharyngeal	____________
C10	Vagus	____________
C11	Spinal root accessory	____________
C12	Hypoglossal	____________

____
ACI or Lab Instructor Initials

Chapter Fourteen

Psychological Disorders

Chapter Outline and Objectives

Introduction

Signs and Symptoms

- ❖ Discuss medical history findings relevant to psychological disorders.
- ❖ Identify signs and symptoms of psychological disorders.
  - Change in Sleep Pattern
  - Changes in Cognitive Status or Function
  - Weight Loss and Loss of Appetite
  - Emotional Lability and Change in Affect (Mood)
  - Unexplainable or Bizarre Symptoms

Pain Patterns

Medical History and Physical Examination

- ❖ Perform physical examination tasks relevant to psychological disorders.

Pathology and Pathogenesis

- ❖ Review pathophysiological mechanisms of psychological disorders.
- ❖ Describe basic psychological concepts such as behavior, mood, orientation, and perception.
- ❖ Discuss, compare, and contrast selected psychological disorders.
  - Substance Abuse
  - Eating Disorders and Disordered Eating
  - Mood Disorders
  - Anxiety Disorders
  - Somatoform Disorders
  - Personality Disorders
  - Psychoses

Pediatric Concerns

- Child Abuse
- Behavioral or Conduct Disorders

This chapter addresses the following competencies from the *Athletic Training Educational Competencies, Fourth Edition*[1]:

Domain	Cognitive	Psychomotor
Acute Care of Injuries and Illnesses	4, 16, 27d, 30	
Medical Conditions and Disabilities	1–3, 18	
Nutritional Aspects of Injuries and Illnesses	16	
Pathology of Injuries and Illnesses	4–6	
Psychosocial Intervention and Referral	10–12	

Introduction

This chapter discusses several general categories of psychological disorders. Disordered eating and substance abuse are the most common psychological issues encountered by athletic trainers. Psychological issues can also affect the course of treatment or the outcome for a musculoskeletal injury. Control of behavior, mood, personality, and cognitive function reside exclusively in the brain. Consequently, pathology in the brain can affect psychological status. Psychological disorders may also simulate or mask symptoms from pathology of other organ-systems.

Signs and Symptoms

Change in Sleep Pattern

Psychological disturbance can affect sleep patterns, either increasing or decreasing sleep duration and quality.

Changes in Cognitive Status or Function

Cognitive changes may be noted by the affected person's acquaintances. Increased passivity or aggressiveness, memory problems, inattention or indifference to environment, disorientation in familiar surroundings, or difficulties with ordinary daily tasks (eg, misplacing or losing things, forgetting to turn off appliances, etc) suggest a possible psychological disorder.

Weight Loss and Loss of Appetite

Psychological conditions such as depression and eating disorders can cause significant weight loss or loss of appetite.

Emotional Lability and Changes in Affect (Mood)

Emotional *lability* refers to frequent, dramatic shifts in mood, such as uncontrollable laughter one minute and crying the next. Conversely, pathological changes in affect (mood) are relatively stable, lasting days or weeks. Relatives or friends, rather than the person, often report these changes. People with depression, however, often report "feeling depressed" if specifically asked. The athletic trainer may notice these subtle changes if they are familiar with the person.

Unexplainable or Bizarre Symptoms

People with psychological disorders may be unable to describe their perceptions in logical, reasonable terms. This does not mean, however, that symptoms or injuries are nonexistent. Occasionally, extreme psychological stress, such as abuse, unstable home environment, extreme emotional or social pressures, causes symptoms that do not correspond with physical examination results. If the clinical presentation is not interpretable, referral to a physician with a report of history and physical examination findings is indicated.

Pain Patterns

A person who has a somatoform or psychosomatic disorder may report inconsistent symptoms that do not match any known referral pattern or nerve distribution. Symptoms of pathology in other organ-systems may be exaggerated, misinterpreted, or ignored by someone who has a psychological condition.

Medical History and Physical Examination

Family and Personal History

Some psychological conditions, such as depression and substance abuse, have genetic components. A family history positive for a diagnosed psychological condition is significant if behavior or mood changes occur.

Known or reported abuse or social disturbances within the immediate family are major warning signals for psychological disorders. As an allied health care professional, the athletic trainer must report suspected abuse to state authorities to protect the abused person. Obtaining legal evidence of abuse is often difficult since abused persons often deny their danger. Indicators of child abuse are discussed later in this chapter.

Many psychotropic medications substantially affect athletic performance and have physical side effects. These medications may affect fine motor coordination and cause weight gain, both of which decrease athletic performance. Furthermore, many of these drugs cause dehydration and hyperthermia,[2] so exercise and fluid intake need to be closely monitored during physical activity.

Physical Examination

Physical examination findings may be inconclusive, confusing, inconsistent, or illogical when a psychological disorder exists. A person's behavior may be an indicator of their psychological status. Persons with significant mental impairment behave

Table 14-1
Mental Status Questions

Mental Function	Question	Acceptable Answers or Interpretation
Judgment	If you found a wallet in the lobby of an office building, what should you do with it?	Turn it in to security, or any other logical answer
Orientation	(Person) What is your name?	The correct name; inability to identify self indicates a serious mental impairment
	(Place) Where are you now?	The correct place; affected with serious injury or impairment
	(Time) What quarter/half are we in? What day of the week is it?	The right answers; affected even with mild injury or impairment
Cognitive	Subtract backward from 100 by 7 (or from 50 by 3)	Should be correct for at least several consecutive subtractions
Memory	List three objects (eg, elephant, hubcap, and pencil) for subject to repeat immediately and at the end of examination	Remembering any less than all three objects indicates a memory deficit

erratically, such as walking in circles or muttering the same phrase over and over, or appear confused or disheveled.[3]

Mental Status Examination

Table 14-1 lists basic screening questions that can be used to examine mental status.[3,4] Inappropriate responses warrant medical examination.

Pathology and Pathogenesis

The most prevalent psychological issues among athletes are substance abuse and disordered eating.[2,5] Other disorders may arise, either as primary (depression, anxiety, behavioral, and affective disorders) or secondary (brain trauma) conditions. Table 14-2 outlines the general categories of psychological pathology and specific disorders within those classes that are discussed in this chapter. Other than medication side effects or significant disability (eg, requiring hospital care), most psychological conditions do not disqualify someone from participation in sports.

Substance Abuse

Substance abuse crosses all gender, socioeconomic, ethnic, and geographical boundaries.[2,5,6] Substance abuse is a pattern of chemical use that interferes with

Table 14-2

Classification Scheme for Psychological Disorders

Category	**Specific Disorders**
Substance abuse	Prescription or illegal drug abuse, alcoholism
Disordered eating	Anorexia nervosa, bulimia nervosa
Mood disturbances	Depression; bipolar disorder; seasonal affective disorder
Anxiety disorders	Phobias; panic disorders; generalized anxiety; obsessive-compulsive disorder; post-traumatic stress and dissociative disorders
Somatoform disorders	Somatization; hypochondria; conversion disorder; malingering; Münchausen's syndrome; chronic pain syndrome
Personality disorders	Antisocial behavior; borderline personality
Psychoses	Schizophrenia; delusional disorders; organic brain syndrome
Child abuse	May coexist with spousal abuse or substance abuse

normal physiological, social, psychological, or emotional function, or the use of a chemical substance for other than its intended purpose. Any substance that can act biochemically has the potential to be abused, including hallucinogenics, stimulants (eg, methamphetamine, ephedrine, caffeine, phenylpropanolamine), depressants, anabolic steroids, analgesics, narcotics, cocaine, marijuana, caffeine, and over-the-counter (OTC) medications. Table 14-3 lists the signs of potential substance abuse.

Alcohol and tobacco are the most frequently used and abused drugs in America.[5] Population health effects of alcohol abuse, including drunk driving accidents, and tobacco abuse, including several pulmonary and oral diseases, are far greater societal problems than abuse of all other substances combined.[6]

Of all drugs, alcohol is the most destructive in terms of prevalence of abuse, social and economic consequences, and medical complications. Anyone drinking alcohol during or before classes, work, or athletic workouts needs immediate intervention and counseling. Such behavior is a sign of uncontrolled alcohol abuse that may lead to alcoholism. Alcoholism, the syndrome of alcohol addiction, is treated with abstinence and counseling programs, but has a very high rate of reoccurrence. Medical problems due to chronic alcohol abuse are due to the combined effects of cellular toxicity and malnutrition and include cerebral atrophy, cirrhosis (scarring) of the liver, peripheral neuropathy, myopathy, hypertension, and pancreatitis. Alcoholism increases the risk of stroke, heart failure, cerebral injury, dementia, cancer, and a host of other cardiovascular and neuromuscular disorders.

Abuse of nicotine in all of its forms (cigarettes, cigars, chewing tobacco, snuff) is also a major health concern. Although direct health effects of nicotine are relatively moderate (acting as a mild stimulant), health risks are greatly increased by chronic exposure to the carcinogens introduced by the methods of delivery, which

Table 14-3

Behavioral Signs Potentially Related to Substance Abuse

- Expresses a feeling or need to limit substance use
- Annoyed by criticism of substance use
- Expresses guilty feelings related to their substance use
- Uses substances in morning (eg, for hangover)
- Uses substances in socially inappropriate situations (eg, during class, practice, work, etc).
- Displays consistent irresponsible behaviors (eg, missed classes, practices, or appointments)
- Increasing academic or legal troubles (eg, declining grades, substance-related arrests)
- Injury as a result of substance use

are typically inhaled smoke or prolonged contact with the oral or nasal epithelium. In addition, since use of most tobacco products are socially acceptable and convenient, nicotine is abused much more frequently than other drugs. The frequency of use greatly increases the number of exposures over time, which increases the risk of developing disease. In addition to cancers of the lung, throat, esophagus, and pancreas, tobacco use increases the risk of emphysema, atherosclerosis, thromboangiitis obliterans, and stroke.

Anabolic steroids, the chemical analogs of the male hormone testosterone, receive frequent media attention for abuse among athletes. Many steroid abusers, however, are not necessarily athletes but young males who use them to enhance their physical appearance. Medically, anabolic steroids are used to maintain body weight among people with chronic, wasting illnesses. Since no legitimate uses exist for healthy individuals, any use is, by definition, abuse.

Testosterone acts on the tissues of the body by increasing protein synthesis (anabolism) and inhibiting protein catabolism. A primary role of testosterone is spermatogenesis; this function is regulated through a complex hormonal feedback system that depends on circulating testosterone levels. Regular steroid abuse produces muscle mass and strength gains, but also causes side effects including infertility, testicular atrophy, gynecomastia (feminization of the male breast), aggressive behavior, increased libido, and enlargement of the clitoris in females.[2,6,7] Chronic abuse causes premature epiphysis closure, liver disorders, heart disease, increased blood lipids, and atherosclerosis.[2,6,7]

A rapid gain of lean body mass is the most obvious physical sign of anabolic steroid abuse.[7] Discolored stripes in the skin called stria, hirsutism, severe acne, hypertension, frequent nose bleeds, and needle marks on the thighs or buttocks may also be observed.[6,7]

Some athletes abuse stimulants (eg, caffeine, ephedrine, amphetamine, nicotine, etc) to increase physiological excitement during competition.[6] These drugs act by stimulating the same receptors as epinephrine (adrenaline). The National Collegiate Athletic Association (NCAA) and International Olympic Committee maintain strict guidelines regarding the use of these agents, including allowable dosage during athletic competition. Stimulants increase energy and elevate mood, but various side effects can occur: hypertension, tachycardia, hyperpnea, arrhythmia, irritability, hyperthermia, convulsions, coma, and even death.[2,6] Many stimulants are widely available as OTC cold and flu medications, various caffeinated beverages, and certain "health" or "energy" supplements. In high enough doses, any of these substances can be toxic and most also act as diuretics.

Diuretics increase urine volume, emetics induce vomiting, and laxatives increase defecation. Athletes in sports requiring weight classification (eg, wrestling) or persons with eating disorders may abuse these substances to lose weight.[8] Abuse of these substances can produce dehydration, electrolyte imbalances, and malnutrition, and can lead to a medical emergency.[2]

Abuse of prescription drugs is also frequent. Opiods (narcotics), which are chemical opium derivatives such as heroin, codeine, and morphine, depress the central nervous system. Opiods are often prescribed as analgesics following an injury or surgery. Abusers of opiods seek the feelings of euphoria (pleasant relaxation) that can occur with adequate doses of these drugs. Acute opiod overdose is a medical emergency.[6] Chronic use increases tolerance to the drug, which requires the person to take an increased dose to achieve the same effects, and physical addiction. Both of these effects are a result of repeated stimulation of opiod receptors that decreases their sensitivity; more stimulation is then needed to produce the same effect (tolerance), and removal of the stimulation produces a physical reaction (physical addiction). Sudden cessation after chronic use leads to withdrawal syndromes that can also be life threatening.

Other depressants, such as barbiturates, sedatives, and sleeping pills, cause effects similar to opiods. Low doses produce intoxication; overdose causes depressed breathing, falling blood pressure, and shock. Tolerance, addiction, and withdrawal also occur with abuse of these drugs.

Abuse of illegal drugs, such as marijuana, hallucinogens, cocaine, and heroin, may also be encountered. Heroin is an opiod, discussed previously. Marijuana produces mild intoxication and hallucination, as well as euphoria, tachycardia, and hypertension.[6] Other hallucinogens, such as LSD, are also frequently abused. The relative toxicity of these drugs is generally low (ie, require large doses for a toxic effect), but their purity may be questionable, as with any drug bought illegally. Hallucinogens affect behavior and cognitive processing, which can increase risk of accidents when performing activities requiring coordination or judgment.

Cocaine, extracted from the coca leaf, is a mild anesthetic, but acts as a stimulant when ingested. It can be absorbed through oral (chewed leaves) or nasal (snorted powder) membranes, intravenous injection, or through the aveloi by inhalation of smoke vapor.[6] Cocaine ingestion causes hypertension, tachycardia, irritability, seizure, cardiac arrhythmia, and coronary artery spasm, sometimes leading to acute myocardial infarction.[6] Smoking marijuana, cocaine, or heroin, can also lead to inflamed, obstructed airways, similar to cigarette smoking.

Risk of cardiac death during exercise is increased by drug use, such as cocaine, anabolic steroids, and alcohol.[9-13] Specifically, cocaine can induce cardiac arrhythmia or coronary artery spasm and anabolic steroids can cause hypertrophic cardiomyopathy.[10,13] Drug abuse can also cause myocardial ischemia, inflammation, or fibrosis, as well as a host of other medical complications.[9,12]

Table 14-4 lists the general signs of intoxication, overdose, and withdrawal. Most cases of mild intoxication, depending on the drug, can be treated by removal to a quiet room, reassurance, and rest to allow the drug to metabolize. If changes of vital signs occur, immediate emergency medical care is needed. Overdose, 911

Table 14-4

General Signs of Intoxication, Overdose, and Withdrawal

Intoxication	Euphoria, decreased voluntary motor control; decreased reflex motor control (pupil, DTR), behavioral changes (stupor to raging), odor (alcohol, smoke, unusual body odor), poor judgment
Overdose (toxicity)	Hypopnea, syncope, stupor, coma, pinpoint pupils, vomiting, shock
Withdrawal	Tremors, headache, nausea, insomnia, irritability, low-grade fever, diaphoresis

indicating acute toxicity, of any drug is a medical emergency. Withdrawal, a condition with physical and psychological effects, occurs stopping use of a physically addicting substance after a period of chronic abuse. Withdrawal from physically addictive drugs (ie, alcohol, opiates, sedatives, and barbiturates) can be life-threatening and should be medically supervised. Treatment of substance abuse requires substantial physical and psychological intervention and social support.

Eating Disorders and Disordered Eating

A distinction exists between a medically diagnosed *eating disorder* and the syndrome of *disordered eating*.[14] Many athletes display behaviors that can be described as disordered eating, including restrictive diets (fad diets or extreme diets), or occasional binge eating (excessive intake of food) and purging (self-induced vomiting or excessive laxative use).

Risk of disordered eating is higher in females (10 to 1 female to male ratio) and increases with perfectionist personality, abnormal attention to body image, participation in sports emphasizing a thin body (eg, gymnastics, figure skating), sports associating low body fat with success (eg, running, swimming), or sports that classify participants by weight category (eg, wrestling, boxing, martial arts).[2,14-17] Long-term dieting (particularly during adolescence), significant emotional trauma (injury, change in coach, family problems, etc), and substantial increases in training have also been identified as factors in disordered eating among elite female athletes.[17] Other psychosocial factors are often associated with disordered eating, such as a conflicted family environment, physical or sexual abuse, inability to handle stress, low self-esteem, and personality disorders.[14,17,18]

Disordered eating often begins as a seemingly harmless dieting, such as eliminating meat or "fattening foods" to lose weight. Over time, however, a self-imposed "forbidden foods" list is created.[14] Simultaneously, exercise increases to excessive levels, often consuming several hours a day. The person may criticize other people's eating habits or begin to purge (induce vomiting) in addition to restricting his or her diet. Alternately, the person may binge (consume large quantities of food) in reaction to severe hunger, then purge in response to feelings of guilt.[14]

Weight loss, dry skin, brittle nails, intolerance to cold, menstrual disorders, orthostatic hypotension, dizziness, and constipation may be early signs of disordered eating. Although the person may never be observed purging, indications of frequent vomiting, such as fatigue, sore throat, abdominal pain, edematous face, and sour breath, may be noticed.[14] Dehydration and inadequate caloric intake increase the risk of injury or illness.[8]

If the disordered eating behaviors persist or progress, the probability of developing an eating disorder increases dramatically. The most common eating disorders among active people are anorexia nervosa and bulimia nervosa.[14,15,18] *Anorexia nervosa* has been noted in 5% to 15% of young females who have amenorrhea and approximately 1% of all females. The reported mortality rate is as high as 10% to 20%.[16,18] The hallmark signs of anorexia nervosa are a severely underweight appearance, inability to recognize self-emaciation, and refusal to maintain body weight within an acceptable range for height and gender.[8,18] Avoidance of weight gain becomes an obsession and a substantial distortion of body image develops. Among females, the chronic malnourishment eventually produces amenorrhea (see Chapter Nine).[8,16,18]

Anorexia nervosa is often episodic (ie, cycles of remission and recurrence), with severity of behavior increasing in each successive episode.[14] Persons with anorexia nervosa may purge, use laxatives, or use diuretics to avoid weight gain. Despite multiple metabolic crises, persons with anorexia often continue to exercise excessively.[14,18] Anorexia nervosa, if untreated, causes electrolytic imbalances, dehydration, endocrine dysfunction, cardiovascular disorders, metabolic collapse, and eventually death from either frank starvation or cardiac failure.[8]

Bulimia nervosa is characterized by "binge and purge" cycles recurring at least twice a week for 3 consecutive months.[16] Binge eating involves bouts of rapid and massive food intake, up to 10,000 or 15,000 calories in less than 2 hours.[14,18] To avoid weight gain, purging occurs shortly after a binge eating episode. Most commonly, purging manifests as self-induced vomiting. Other purgative behaviors include laxative and diuretic abuse (although neither actually affects caloric absorption), excessive exercise, or self-imposed fasting.[8,14,16,18] Purging is associated with many complications, including electrolyte imbalances, gastrointestinal disturbance, renal complications, and seizures.[8,19]

In contrast to anorexia nervosa, persons with bulimia nervosa often have normal body weight and do not develop amenorrhea. They express concern about their "lack of control" over eating or food, whereas persons with anorexia exhibit very strict control of their eating habits. An estimated 1% to 3% of young women have bulimia nervosa, and the mortality rate is considerably lower than that of anorexia nervosa.

Abrasions or lacerations on the back of the hand or knuckles (Russell's sign) may be the most obvious physical sign of bulimia nervosa.[19] These lesions are created during self-induced vomiting as the upper incisors cut into the dorsum of the hand.[19] Associated physical findings are erosions of the posterior surface of the frontal teeth and inflamed parotid glands (anterior and inferior to the ears).[8,19]

Treatment of eating disorders has two components: recognition and intervention.[16] Recognizing eating disorders may be difficult unless behaviors are directly observed. Table 14-5 lists warning signs of disordered eating syndromes.[8,14,16,20,21] Intervening when disordered eating is suspected can also be difficult, requiring a desire to understand rather than accuse.[14] Presenting evidence of the behaviors and expressing concern for health are appropriate first interventions.[14] Involving family members or friends in a nonconfrontational manner may be necessary. If an eating disorder is suspected, prompt referral to a physician and a multidisciplinary treatment program are required.[16,18,22]

Table 14-5 Warning Signs for Eating Disorders
• Obsession with calories and body weight
• Expression of "being fat" when not obese
• Consuming inappropriate amounts of food, high or low
• Compulsive exercise
• Expresses concern about other people's eating habits
• Greater than 5% change in body weight in 4 weeks
• Sudden changes in mood or personality

Prevention programs, particularly among young female athletes, may be useful. Effects of disordered eating on health and athletic performance should be presented.[15] In addition, education of coaching staff to avoid comments or behaviors that may inadvertently reinforce disordered eating may be appropriate, such as daily weigh-ins, unrealistic expectations for weight loss, and inappropriate weight loss plans.[16] The American College of Sports Medicine (ACSM) and the NCAA provide information for such programs.[23,24]

Mood Disorders

The major "mood disorders" (formerly called "affective disorders"), include depression, bipolar disorder, and seasonal affective disorder.

Depression

Prevalence of depression, a medical condition wherein feelings of grief or sadness impair physical and social function, is estimated to be between 10% and 20%.[25] Signs and symptoms include a loss of pleasure, changes in body weight (gain or loss), disturbed sleep pattern, fatigue, inability to concentrate, and suicidal thoughts or expressions.[25] Behavioral manifestations include isolation from family and friends, sudden changes in academic or athletic performance, interpersonal conflicts, and increased complaints of medical problems.[25] Depression is a major risk factor for suicide. Table 14-6 lists other suicide risk factors.[26-28]

Depression has been linked to a relatively low level of the neurotransmitter serotonin in the brain. Current pharmacological treatment focuses on increasing the activity of serotonin. Counseling and behavioral interventions may also be indicated.

Bipolar Disorder

Recurrent cycles of depression and elation ("mania"), both severe enough to impair normal daily life, characterize bipolar disorder.[3] The signs and symptoms of the depression phase are similar to those listed above. The elation or "manic" phase produces hyperactive motor and speech patterns, and insomnia. During the manic phase the person may be very productive. Eventually, however, this overstimulated state interferes with judgment and social interactions.[3]

The etiology of bipolar disorder is unclear, but may be related to serotonin or dopamine action in the brain, genetics, and environmental factors. Treatment

Table 14-6

Signs of Increased Suicide Risk

• Depression	• Substance abuse
• Previous suicide attempt	• Recent personal loss
• Family history of suicide	• Expression of hopelessness
• Social isolation	• Impulsive or secretive behavior

involves mood-stabilizing medication to control both the manic and the depressive phases, psychotherapy, and behavioral interventions.

Seasonal Affective Disorder

Seasonal affective disorder describes depression that occurs only during particular seasons, most commonly winter.[29,30] The relative decrease in sunlight affects the body's internal metabolic rhythm (circadian rhythm) and the production of serotonin, which works in the mood centers of the brain. The condition completely resolves in the other seasons. Increased sleep, food intake, weight gain, irritability, and mild physical fatigue occur in seasonal affective disorder.[29,30] Four times more common among females, seasonal affective disorder occurs most often in early adulthood and decreases with age. It often occurs in the more northern latitudes because of the pronounced seasonal sunlight and weather changes. As with depression, seasonal affective disorder may affect performance.[29]

Depression, seasonal or otherwise, requires referral to a physician or psychological health consultant. Artificial light exposure of a certain intensity and duration is often used as treatment, although medication or psychotherapy may be used to augment treatment.[29,30]

Anxiety Disorders

Perceived physical, mental, or emotional stress can cause a normal reaction called anxiety, a state of intense worry. Pathological anxiety, however, changes behavior or interferes with normal social function. Some types of anxiety disorders are: phobias, obsessive-compulsive disorders, and dissociative disorders.[3]

Phobias

An abnormal fear of a specific object or situation that does not cause anxiety in the average person is called a phobia.[3] Phobias are thought to result from adverse experiences during growth or stressful or emotional periods of life. For example, athletes may experience performance anxiety, where the phobia becomes so intense that performance is impaired or avoided. Other common phobias include fear of darkness, heights, strangers, closed or crowded spaces, and germs or dirt. Clinical indications of a phobia (other than anxiety) may include physical avoidance of a situation or object, increased psychoemotional stress upon mention or thought of a situation or object, or an unusual attachment to a "protective" person or place.[25] Treatment involves counseling, gradual, controlled exposure to the precipitating factor, and medication.

Generalized anxiety disorder, another example of phobia, is characterized by incessant worry about future events, self-conscious mannerisms, a perfectionist attitude, and a desire for constant reaffirmation from others.[25] Panic attacks, episodes of frequent and intense anxiety, impair daily life.

Obsessive-Compulsive Disorder

Recurrent thoughts that focus on an irrational or unreasonable fear constitute an obsession. Compulsions are behaviors that are ritually repeated, sometimes hundreds of times a day.[31] Persons with obsessive-compulsive disorder display related obsessions and compulsions, such as a compulsion to recheck the lock on a door because of an obsession with being robbed. When these behaviors interfere with daily life, the condition may require treatment with medication and counseling. Depression often coexists in persons with obsessive-compulsive disorder.[31] A deficiency of serotonin may be related to development of obsessive-compulsive disorder, although the disease is thought to be multifactorial. Treatment involves psychotherapy to modify behaviors and medication to increase serotonin levels. Familial involvement in therapy is recommended.

Dissociative Disorders

Dissociative disorders occur when a person's identity or behaviors suddenly change so radically that "association," or memory, of their "former self" is temporarily lost.[26] People with dissociative disorders often have no awareness of their various identities. Dissociative disorders can be induced by extreme physical-behavioral stress such as prolonged physical or mental abuse, severe injury, or extreme emotional states, thus constituting a form of post-traumatic stress syndrome.[32]

In such situations, the mind separates intolerable thoughts and experiences from the primary identity by forming alternate identities. The alternate identities experience and remember the situation, thus sparing the primary identity. Complete amnesia for a single event or period of time may exist, or entirely separate personalities may develop if the offending experiences are recurrent or unresolved (eg, physical or sexual abuse, overwhelming debt). Treatment of dissociative disorder is complex, involving medication and extensive psychotherapy in order to reintegrate the personalities into a single identity. Addressing the experiences that led to dissociation is a focus of treatment.[32]

Somatoform Disorders

Somatoform disorders are perceived or imposed physical disorders that are produced by mental or emotional disturbances. The person unconsciously seeks attention and comfort for an imagined, exaggerated, or artificially imposed physical problem. Complaints are often vague, exaggerated, inconsistent, and recurrent.[25] A stressful family or home environment may be a factor in these syndromes. Risk factors include overprotective spouse or parents, frequent but unresolved family conflicts, a major life event (divorce, death of a family member), or physical or sexual abuse.[25] An athletic trainer should never assume a somatoform disorder exists. If the person's comments or behavior suggest a psychological issue, medical referral with complete documentation is indicated.

Personality Disorders

Personality disorders may appear as recurrent antisocial behaviors, such as violence or crime.[25] Often the behavior continues to escalate in frequency and severity despite disciplinary efforts. A type of personality disorder is "borderline" personality, or abnormal dependence on other people for personal psychoemotional stability. Similar to other major psychological illnesses, unstable or abusive family environment can contribute to development of an unstable personality. Many personality disorders are thought to be a result of inherited traits and psychosocial factors, such as abuse or neglect. Treatment involves psychotherapy; medications are less effective because, to date, no consistent biochemical changes have been noted.

Psychoses

Psychoses are disorders of orientation to physical surroundings. The ability to perceive and interpret experiences and surroundings is impaired. Persons who have psychotic disorders may hallucinate (visual, auditory, or sensory) or display a complete lack of logical order to their thoughts and actions. Psychoses are extremely disabling and therefore rarely encountered in competitive athletics. Psychoses may be caused by a number of medical conditions, neurotoxicity, drug toxicity or withdrawal, increased electrical activity in the brain, or abnormally high levels of dopamine. Treatment is focused at eliminating the underlying cause.

Pediatric Concerns

Child Abuse

Child abuse is a familial or social disorder, meaning that the entire family is affected by the illness. Any behavior that interferes with a child's development, particularly when that behavior changes the child's personality, is child abuse.[3] In many cases, an abused child acts more like an adult and becomes a "caretaker" for other family members.[3] Aggressive behavior appears and increases, but the abused child may seem unaware of, or indifferent to, the effects of violence.[3] The family in which abuse occurs often isolates itself socially and physically, avoiding contact with relatives and authority figures. The parents often express very high expectations for the child, paradoxially relying on the child to provide them emotional support.[3,33]

Various manifestations of child abuse include physical, sexual, emotional, or neglect (withholding physical and emotional support), with neglect being the most commonly reported. Neglect is associated with parental substance abuse or depression, which affects the parent's ability to care for both him- or herself and his or her family.[33]

The family dynamic can be very complex in the case of an abused child, usually including one abusive parent and one who "looks the other way," is abused themselves, or is completely passive in family interactions. More than one sibling may be abused, and often the abusive parent was abused as a child and consequently failed to develop emotional maturity.[33] In addition, an abused child may be hyperactive, impulsive, or handicapped, thus requiring more emotional support than the parents are capable of providing. The abusive parent resents the dependency of the disabled child, which reinforces the abusive behavior.

Identifying child abuse is complicated. Suspicion should be raised under certain circumstances. A parent or child unable or unwilling to report how an injury occurred, or an injury that is inconsistent with the history may be early indications.[33] Signs of abuse include skin injuries (cuts, bruises, burns) hidden under clothing, abdominal trauma, face and head trauma, or a fracture without a reasonable history. Most suggestive of abuse are multiple injuries in various stages of healing.[33]

Signs of neglect include malnutrition, fatigue, poor hygiene, poor school attendance, and trouble with peer social interactions.[33] Discussions with the child and parents should be calm and supportive, attempting to elicit information and expressing concern for injuries rather than making accusations.[33] Treatment may involve medical treatment of injuries, removing the child from the family, family counseling, and long-term family therapy.[33]

Health care workers are required by law to report suspected abuse to local child and family protection agencies, but may feel reluctant to do so without "hard evidence." Careful documentation is essential, including history, physical examination findings, and notes of parental meetings or discussions if possible. State and local laws outline the reporting of child abuse. These regulations often include what required information and specific situations obligate reporting to a protective agency.

Behavioral or Conduct Disorders

Behavioral or conduct disorders among children and adolescents may be indicative of psychological or social disturbances.[3,25] Recurrent, escalating violent or antisocial behavior (fighting, vandalism, setting fires, stealing, etc) may be a result of an unstable or abusive home environment, poor adult role models, lack of parental empathy or contact, or substance abuse by the family or child.[3,25]

The child develops a limited sense of responsibility or consequences of behavior and a decreased ability to learn from experience.[25] When confronted, the child may blame their behavior on others (eg, "they left me no choice").[25] Treatment with medication decreases aggressive behavior. Various psychosocial interventions, including family psychotherapy, peer groups programs, and psychological counseling, address other contributing psychosocial issues.[25]

Summary

Psychological disorders, while relatively common, may be difficult to detect and may or may not interfere with physical performance. Mental, social, or emotional impairment is often as disabling as physical impairment. Understanding psychological disorders may assist athletic trainers when they work with persons who have these conditions. Changes in mood or behavior may accompany onset of a psychological disorder. Unstable family or home life also contributes to development of many psychological conditions. Disordered eating, substance abuse, and child abuse are psychological conditions that may be encountered in sports medicine settings.

Case Study

The university where you work has had several recent cases of drug overdoses and injuries related to intoxication. One of the injuries was a basketball player who jumped from a second-story balcony during a party while drunk. As part of a university-wide program, you have been asked to present a lecture to the athletes and coaches on how to recognize potential signs of substance abuse. The university would also like you to include how to recognize potential abuse of performance-enhancing drugs in your presentation to the athletes.

Critical Thinking Questions

1. What types of substance abuse will you review? Alcohol? Nicotine? What types of performance-enhancing drugs might you include?
2. What signs will you tell the athletes and coaches to look for? What types of behavioral or other problems might be related to substance abuse?
3. What will you advise the athletes and coaches to do if they suspect someone is abusing drugs?
4. What other steps or actions might you take to assist the athletic department and university to eliminate substance abuse from its campus?

References

1. National Athletic Trainers' Association. *Athletic Training Educational Competencies.* 4th ed. Dallas, TX: National Athletic Trainers' Association, 2005.
2. Macleod AD. Sport psychiatry. *Aust N Z J Psychiatry.* 1998;32:860-866.
3. Good WV, Nelson JE. *Psychiatry Made Ridiculously Simple.* 2nd ed. Miami, FL: MedMaster, Inc; 1991.
4. Goldberg S. *The Four-Minute Neurologic Exam.* Miami, FL: MedMaster, Inc; 1987.
5. Blood KJ. Non-medical substance use among athletes at a small liberal arts college. *Athletic Training.* 1990;25:335-338.
6. Felter RA, Fitzgibbon J. Drug-related emergencies in athletes. *Clin Sports Med.* 1989;8:129-138.
7. Potteiger JA, Stilger VG. Anabolic steroid use in the adolescent athlete. *J Athl Training.* 1994;29:60-64.
8. Stephenson JN. Medical consequences and complications of anorexia nervosa and bulimia nervosa in female athletes. *Athletic Training.* 1991;26:130-135.
9. Basilico FC. Cardiovascular disease in athletes. *Am J Sports Med.* 1999;27:108-121.
10. Franklin BA, Fletcher GF, Gordon NF, Noakes TD, Ades PA, Balady GJ. Cardiovascular evaluation of the athlete: issues regarding performance, screening and sudden cardiac death. *Sports Med.* 1997;24:97-119.
11. Futterman LG, Myerburg R. Sudden death in athletes: an update. *Sports Med.* 1998;26:335-350.
12. Maron BJ. Cardiovascular risks to young persons on the athletic field. *Ann Intern Med.* 1998;129:379-386.
13. O'Connor FG, Kugler JP, Oriscello RG. Sudden death in young athletes: screening for the needle in a haystack. *Am Fam Physician.* 1998;57:2763-2770.
14. Johnson MD. Disordered eating in active and athletic women. *Clin Sports Med.* 1994;13:355-369.
15. Dick RW. Eating disorders in NCAA programs. *Athletic Training.* 1991;26:136-147.
16. Grandjean AC. Eating disorders: the role of the athletic trainer. *Athletic Training.* 1991;26:105-112.
17. Sundgot-Borgen J. Risk and trigger factors for the development of eating disorders in female elite athletes. *Med Sci Sports Exerc.* 1994;26:414-419.
18. Johnson C, Tobin DL. The diagnosis and treatment of anorexia nervosa and bulimia among athletes. *Athletic Training.* 1991;26:119-128.
19. Daluiski A, Rahbar B, Meals RA. Russell's sign: subtle hand changes in patients with bulimia nervosa. *Clin Orthop.* 1997;343:107-109.
20. Teitz CC, Hu SS, Arendt EA. The female athlete: evaluation and treatment of sports-related problems. *J Am Acad Orthop Surg.* 1997;5:87-96.
21. West RV. The female athlete: the triad of disordered eating, amennorrhea, and osteoporosis. *Sports Med.* 1998;26:63-71.
22. Woscyna G. Nutritional aspects of eating disorders: nutrition education and counseling as a component of treatment. *Athletic Training.* 1991;26:141-147.
23. Otis CL, Drinkwater B, Johnson M, Loucks A, Wilmore J. American College of Sports Medicine position stand. The female athlete triad. *Med Sci Sports Exerc.* 1997;29:i-ix.

24. NCAA Committee on Competitive Safeguards and Medical Aspects of Sport. *Guideline 2F: Nutrition and Athletic Performance.* Indianapolis, IN: National Collegiate Athletic Association; June 2002.
25. Post D, Carr C, Weigand J. Teenagers: mental health and psychological issues. *Prim Care.* 1998;25:181-192.
26. Bilkey WJ, Koopmeiners MB. Screening for psychological disorders. In: Boissonnault WG, ed. *Examination in Physical Therapy Practice: Screening for Medical Disease.* 2nd ed. New York, NY: Churchill Livingstone; 1995:277-301.
27. Schapira K. Suicidal behavior. In: Beers MH, Berkow R, eds. *The Merck Manual of Diagnosis and Therapy.* 17th ed. Whitehouse Station, NJ: Merck Research Laboratories; 1999:1544-1549.
28. Smith AM, Milliner EK. Injured athletes and the risk of suicide. *J Athl Training.* 1994;29:337-341.
29. Rosen LW, Smokler C, Carrier D, Shafer CL, McKeag DB. Seasonal mood disturbances in collegiate hockey players. *J Athl Training.* 1996;31:225-228.
30. Saeed SA, Bruce TJ. Seasonal affective disorders. *Am Fam Physician.* 1998;57:1340-1346.
31. Goodman CC. Biopsychosocial concepts related to health care. In: Goodman CC, Boissonnault WG, eds. *Pathology: Implications for the Physical Therapist.* Philadelphia, PA: WB Saunders Co; 1998:9-43.
32. Kluft RP. Dissociative disorders. In: Beers MH, Berkow R, eds. *The Merck Manual of Diagnosis and Therapy.* 17th ed. Whitehouse Station, NJ: Merck Research Laboratories; 1999:1519-1525.
33. Sayre JW. Child abuse and neglect. In: Beers MH, Berkow R, eds. *The Merck Manual of Diagnosis and Therapy.* 17th ed. Whitehouse Station, NJ: Merck Research Laboratories; 1999:2300-2303.

Online Resources

Alcoholics Anonymous
www.aa.org

Cocaine Anonymous
www.ca.org

Drug Free America Foundation, Inc
www.dfaf.org/forum.php

Mental Health Foundation
www.mentalhealth.org

Narcotics Anonymous
www.na.org

National Association of Anorexia Nervosa and Associated Disorders (ANAD) (referrals to treatment and information)
847-831-3438
www.anad.org

National Center for Drug Free Sport, Inc
www.drugfreesport.com/home.asp

National Eating Disorder Referral and Information Center
858-481-1515
www.edreferral.com

National Eating Disorders Association
www.edap.org/p.asp?WebPage_ID=337

National Suicide Hotlines
1-800-784-2433
http://suicidehotlines.com (also provides a link for hotlines in each state)

Toll-Free Resources

National Adolescent Suicide Hotline
1-800-621-4000
National Foundation for Depressive Illness, Inc
1-800-248-4344
National Youth Crisis Hotline (reporting child abuse and help for runaways)
1-800-448-4663
Nationwide Crisis Hotline
1-800-333-4444
United Way Helpline
1-800-233-HELP (1-800-233-4357)

Chapter Fifteen

Differentiation of Signs and Symptoms

Chapter Outline and Objectives

Introduction

Medical Emergency

- Identify signs and symptoms of medical emergencies.

Evaluating Seriousness of Condition

- Discuss signs and symptoms of systemic pathology that are similar to musculoskeletal pathology.
- Describe the process of developing differential diagnoses for pathology involved each of the major bodily systems.

Assessment Algorithms for Key Symptoms

- Use evaluation and management algorithms to formulate clinical decisions including medical referral decisions.

This chapter addresses the following competencies from the *Athletic Training Educational Competencies, Fourth Edition*[1]:

Domain	Cognitive	Psychomotor
Acute Care of Injuries and Illnesses	16, 30	
Medical Conditions and Disabilities	6, 7, 11–14, 16–18, 20	

Introduction

This chapter summarizes information in the preceding chapters into a clinical assessment scheme. Understanding pathophysiological mechanisms and clinical presentations of various diseases is important. It is equally important, however, to differentiate a medical emergency from less severe illnesses, as well as to differentiate musculoskeletal injury from systemic illness or disease. This chapter reviews what conditions or situations constitute a medical emergency, which would supercede the need to differentiate the system of origin. It next provides a method to evaluate illness or injury by the relative seriousness of the condition. Third, several tables list conditions of the various organ-systems that may produce signs and symptoms similar to musculoskeletal conditions. Last, algorithms organized by primary sign or symptom are presented as guides to assessment and clinical decision-making. If a topic is not fully understood, rereading the related chapters or sections is recommended. In addition, several medical references that were consulted frequently during development of this chapter can provide additional information.[2-10]

Medical Emergency

Several conditions, listed in Table 15-1, constitute a medical emergency, thus requiring rapid activation of emergency medical services (EMS) and transport to a medical facility. These conditions do not require a full differential assessment since the course of action would not change. Delay of appropriate treatment, however, may cause permanent tissue damage or death. The role of the athletic trainer in these situations, after recognition of the emergency, is to provide life support or basic first aid until EMS arrives or provide transportation to a medical facility. Monitoring vital signs, treating for shock, splinting suspected fractures, and controlling severe bleeding are appropriate actions after EMS is activated. Noting the time of the incident and any known mechanism of injury may also be useful to medical personnel. Emergency plans should be established before the season or school year and reviewed regularly by sports medicine and coaching personnel.

Evaluating Seriousness of Condition

This section presents a framework for assessment to determine the relative severity of a condition, thus facilitating clinical decision making (ie, referral to emergency, urgent, or standard/routine medical care). The section is organized from most to least serious situation, which assumes the medical emergencies in Table 15-1 have been excluded during the primary assessment. Table 15-2 summarizes the assessment process when determining the seriousness of the condition.

The first and most serious pathological signs are abnormalities of the major life-sustaining functions, such as breathing and maintaining circulation. Heart rate, respiration rate, blood pressure, or body temperature (vital signs) outside the normal ranges, either high or low (Table 15-3), require prompt medical referral. Baseline values should be obtained during preparticipation examination for athletes. Significant changes from these baseline values demand medical explanation. Noticeable changes (ie, steady increase or decrease) over several minutes or hours

Table 15-1
Medical Emergencies: Immediately Activate EMS

Condition	Signs and Symptoms	Management (Activate EMS)
Rapid changes (within minutes) in vital signs	Significant changes in BP, HR, RR, body temperature	ABCs, monitor vital signs until EMS arrives
Shock	Systolic BP <90 mmHg, tachycardia and hyperpnea, pallor, diaphoresis, cyanosis, altered cognition, lethargy	Elevate feet, ABCs, monitor vital signs
Nontraumatic syncope or unconsciousness	Complete loss of consciousness lasting over 1 minute	ABCs, monitor vital signs, mental and neurological tests if wakens (urgent referral if reported by subject but not observed by examiner)
Profuse bleeding or bleeding from mucous membranes or orifices	Large volume of bleeding that persists longer than 1 or 2 minutes	Treat for shock, apply pressure points if applicable
Abdominal rigidity or severe pain	Tenderness to palpation, unusual distention, palpable organs/mass	Assess for other systemic signs; monitor vital signs
Prolonged or unexplained severe vomiting or diarrhea	Accompanied by syncope, hematemesis, fever	Prevent dehydration, treat for shock, monitor vital signs
Known or suspected poisoning	History of exposure, severe vomiting, headache, dyspnea, hypotension, altered consciousness, syncope, loss of motor coordination or control	Call poison control or read packaging if available
Seizure	No known history of epilepsy or previous seizure	Protect head, ABCs, remove to quiet area after seizure

ABCs=monitor airway, breathing, and circulation.

may indicate rapidly progressing pathology. Many pathological conditions eventually affect these vital body functions, making them useful indicators of potentially serious pathology.

Next, evaluation of brainstem (smell, vision, facial sensation and movement, hearing, taste, speech, swallowing) and neurological function (reflexes, coordination, ataxia, balance, sensation) is conducted. The brain and nervous system, like the heart and lungs, are very sensitive to changes in the internal environment of

Table 15-2

Hierarchy of Assessment for Seriousness of Condition

1. Vital signs	Changes in heart rate, respiration rate, blood pressure, body temperature
2. Brainstem and neuromotor	Smell, vision, hearing, taste, swallowing, speech, tactile sensation, reflexes, coordination, balance
3. Endocrine and metabolic	Dehydration, lethargy, fatigue, altered cognition, edema, loss or gain in body weight
4. Daily functions	Sleep, eating, urination, defecation, sexual function

Table 15-3

Abnormally High and Low Values for Vital Signs in Adults

Vital sign	High	Normal	Low
Heart rate (at rest)	>100 bpm	70 to 100 bpm	<60 bpm
Respiration rate (at rest)	>20 bpm	10 to 15 bpm	<10 bpm
Blood pressure	>140 systolic >90 diastolic	100 to 140 systolic 70 to 90 diastolic	<90 systolic <70 diastolic
Body temperature	>100°F	97° to 99°F	<96°F

the body. Thus, impairment of neurological status usually indicates a significant pathological process. Furthermore, the neurological system allows perception and interaction with the environment. If these functions are impaired, the person may be unable to walk, drive, or perform other tasks safely. Rapid changes (minutes to hours) in neurological function suggests a serious medical condition.

At the next level of severity, signs of endocrine or metabolic disorders are often subtle and therefore require careful examination. Fortunately, most endocrine-metabolic conditions develop more slowly than cardiopulmonary or neurological disorders. Potential indicators include gradual changes in body temperature, signs of dehydration (dry tongue, decreased skin turgor, tachycardia, postural hypotension), lethargy or fatigue, altered cognition, peripheral neuropathies (sensory or motor, usually bilaterally distributed), presence of edema, or a significant (more than 5% change) loss or gain in body weight. Certain metabolic conditions constitute a medical emergency, such as diabetic ketoacidosis (see Chapter Ten), but most develop slowly over several days. If untreated, however, the long-term consequences can be debilitating and permanent.

Last, changes in regulation or pattern of "normal" day-to-day functions, such as sleep (insomnia, hypersomnia, or sleep disrupted by symptoms), eating (loss of

Table 15-4
Cardiovascular and Pulmonary Disorders

Condition	Confounding Symptom	Differentiating Signs and Symptoms
Cardiac ischemia or valve stenosis	Left arm pain	Chest pain that worsens with activity; dyspnea, diaphoresis, or syncope; over age 35
Sickle cell anemia	Leg pain	Abdominal pain, enlarged abdominal organs, nosebleeds, fever, headache; African-American male
Thoracic outlet syndrome or vascular occlusive disorder	Arm (or leg) pain	Pain worsens during activity and is relieved by rest; edema, paraesthesia, fatigue in limb with exercise, distal cyanosis
Aortic aneurysm	Sudden severe or intermittent moderate back pain	Pain with mild activity or at rest; palpable, pulsating mass in abdomen; auscultated bruit in abdomen; nausea, cough, or paraesthesia
Pneumothorax	Back or trunk pain	History of chest trauma, chest pain, severe dyspnea, tachypnea, hyperresonance upon percussion of thorax, absent breath sounds
Spleen injury	Left shoulder pain (Kehr's sign)	Painful or rigid LUQ to palpation, nausea, history of left thorax or abdominal trauma

A "confounding symptom" is one that may be confused for a musculoskeletal injury or condition.
LUQ=left upper abdominal quadrant.

appetite or sudden polyphagia), urination or defecation (frequency and volume), and social and sexual function are yet more subtle and difficult to detect. A pathological condition, if serious enough, affects daily life. These effects may be the earliest indicators of a slowly developing chronic disease (e.g., cancer, degenerative neurological disorders), but are difficult to observe due to their insidious and personal nature. Taking a careful medical history is required to assess this information accurately. Any change in these activities that the person mentions is significant, particularly if accompanied by other systemic signs and symptoms.

Tables 15-4 through 15-8 list pathological conditions by organ-system that present signs or symptoms similar to musculoskeletal conditions. Table 15-9 lists psychological red flags that require urgent medical evaluation. Table 15-10 provides possible pathology by body region of symptoms, which could lead to confusion when differentiating musculoskeletal from systemic conditions.

Table 15-5
Gastrointestinal and Hepatic Disorders

Condition	Confounding Symptom	Differentiating Signs and Symptoms
Peptic ulcer	Thoracic, chest, or neck pain	Pain changes after eating, worse at night, loss of appetite or vomiting may occur; history of NSAID use, alcohol abuse, tobacco use, or psychological stress
Appendicitis	Back or right hip pain	Progressive worsening of condition, nausea, may be fever or fatigue, rebound tenderness of RLQ
Hernia	Anterior hip or thigh pain	Pain worse with activity, Valsalva maneuver, or certain postures; tenderness or palpable mass at inguinal or femoral canal
Liver injury	Right shoulder pain	Painful or rigid RUQ to palpation, nausea, vomiting, history of right trauma to thorax or abdomen
Gallstones (cholelithiasis)	Right shoulder pain	Painful or rigid RUQ to palpation, nausea, vomiting, history of intolerance to fatty foods

A "confounding symptom" is one that may be confused for a musculoskeletal injury or condition. NSAID=nonsteroidal anti-inflammatory drug, RLQ=right lower abdominal quadrant, RUQ=right upper abdominal quadrant.

Assessment Algorithms for Key Symptoms

The algorithms provided at the end of this chapter should be used to assist the clinical decision-making process. They are not intended to replace a physician's medical examination and diagnosis. If a person's signs and symptoms are suggestive of systemic pathology listed in the algorithms, the index of suspicion is raised enough to warrant medical referral. This does not mean the condition exists, only that it cannot be excluded without medical examination and testing. If in doubt, refer immediately. Record all pertinent findings in your referral report. Document your recommendation for referral in your medical record, and when and to whom (ie, the athlete, parents, spouse, etc) instructions were provided. The presence of conditions and signs and symptoms in Table 15-1 always take precedence and should be excluded by primary assessment before performing additional evaluation. Any person who exhibits syncope, rapidly changing vital signs, or appears to be in shock should be transported by EMS immediately.

The algorithms outline a clinical assessment process for non-orthopedic pathology, but they do not substitute for sound judgment and experience. The usual sec-

Table 15-6

Renal, Urogential, and Endocrine Disorders

Condition	Confounding Symptom	Differentiating Signs and Symptoms
Kidney injury	Back or flank pain	History of trauma to abdomen or back, hematuria, painful percussion at CVA, edema of flank
Kidney stone (urolithiasis)	Back or groin pain	Nausea and vomiting, pallor, tachycardia, stable vital signs, positive family history
Prostatitis	Back pain	Pain unchanged by posture; nocturia, increased urgency and frequency of urination, difficulty initiating urine stream, male over age 50
Endometriosis	Back pain	Painful and heavy menstruation, painful sexual intercourse, female over age 30
Pregnancy	Back (or joint) pain	Amennorrhea, abdominal pain, recurrent nausea, weight gain, distal extremity edema, female beyond menarche; shock if ruptured ectopic pregnancy
Endocrine disorders	Widespread myalgia and arthralgia (depending on gland and hormone affected)	Weakness and atrophy, spasms, tachycardia/bradycardia, fatigue, paraesthesias, dry or diaphoretic skin, slow healing

A "confounding symptom" is one that may be confused for a musculoskeletal injury or condition. CVA=costovertebral angle.

ondary assessment procedure of medical history, inspection, palpation, and special testing should be followed, but adjusted appropriately for the apparent nature and urgency of the condition. The information collected during the secondary assessment allows application of the algorithms and potentially better clinical decisions.

Algorithms work like flow charts. First, locate the algorithm titled with the key symptom of the patient's complaint (eg, "Abdominal Pain"). Beginning in the uppermost left corner, a list of "accompanying" signs or symptoms flows down the left side of the table, approximately in decreasing order of severity. If the secondary signs and symptoms are not present, follow the "NO" down to the next sign or symptom. When one of these signs or symptoms matches the patient's condition, following the word "YES" (ie, moving to the right on the table) provides a list of potential condition or conditions, with additional "confirmatory" signs and symptoms for the particular condition enclosed in parentheses. The recommended action for that condition is immediately to the right. The three actions are: "ER" for emergency, indicat-

Table 15-7

Neurological and Psychological Disorders

Condition	Confounding Symptom	Differentiating Signs and Symptoms
Spina bifida occulta	Back pain	Patch of hair over spine, absent spinous process upon palpation, normal neurological tests
Multiple sclerosis	Weakness or incoordination	Intermittent sensory and reflex changes, visual disturbance, unusual fatigue (particularly in heat); over age 20
Reflex sympathetic dystrophy	Severe localized pain	History of injury with joint immobilization, edema, decreased range of motion, skin and nail changes, increased skin temperature
Amyotropic lateral sclerosis	Weakness	Bilaterally symmetric weakness, hyperactive reflexes; over age 30
Guillain-Barré syndrome	Leg and back weakness and pain	Rapid progression (hours), headache, fever, history of recent viral infection, loss of reflexes
Myasthenia gravis	Sudden severe muscle fatigue	Rapid progression (hours), diplopia, dysarthria, dysphagia, dyspnea, normal reflexes; over age 20
Muscular dystrophy	Hip and shoulder weakness	Slowly progressive (years), frequent falls, difficulty rising from ground or with stairs, waddling gait; age 8 to 12 years at onset
Child abuse	Multiple skin wounds, frequent unexplained injury, or multiple injuries in various stages of healing	Inconsistent or unreasonable history of injury, behavioral problems, difficulty interacting with peers, avoidance behaviors by child and family, substance abuse in family

A "confounding symptom" is one that may be confused for a musculoskeletal injury or condition.

ing activation of EMS or other emergency plan; "Urgent" for conditions that are not emergencies but require medical attention in the next 24 to 36 hours; and "Standard" for conditions that require medical examination at the next earliest convenience (eg, the next visit of the team physician), but within the week.

Some of the algorithms have the left column divided into subsections that specify a region of the body, an event, gender, or pattern of symptoms that assist in differentiating between conditions. For instance, pregnancy is listed only under female. These left column subheadings are underlined for easier reference.

The word "AND" in all capital letters indicates that the signs or symptoms preceding and following both have to be present before proceeding to the "YES" path-

Table 15-8
Infections, Immune Disorders, and Cancer

Condition	Confounding Symptom	Differentiating Signs and Symptoms
Meningitis	Severe neck pain	Headache, fever, neck rigidity, history of recent URI, vomiting, skin rash on head, altered mental status, rapid progression (hours)
Septic arthrosis and osteomyelitis	Joint or localized bone pain	Signs of acute inflammation, history of recent injury or surgery in the body region, fever (osteomyelitis), rapid progression (septic arthosis)
Rheumatoid arthritis/ Juvenile rheumatoid arthritis	Bilateral hand or foot pain	Mild inflammation of affected joints, morning stiffness; adolescent age (JRA)
Urogenital cancers	Back or hip pain	Mild systemic signs, abdominal pain, abnormal urinary or sexual function (or menstruation in females); palpable mass (testicular or breast), testicular, male 15 to 35; prostate male over 50; cervical, ovarian, uterine female over 45; breast female over 45
Lung cancer	Shoulder, arm, or neck pain	History of smoking, dyspnea, hemoptysis, pneumonia; over age 35
Leukemia or lymphoma	Deep "bone" pain	Frequent bleeding episodes, systemic signs, recurrent infection, anemia, lymphadenopathy, vomiting; most over age 10
Bone cancers	Dull, aching bone pain or tender bone mass	Impaired or painful joint function, signs of local inflammation, or systemic signs

A "confounding symptom" is one that may be confused for a musculoskeletal injury or condition.

way. If both are not present, continue down the left column (following the "NO"). The word "OR" in all capital letters indicates that at least one of the list of signs or symptoms separated by "OR's" must be present to proceed to the "YES" pathway. All signs or symptoms preceding or following "OR" do not have to be present.

Bold words in the algorithms indicate a separate algorithm exists specifically for that sign or symptom. If a clinical decision is not reached by consulting one algorithm, another algorithm for an associated sign or symptom that coincides with the patient's complaints can be used.

Table 15-9

Psychological Red Flags

- Disorientation
- Hallucination
- Debilitating apathy or lethargy
- Severe agitation
- Sudden cognitive deficit
- Violent behavior
- Acquired memory deficit
- Confusion
- Permanent or rapidly alternating changes in affect (mood)
- Antisocial or avoidance behavior
- Behavior is dangerous to themselves or others

Require urgent (within a day) or emergency medical referral.

Table 15-10

Possible Systemic Pathology by Body Region

Location of Symptoms		Possible Systemic Pathology
Arm pain	Left	Cardiac ischemia, spleen injury, lung cancer
	Right	Liver injury, gallbladder disorder, lung cancer
Leg or groin pain		Sickle cell anemia, appendicitis (right hip), hernia
Back or thoracic pain		Aortic aneurysm, pneumothorax, peptic ulcer, appendicitis, kidney disorder, prostatitis, endometriosis, pregnancy, spina bifida occulta, urogenital cancer
Neck pain		Meningitis, lung cancer
Multiple joints or sites		Endocrine disorder, child (or domestic) abuse, rheumatoid arthritis
Weakness or fatigue		Multiple sclerosis, amyotropic lateral sclerosis, Guillain-Barré syndrome, myasthenia gravis, muscular dystrophy

References

1. National Athletic Trainers' Association. *Athletic Training Educational Competencies.* 4th ed. Dallas, TX: National Athletic Trainers' Association, 2005.
2. Andreoli TE, Carpenter CCJ, Plum F, Smith Jr. LH, eds. *Cecil Essentials of Medicine.* 2nd ed. Philadelphia, PA: WB Saunders Co; 1990.

3. Beers MH, Berkow R, eds. *The Merck Manual of Diagnosis and Therapy.* 17th ed. Whitehouse Station, NJ: Merck Research Laboratories; 1999.
4. Bickley LS, Hoekelman RA. *Bates' Guide to Physical Examination and History Taking.* 7th ed. Philadelphia, PA: Lippincott Williams & Wilkins; 1999.
5. Daly S, Holmes PA, Blake GJ, Charnow JA, eds. *Professional Guide to Signs and Symptoms.* Springhouse, PA: Springhouse Corp; 1993.
6. DeGowin RL, Brown DD. *DeGowin's Diagnostic Examination.* 7th ed. New York, NY: McGraw-Hill; 2000.
7. Gould BE. *Pathophysiology for the Health-Related Professions.* Philadelphia, PA: WB Saunders Co; 1997.
8. Jamison JR. *Differential Diagnosis for Primary Practice.* London: Churchill Livingstone; 1999.
9. Shaw M, Roy CM, Bartelmo JM, et al, eds. *Pathophysiology Made Incredibly Easy.* Springhouse, PA: Springhouse Corp; 1998.
10. Underwood JCE, ed. *General and Systemic Pathology.* 2nd ed. New York, NY: Churchill Livingstone; 1996.

Abbreviations for Algorithms

BP	Blood pressure	RLQ	Right lower (abdominal) quadrant
CA	Cancer	r/o	Rule out (exclude from possibility)
DVT	Deep vein thrombosis	RUQ	Right upper (abdominal) quadrant
EIB	Exercise-induced bronchospasm	S&S	Signs and symptoms
GI	Gastrointestinal	STD	Sexually transmitted disease
HA	Headache	TB	Tuberculosis
Hx	History or history of	URI	Upper respiratory infection
LLQ	Left lower (abdominal) quadrant	UTI	Urinary tract infection
LUQ	Left upper (abdominal) quadrant		

ABDOMINAL PAIN

Accompanying Signs or Symptoms		*Potential Condition (and Confirmatory S&S)*	*Action*
Fever	YES	See separate algorithm	
NO			
Vomiting or diarrhea?	YES	See separate algorithm	
NO			
Rigidity OR rebound tenderness OR positive "jar" test OR signs of shock	YES	Peritonitis, abdominal hemorrhage (eg, perforated ulcer, ruptured appendix)	ER
NO			
Progressively worse AND distention OR rigidity OR worse when rising from supine	YES	Peritonitis, abdominal hemorrhage (eg, perforated ulcer, ruptured appendix)	ER
NO			
Absence of bowel sounds (>3 min)	YES	Bowel obstruction (visible peristalsis, "tinkling" in proximal bowel, silence in distal bowel, status rapidly deteriorates)	ER

If none of the above, assess by the location of symptoms in the abdomen.

ABDOMINAL PAIN (CONTINUED)

Accompanying Signs or Symptoms		*Potential Condition (and Confirmatory S&S)*	*Action*
Epigastric or general abdominal			
Severe pain and hx Marfan syndrome? NO	YES	Aortic aneurysm (pulsing pain, does not decrease, cardiac signs)	ER
Decreasing blood pressure, syncope, **chest pain**, or **dyspnea**? NO	YES	Cardiovascular event (tachycardia, hyperpnea)	ER
Chronic, recurs after meals? NO	YES	Peptic ulcer	Standard
Chronic, gnawing, night pain, vague location? NO	YES	Pancreatitis or pancreatic tumor	Urgent
Burning, worse with caffeine, spices, alcohol, when supine? NO	YES	Esophageal reflux, peptic ulcer	Standard
Distention, borborygmi, usually after ingestion of dairy products	YES	Lactose intolerance	Standard
Suprapubic female (postmenarche)			
Amenorrhea and unusual vaginal discharge? NO	YES	Miscarriage (known pregnancy) OR ruptured ectopic pregnancy OR ruptured ovarian/uterine cysts (both progress to shock)	ER ER
Amenorrhea, nausea, recent weight gain? NO	YES	Pregnancy	Standard
Unusual vaginal discharge? NO	YES	Ovarian/uterine cysts, STD, UTI	Urgent
Currently menstruating, referred to back/thighs, no fever? NO	YES	Menstrual cramps (young or nonparous females)	Standard
Recurrent, worse with menstruation?	YES	Endometriosis (if unusual vaginal discharge, Urgent)	Standard
Either gender			
Dysuria or **Hematuria**? NO	YES	See separate algorithm	

ABDOMINAL PAIN (CONTINUED)

Accompanying Signs or Symptoms		*Potential Condition (and Confirmatory S&S)*	*Action*
With groin pain and **vomiting**? (NO)	YES	Strangulated hernia	ER
With flank or groin pain, incapacitating in intensity, and recurring at regular intervals?	YES	Kidney stone (usually **hematuria** or **vomiting**)	ER
Right upper quadrant			
Trauma to right side/flank AND palpable rib fracture OR positive compression test (NO)	YES	Possible liver, kidney damage	ER
AND tender, rigid RUQ, without hematuria (NO)	YES	Ruptured liver (falling BP, shock, right shoulder pain)	ER
AND tender, rigid RUQ, with hematuria (NO)	YES	Ruptured or contused right kidney	ER
No history of trauma Severe cramping and rigidity with intermittent full relief? (NO)	YES	Cholelithiasis (right shoulder pain, pain worse with deep breath, pain with percussion RUQ)	ER
Diffuse, vague pain, tender RUQ AND positive hammering RUQ? (NO)	YES	Cholecystitis, hepatitis (right shoulder or scapula pain)	Urgent

Recheck for fever, vomiting, diarrhea, rebound tenderness, rigidity, distention, and bowel sounds (see top of chart); if still negative, see "epigastric or general abdominal" and "suprapubic" above.

Accompanying Signs or Symptoms		*Potential Condition (and Confirmatory S&S)*	*Action*
Left upper quadrant			
Trauma to left side/flank AND palpable rib fracture OR positive compression test (NO)	YES	Possible spleen, kidney damage	ER
AND tender, rigid LUQ, without hematuria? (NO)	YES	Ruptured spleen	ER

ABDOMINAL PAIN (CONTINUED)

Accompanying Signs or Symptoms		*Potential Condition (and Confirmatory S&S)*	*Action*
AND tender, rigid LUQ, with hematuria?	YES	Ruptured or contused left kidney	ER
NO			

Recheck for fever, vomiting, diarrhea, rebound tenderness, rigidity, distention, and bowel sounds (see top of chart); if still negative, see "epigastric or general abdominal" and "suprapubic" above.

Accompanying Signs or Symptoms		*Potential Condition (and Confirmatory S&S)*	*Action*
<u>Right lower quadrant</u>			
Vomiting, pain originated in epigastric region?	YES	Appendicitis in "intermediate" stage (tender McBurney's sign, positive rebound) OR inflammatory bowel disease OR ("Meckel's") diverticulitis (ER since these conditions cannot be differentiated through clinical examination alone)	ER
NO			
Vomiting, positive rebound, positive "jar," rigidity	YES	Perforated appendix (shock, fever) OR perforated ulcer (drains to RLQ)	ER
NO			

Recheck for fever, vomiting, diarrhea, rebound tenderness, rigidity, distention, and bowel sounds (see top of chart); if still negative, see "epigastric or general abdominal" and "suprapubic" above.

Accompanying Signs or Symptoms		*Potential Condition (and Confirmatory S&S)*	*Action*
<u>Left lower quadrant</u>			
Tender LLQ, no rigidity	YES	Diverticulitis or inflammatory bowel disease (usually hx of difficult defecation, alternating constipation and diarrhea)	Urgent
NO		If a fever is also present	ER
Nontender mass in LLQ And reports straining to defecate small stools	YES	Constipation	Standard
NO			

Recheck for fever, vomiting, diarrhea, rebound tenderness, rigidity, distention, and bowel sounds (see top of chart); if still negative, see "epigastric or general abdominal" and "suprapubic" above.

BONE OR JOINT PAIN—NONTRAUMATIC

Accompanying Signs or Symptoms		*Potential Condition* (and Confirmatory S&S)	*Action*
Fever	YES	See separate algorithm	
NO			
Skin rash, **lymphadenitis**, fatigue, night pain, OR any other systemic signs?	YES	Metabolic bone disease or tumor	Urgent
NO			
Multiple joints involved AND significant morning stiffness?	YES	Rheumatoid arthritis, juvenile RA (age <20 years)	Standard
NO			
Recent injury OR orthopedic surgery in region			
AND mild inflammation?	YES	Osteomyelitis (usually **fever**)	Urgent
AND severe inflammation, rapid onset?	YES	Septic arthrosis (may not be a **fever**)	ER/Urgent
NO			
Excruciating, severe inflammation, rapid onset, but no trauma?	YES	Gout (progressively worsens)	Urgent
NO			
Signs of neurological or vascular impairment (paresthesia, pallor, pulses or reflexes, OR specific motor weakness)			
AND rapid onset after injury or prolonged exercise?	YES	Acute compartment syndrome	ER
AND recurrent with exercise, completely resolves with rest?	YES	Chronic compartment syndrome	Standard
AND constant pain, slowly progressing in intensity?	YES	Impingement or entrapment	Standard
NO			
Night pain, nearly complete relief with NSAIDs, age <30?	YES	Osteoid osteoma, osteoblastoma	Urgent
NO			
Tender mass palpable on bone			
AND inflamed, impaired joint, age <30?	YES	Osteosarcoma	Urgent
NO			

BONE OR JOINT PAIN—NONTRAUMATIC (CONTINUED)

Accompanying Signs or Symptoms		*Potential Condition (and Confirmatory S&S)*	*Action*
AND inflamed, impaired joint, age >30? NO	YES	Chondrosarcoma	Urgent
AND inflamed, impaired joint, fever, age <20? NO	YES	Ewing's sarcoma	Urgent
AND in spine, ribs, pelvis, systemic signs, and age >30? NO	YES	Multiple myeloma	Urgent

Perform assessment for musculoskeletal condition or other systemic involvement (by location of symptoms) and refer appropriately.

CHEST PAIN

Accompanying Signs or Symptoms		*Potential Condition (and Confirmatory S&S)*	*Action*
Fever? NO	YES	See separate algorithm	
Pain ≥15 min AND age ≥35 years? OR no improvement with rest? OR history of heart disease, diabetes, Marfan's? NO	YES	Myocardial infarction or cardiac event (diaphoresis, left arm pain, **nausea**, denial, syncope, or anxiety)	ER
Dyspnea, hemoptysis, cyanosis with sudden onset? NO	YES	Pneumothorax (auscultation, percussion abnormal, tracheal deviation) or pulmonary embolism (hx suggests DVT; falling BP)	ER
Syncope (hx or observed)? OR Unequal femoral or brachial pulses? NO	YES	Cardiac event or aortic dissection	ER
Tachycardia, hyperpnea, gasping breaths?	YES	Tracheal or bronchial spasm (recent toxic exposure, hx asthma)	ER
AND pruritis (itching)? NO	YES	Anaphylaxis (allergic reaction)	ER
Recent or current infection (GI, URI, etc) NO	YES	Pericarditis, endocarditis, pleurisy (fever, auscultated friction rub, systemic signs)	ER

CHEST PAIN (CONTINUED)

Accompanying Signs or Symptoms		*Potential Condition (and Confirmatory S&S)*	*Action*
Dyspnea only with exertion? NO	YES	Ischemic heart failure	Urgent
Palpitations with exertion? NO	YES	Arrythmia	Urgent
Purulent **cough** AND abnormal auscultation? NO	YES	Pneumonia or pulmonary infection (usually accompanied by fever)	Urgent
Dysphagia that changes with meals, while reclining? NO	YES	Upper GI; dyspepsia, gastric reflux (intermittent, recurrent, pain referring to left chest or arm)	Standard
Palpable mass in chest muscle/skin? NO	YES	Breast tumor or other neoplasm	Standard
Single dermatome distribution? NO	YES	Nerve root irritation	Standard
Tender palpation of ribs, pectoralis, or costal cartilage?	YES	Musculoskeletal injury (hx trauma, heavy lifting, previous episode)	Standard

COUGH

Accompanying Signs or Symptoms		*Potential Condition* (and Confirmatory S&S)	*Action*
Fever NO	YES	See separate algorithm	
Cyanosis NO	YES	Airway obstruction, respiratory distress	ER
Dyspnea? NO	YES	See separate algorithm	
Productive cough Hemoptysis AND abnormal auscultation AND **chest pain** or **dyspnea**?	YES	Pneumonia, TB, pulmonary embolism (systemic signs)	ER
AND weight loss, OR hx smoking, OR hx cancer? NO	YES	Lung cancer, lung metastases (CA warning signs, hx cancer)	Urgent

COUGH (CONTINUED)

Accompanying Signs or Symptoms		*Potential Condition (and Confirmatory S&S)*	*Action*
Hemoptysis AND normal auscultation?	YES	Lung cancer, lung metastases (CA warning signs, hx of cancer)	Urgent
NO		Throat, nasopharynx, bronchial injury (hx trauma)	Urgent (if airway is clear)
Purulent sputum AND abnormal auscultation?	YES	Pulmonary infection, pneumonia, bronchitis, bronchiectasis (fever usually present)	Urgent or ER
NO			
Purulent sputum AND normal auscultation?	YES	Pulmonary or nasopharangeal infection (tonsillitis, pharyngitis)	Urgent
NO			
Clear or mucoid sputum?	YES	URI, asthma, allergy, coryza (auscultation normal, no fever)	Standard
AND abnormal auscultaton?	YES	Manage as "purulent sputum with normal auscultation," above	Urgent
NO			
Nonproductive cough			
Back or **chest pain**?	YES	Aortic aneurysm (pulsing SC joint, syncope, changing vital signs, or hx/morphology of Marfan syndrome)	ER
NO			
Lymphadenitis (cervical)?	YES	Nasopharyngeal infection	Urgent
AND systemic signs?	YES	Lung cancer or pulmonary infection (auscultation abnormal)	Urgent
NO			
HA, sore throat, sneezing, rhinorrhea, low fever?	YES	Coryza or URI (auscultation normal)	Standard
NO			
Recurs after exercise only?	YES	EIB (clear in 20 minutes, postexercise cough)	Standard
NO			
Hx of allergy, asthma?	YES	Asthma, bronchospasm (expiratory wheezing, tight chest; see also **dyspnea**)	Standard
NO			
Hx of smoking?	YES	Smoker's cough (morning cough worse)	Standard

Automatic ER if: ABCs impaired, cyanosis, sudden and severe onset.
Urgent or ER if: vital signs stable, fever <101°F, and no respiratory distress (cyanosis, anxiety); urgent referral is appropriate.

DIARRHEA

Accompanying Signs or Symptoms		*Potential Condition (and Confirmatory S&S)*	*Action*
Fever? NO	YES	See separate algorithm	
Abdominal pain AND rigidity, OR distention OR ileus NO	YES	Bowel obstruction, perforation	ER
Red blood in stool AND pus in stool, **abdominal pain**? NO	YES	Dysentery (**fever** usually present) or ulcerative colitis (severe dehydration=ER)	Urgent
AND **vomiting**, abdominal cramps beginning 1 to 6 hrs after eating? NO	YES	Food poisoning	Urgent
AND perianal/rectal trauma NO	YES	Rectal or perianal tissue injury	Urgent
AND hx hemorrhoids? NO	YES	Thrombosed hemorrhoid	Standard
Melena (black, tarry stool)? NO	YES	Ulcer or other upper GI bleeding (cyclic **abdominal pain** after meals) OR ingestion of cherries, iron, bismuth within previous 24 hrs	Urgent None (if clears)
Acute, nonbloody, loose stool AND **vomiting**, pain umbilical, ORMcBurney's, OR rebound tenderness, OR positive "jar" sign? NO	YES	Appendicitis, peritonitis	ER
AND **vomiting**, myalgia, but no **abdominal pain**, tenderness, rigidity? NO	YES	Viral gastroenteritis (should resolve in <48 hrs, usually a fever; maintain hydration)	Standard
AND recurrent **vomiting**? NO	YES	Food poisoning (symptoms usually occur within 6 hrs of eating)	Standard
AND hx alcohol or drugs (antibiotics, vitamin C, laxatives) in previous 24 hrs? NO	YES	Pharmacologically increased peristalsis (screen for substance abuse; eating disorder if laxatives are abused)	Standard

DIARRHEA (CONTINUED)

Accompanying Signs or Symptoms		*Potential Condition (and Confirmatory S&S)*	*Action*
Chronic, nonbloody, loose stool AND fatty/greasy stool (NO)	YES	Pancreatitis (hx of alcohol abuse or cholelithiasis)	Urgent
AND **abdominal pain**, weight loss, borborygmi (audible peristalsis) (NO)	YES	Inflammatory bowel disease	Urgent
AND abdominal cramps, anxiety, but no weight loss? (NO)	YES	Irritable bowel syndrome	Standard
AND abdominal cramps, but no tenderness or rigidity?	YES	Food allergy (seafood, milk, cereal, MSG), only when ingesting offending food	Standard

DYSPNEA

Accompanying Signs or Symptoms		*Potential Condition (and Confirmatory S&S)*	*Action*
Chest pain? (NO)	YES	See separate algorithm	
Fever? (NO)	YES	See separate algorithm	
Inspiratory stridor (NO)	YES	Airway obstruction (unable to speak) OR exercise-induced anaphylaxis (croupy cough, signs of shock)	ER
Onset after chest trauma?	YES		ER
Asymmetrical chest movement?	YES	Flail chest injury	
Deviated trachea?	YES	Pneumothorax, atelectasis (auscultation and percussion abnormal)	
Subcutaneous air (crepitus)	YES	Pseudomediastinum, pneumothorax	
Positive compression test? (NO)	YES	Rib fracture	
Cyanosis, tachypnea, accessory muscle use, difficult speech (NO)	YES	Respiratory distress syndrome (auscultation abnormal)	ER
Productive **cough** AND auscultation abnormal AND			

DYSPNEA (CONTINUED)

Accompanying Signs or Symptoms		*Potential Condition (and Confirmatory S&S)*	*Action*
Fever?	YES	Pulmonary infection	ER
Chest pain?	YES	Endocarditis, heart failure	ER
Neither?	YES	Potential heart failure (hx cardiac?)	ER
NO			
Expiratory wheezing?	YES	Bronchospasm: asthma (hx asthma, panting speech, can't hold breath)	Urgent
NO		Bronchospasm: exercise-induced (hx postexercise cough, condition resolves 20 to 30 min)	Urgent
Hyperventilation, able to speak	YES	Anxiety attack (normal auscultation; resolves with psychoemotional calming)	Standard

DYSURIA OR HEMATURIA

Accompanying Signs or Symptoms		*Potential Condition (and Confirmatory S&S)*	*Action*
Fever?	YES	See separate algorithm	
NO			
Recent flank, back, or abdominal trauma?	YES	Renal or bladder injury (progresses to shock)	ER
NO			
Hx hemophilia OR sickle cell disease OR other blood disease?	YES	Clotting disorder	ER
NO			
Age >55 AND positive urine dipstick?	YES	Renal or urinary tract disease	Urgent
NO			
Flank, back, or **abdominal pain** <u>Age <15</u> AND **fever**, hypertension?	YES	Nephroblastoma	Urgent
NO			
<u>Age >15</u> AND constant, excruciating, "colic" type pain?	YES	Kidney stone (disabling pain, **vomiting**)	ER
NO			
Mild to moderate?	YES	UTI, STD, renal infection (**fever**)	Urgent
NO			
Cloudy or purulent urine?	YES	UTI, STD	Urgent
NO			

DYSURIA OR HEMATURIA (CONTINUED)

Accompanying Signs or Symptoms		*Potential Condition (and Confirmatory S&S)*	*Action*
Nocturia, male, age >40? NO	YES	Prostatitis, prostate disease	Urgent
Genital or perianal trauma? NO	YES	Urethral injury, bladder injury	ER/Urgent
Prolonged, strenuous exercise, such as long-distance running? NO	YES	Bladder or renal microtrauma or ischemic damage (occurs only after exercise)	Standard
Medications (NSAIDs, birth control pills, anticoagulant therapy)?	YES	Renal side effects	Urgent

FEVER

Accompanying Signs or Symptoms		*Potential Condition (and Confirmatory S&S)*	*Action*
Fever over 104°F NO	YES	Heat stroke, heat exhaustion (altered consciousness, collapse; over 106°F immediately life threatening)	ER
High-grade (102°F) AND any of the signs or symptoms listed below			ER

(Note: Most high-grade fevers cause malaise, pallor, tachycardia, hyperpnea, weakness, and loss of appetite in addition to other signs and symptoms)

Syncope, altered consciousness	YES	Endocarditis, myocardial infarction, sepsis/septemia, neurological infection
Severe headache, rigid neck	YES	Meningitis (positive Kernig or Brudzinski tests)
Abdominal pain, rigidity	YES	Peritonitis
Vomiting or **diarrhea**	YES	Gastroenteritis, GI infection, food poisoning
Cough with purulence OR abnormal auscultation	YES	Pneumonia or other pulmonary infection
Chest pain AND **dyspnea**, cyanosis, or syncope	YES	Cardiac event or infection
Joint pain and loss of motion	YES	Septic arthrosis, metabolic arthrosis, leukemia
Dysuria, increased urgency	YES	Urinary infection, renal infections

FEVER (CONTINUED)

Accompanying Signs or Symptoms		*Potential Condition (and Confirmatory S&S)*	*Action*
Unusual bleeding or bruising, or nontender lymphadenitis	YES	Leukemia, lymphoma	
NO			
High-grade (102°F) without any of the signs or symptoms above	YES	Infection (check temperature every 2 to 4 hrs; if sustained 102°F=ER)	Urgent
NO			
Low-grade (99°F to 101.9°F) AND sustained >48 hrs duration	YES	A number of conditions, including anemia, endocrine crisis, immune compromise, cancer (assess for other signs)	Urgent
NO			
Low-grade AND <48 hrs duration AND dysuria, increased urgency	YES	Urinary tract infection	Urgent
NO			
Low-grade AND <48 hrs duration AND severe postoperative joint pain, erythema, sudden loss in motion	YES	Postoperative infection	Urgent (contact surgeon's office)
NO			
Low-grade AND <48 hrs AND nonproductive cough, rhinorrhea, normal auscultation	YES	Upper respiratory infection, coryza (48 hrs duration)	Standard
NO			
Any recurrent fever (consecutive days or nights, cyclic)	YES	Malignancy, other chronic conditions	Urgent

LYMPHADENITIS

Accompanying Signs or Symptoms		*Potential Condition (and Confirmatory S&S)*	Action
Fever? NO	YES	See separate algorithm	
Age <20 (any location)? NO	YES	Infection	Urgent
<u>Location</u>			
Cervical, unilateral? NO	YES	Infection of head, eye, ear, nose, mouth, etc (local S&S to confirm)	Urgent
Cervical, bilateral, AND tender to palpation? NO	YES	Mononucleosis	Urgent
AND not tender to palpation? NO	YES	Hodgkin's lymphoma, metastases	Urgent
Axillary or inguinal? NO	YES	Infection distal to nodes (arms or legs)	Urgent
General lymphadenitis AND fatigue, pallor, arthralgia? NO	YES	Rheumatoid arthritis, rheumatic disease	Standard
AND unusual bleeding? NO	YES	Leukemia	ER/Urgent
None of the above	YES	Infection	Standard

VOMITING AND NAUSEA

Accompanying Signs or Symptoms		*Potential Condition (and Confirmatory S&S)*	*Action*
Fever? NO	YES	See separate algorithm	
Chest pain? NO	YES	See separate algorithm	
Recent head trauma? NO	YES	Rising intracranial pressure (rising BP, decreased HR, usually projectile vomitting without nausea)	ER
Hematemesis (bright red vomiting)? NO	YES	Peptic ulcer, gastritis, esophageal varices (varicose veins)	ER
Substantial **abdominal pain** AND rigidity, distention, progressively worse? NO	YES	Peritonitis	ER

VOMITING AND NAUSEA (CONTINUED)

Accompanying Signs or Symptoms		*Potential Condition (and Confirmatory S&S)*	*Action*
AND fecal odor in vomitus, absent bowel sounds? NO	YES	Bowel obstruction	ER
ANDupper abdomen pain and right shoulder pain? NO	YES	Cholecystitis, cholelithiasis	ER
Back or flank pain AND acute hematuria? NO	YES	Kidney stone	ER
AND chronic nocturia, pallor? NO	YES	Renal disorder	ER
Headache AND rigid neck, rising **fever**? NO	YES	Meningitis (rapid collapse)	ER
AND photophobia, phonophobia, no systemic signs? NO	YES	Migraine headache (hx recurrence)	Standard
Cyclic pain with diarrhea OR loss of appetite OR borborygmi? NO	YES	Food poisoning (hx of eating in restaurant, undercooked food, etc) or gastroenteritis (monitor hydration status)	Urgent
Female, amenorrhea, weight gain, polyuria? NO	YES	Pregnancy (recurrent vomiting in morning; ER if signs of shock)	Standard
After use of alcohol, aspirin, caffeine, drugs? NO	YES	Gastritis, peptic ulcer, drug toxicity (urgent or ER if suspected drug over-dose; counseling if illicit drugs or alcohol abuse)	Standard
Low body weight, obsession with weight or calories, Russell's sign on hands/knuckles, self-induced vomiting	YES	Disordered eating/eating disorder (body image disturbance, inadequate food intake; secretive; mood or personality disturbances, excessive exercise, compulsiveness about eating habits)	Urgent

Glossary

Phonetic pronunciation of medical terms are in [brackets]. Dashes (-) indicate separation of syllables. CAPS indicate the syllable(s) that is stressed in speech. (Some of the very common medical terms do not include phonetics.) For unfamiliar terms, practice pronunciation by reading the phonetic syllables slowly, then repeating them more rapidly until they sound like a single word.

allergy localized, cell-mediated immune reaction to a toxin (ie, an antigen)
alopecia [al-oh-PEE-she-ah] lack of hair in a body region that normally has hair
amenorrhea [a-MEN-o-REE-uh] lack of menstruation for 3 consecutive months, or less than 3 menstrual cycles per year; primary amenorrhea occurs when menarche (initiation of menstruation) has not occurred by the age of 16 years
anaphylaxis [ann-uh-fuh-LACK-sis] generalized inflammatory response, including vascular, pulmonary, and dermatologic systems
anasarca [ann-uh-SAR-kah] generalized edema; fluid in the interstitial spaces
anemia [a-NEE-mee-uh] a condition defined as a very low number of circulating red blood cells relative to a person's gender and age group
angina [ann-JIY-nuh] distinctive type of chest pain that radiates to the arm, neck, jaw, or back, usually lasting 2 to 10 minutes
anorexia [ann-oh-RECK-see-uh] loss of appetite; occurs with a number of physical, medical, or psychological conditions
anoxia [ann-OCK-see-uh] lack of oxygen
antigen a foreign substance that initiates an immune response upon contact with tissue
anuria [ann-oo-REE-uh] absence of urination
anxiety a state of intense worry
arachnodactyly [uh-rack-no-DACK-tee-lee] long, thin fingers ("spider-like")
arrythmia [ah-RITH-mee-uh] interruption of the heart's electrical system, causing an irregular heartbeat
arteriosclerosis [ar-TEER-ee-oh-skleh-ROH-sis] hardening of the arteries
arthralgia [ar-THRAL-jee-uh] joint pain
ascites [ah-sy-TEEZ] abnormal accumulation of fluid in the peritoneal space of the abdomen
ataxia [uh-TACK-see-uh] inability to control voluntary movements
atelectasis [at-uh-LECK-ta-sis] complete removal of air of a segment of lung tissue
atherosclerosis [ATH-er-oh-skleh-ROW-sis] lipid deposits on interior of blood vessels causing a narrowing of the vascular lumen
atopy [AT-o-pee] allergy producing symptoms upon exposure to an offending antigen
atrophy [AT-row-fee] decrease in cell and tissue size, caused by a decrease in metabolic supply or metabolic demand

auscultation [AWS-kuhl-TAY-shun] use of a stethoscope to listen for sounds originating in, or conducted by, the body

benign [beh-NINE] mild, relatively harmless (opposite of malignant)

bioavailability the amount of a drug that is available to the body's tissues, which is typically less than the ingested dose

blood-brain barrier impermeable membrane of the brain's vascular system that prevents diffusion of certain compounds into the central nervous system

bradycardia [brayd-ee-KAR-dee-uh] heart rate relatively slower than normal, usually less than 60 beats per minute; may occur at rest in healthy athletes as a result of training

bronchiectasis [brahng-kee-ECK-tah-sis] abnormal increase in diameter of bronchus and consolidation of smaller bronchi due to disease process

bronchophony [brahng-KOFF-oh-nee] abnormal auscultation; spoken sounds are clearly heard

bruit [BREW-ay] abnormal sound upon auscultation, particularly one detected over an artery

cancer proliferation of undifferentiated cells replacing normal cells at a high rate of division; malignant dysplasia

carcinogen [KAR-sih-noh-jin] substances known to cause cancer in human tissue

cardiac hypertrophy abnormal enlargement of all or part of the heart structures

cardiac output the product of stroke volume and heart rate; the amont of blood ejected by the heart in 1 minute

catabolism metabolic breakdown of cells and tissues

cerumen [sih-ROO-min] waxy substance secreted in the external auditory canal

chief complaints symptoms causing an injured or ill person to seek medical attention

cilia [SIHL-ee-uh] small hair-like projections, particularly on cells lining the airway

claudication [KLAW-dih-KAY-shun] impairment of gait (ie, limping) caused by vascular pathology

clinical decision making determining the best medical course of action for a patient, based on history, signs, and symptoms

clinical diagnosis the identification of an injury, illness, or disease based primarily on medical history and physical examination, without laboratory tests or imaging studies

clinical pathology the medical practice of pathology as it pertains to the care of patients

clonus [KLOH-nus] abnormal reflex elicited by sudden flexion or extension of a distal joint and demonstrated by rapid oscillations

coexisting condition a medical condition in addition to the one for which the patient is seeking care (see also **comorbidity**)

colic [KAH-lick] a very sudden attack of severe abdominal pain, characteristic of spasm of an obstructed abdominal organ (adj. colicky)

coma [KOH-ma] a complete, profound, and persistent loss of consciousness from which a person cannot be aroused (compare with **lethargy**)

communicable describes a disease that can be passed directly from person to person, person to animal, or animal to person

comorbidity the simultaneous existence of two or more pathological conditions in one person (see also **coexisting condition**)
concussion collision of the brain with the cranium, causing temporary interruption of neural function
contagious [kon-TAY-jus] describes a disease that can be directly passed from person to person
contrecoup concussion occurring opposite to the side of impact to the head
cor pulmonale [KOR PUL-moh-NAHL-ee] right ventricular hypertrophy resulting from increased pulmonary tension, eventually leading to congestive heart failure
coryza [koh-RIH-zah] "common cold" or rhinitis; accompanied by nasal drainage, sore throat, sneezing, sinusitis
cough forceful, often involuntary expiratory effort, usually to clear the airway of sputum or other substances or objects
croup [kroop] high, resonant cough, often described as "barking," accompanied by loud, labored breathing, usually associated with laryngeal obstruction
cyanosis [sigh-ah-NO-sis] bluish tint to the skin; characterized as either peripheral (in the extremities) or central (present throughout the body, particulary the lips, tongue, and face); caused by insufficient oxygenation of the blood

dermatome area of cutaneous sensation supplied by one spinal nerve root
diagnosis definitive identification of an injury, illness, or disease
diagnostic reasoning identifying and interpreting signs and symptoms to obtain a diagnosis
diaphoresis [DIE-uh-four-EE-sis] profuse sweating not caused by physical exertion
diarrhea [die-uh-REE-uh] more than three bowel movements per day, or an unexpected increase in frequency of bowel movements
diastole [die-AS-toe-lee] passive filling phase of the cardiac contraction cycle
differential diagnosis determination of which specific disease a patient has
differentiation sorting and interpretation of signs, symptoms, and other information
diplopia [die-PLOH-pee-uh] blurred or "double" vision
disease disruption of homeostasis caused by cellular damage or abnormal organ function
dysarthria [dis-AR-three-uh] difficulty speaking
dyspareunia [dis-pa-RUE-nee-uh] painful intercourse
dysphagia [dis-FA-jee-uh] difficulty swallowing
dysplasia [dis-PLAY-zee-uh] change of normal cells to several abnormal types with increased rate of division
dyspnea [DISP-nee-uh] difficulty breathing or "shortness of breath"
dysuria [dis-YOU-ree-uh] painful or difficult urination

ecchymosis [EK-ee-MO-sis] very dark red, blue, or black discoloration of the skin, caused by blood cells in the interstitial space; a "bruise"
edema [uh-DEE-muh] collection of fluid in a body cavity or interstitial space
egophony [eh-GOF-oh-nee] abnormal auscultation; spoken sound is transmitted in a high pitch
embolism [EM-bo-liz-im] sudden obstruction of a blood vessel by an embolus

embolus [EM-bo-lis] an abnormal particle or object (air bubble, blood clot) freely floating in the blood
emesis [EM-eh-sus] vomiting
endocardium connective tissue sac that surrounds and invests the structures of the heart
endothelium cells lining the cardiovascular system, including the heart, arteries, and veins (see also **epithelium**)
enteric coating a protective covering on a pill that delays medication release until the pill reaches the small intestine
epistaxis [ep-uh-STACK-sis] nosebleed
epithelium cells lining the interior cavities and exterior surfaces of the body (see also **endothelium**)
erythema [er-ih-THEE-mah] reddening of the skin, usually a result of inflammation
etiology [eh-tee-AHL-oh-jee] the study of pathogenesis, including theories of illness and disease
euphoria [yew-FOH-ree-uh] a sensation of pleasant relaxation or well-being
exacerbated [EKS-as-ur-BAY-tihd] increase in intensity or severity of a disease

fatigue state of metabolic imbalance that occurs when energy demands exceed energy supply
fever systemic increase in body temperature; "low-grade" fever is less than 102°F; "high-grade" fever is equal or greater than 102°F

glucosuria [glue-koh-SUE-ree-uh] presence of glucose in the urine
goiter [GOY-tur] an abnormally enlarged thyroid gland
gonads organs of reproduction
gynecomastia [GUY-nih-coh-MASS-tee-ah] feminization of the female breast, including development of mammary glands

heart failure inability of the heart to maintain normal cardiac output
hematemesis [HEE-mih-TIM-ee-sis] bloody vomitus
hematochezia [HIM-ah-toh-KEE-zee-ah] presence of blood in the feces or during defecation
hematoma [HEE-mah-TOH-mah] collection of blood outside the vascular system
hematuria [HEE-muh-TUR-ee-uh] blood in the urine, in either microscopic or grossly visible amounts
hemoglobinuria [HEE-moh-gloh-bih-NEW-ree-uh] hemoglobin in the urine, producing a reddish tint
hemoptysis [hih-MOP-tih-sis] coughing or spitting bloody sputum
hemorrhage [HIM-ih-ridj] sudden loss of blood (either internally or externally) resulting from damage to the vascular system
hemorrhoids [HIM-ih-roydz] varicose veins in the rectum or on the anus
hemospermia [HIM-uh-to-SPERM-ee-uh] blood in the male ejaculate
hemostasis [HEE-mo-stay-sus] a vascular response to control blood loss after injury
hepatomegaly [hih-PAT-uh-MEG-uh-lee] pathologic enlargement of the liver
hernia [HER-nee-ah] a condition in which an organ or part of an organ protrudes through a defect in the wall of the body cavity that normally contains that organ

hirsutism [HIR-sue-tiz-um] appearance of course hair on the chest and face of females, caused by abnormal concentrations of androgens from endocrine disorders or anabolic steroid abuse

homeostasis [HOH-mee-oh-STAY-sis] a healthy state of biochemical dynamic equilibrium within the body's internal environment

host an organism harboring an infectious agent

hydrocele [HI-droh-seel] fluid-filled sac in the scrotum

hypercapnia [hi-pur-KAP-nee-uh] increased carbon dioxide levels in the blood

hyperhydrosis [hi-pur-hi-DRO-sis] excessive global or localized sweating (eg, the palms of the hands)

hyperlipidemia [hi-pur-lip-ih-DEEM-ee-ah] excessive fat (lipids) in bloodstream

hyperplasia [hi-pur-PLAY-see-ah] increase in the total number of cells in a given tissue

hyperpnea [hi-PERP-nee-uh] rapid ventilation rate

hypertension high blood pressure; usually systolic over 140 mmHg or diastolic over 90 mmHg

hyperthermia central body temperature above 105°F or 39°C

hypertrophy [hi-PUR-tro-fee] increase in cell size, causing an associated increase in tissue size, resulting from increased metabolic demand

hyperventilation increase in ventilatory rate without an increase in ventilatory depth

hypervolemia [HI-pur-voh-LEE-mee-ah] abnormally high retention of fluid in the bloodstream; eventually produces hypertension

hypotension low blood pressure; usually systolic below 95 mmHg or diastolic below 60 mmHg

hypothermia central body temperature below 94°F or 34.4°C

hypoxemia [HI-pock-SEE-mee-ah] reduced oxygen saturation in arterial blood

hypoxia [hi-POK-see-ah] reduced availability of oxygen to the tissues

icterus [ICK-tur-us] yellow discoloration of the sclera, skin, and mucous membranes; also called **jaundice**

idiopathic [ID-ee-oh-PATH-ick] without a known etiology; occurring spontaneously

ileus [ILL-ee-us] paralyzed section of bowel, usually a result of obstruction or infarction

impotence [IM-poh-tense] also called erectile dysfunction; inability to achieve or maintain an erection

incontinence loss of the ability to control either urination or defecation

incubation time interval between infection and appearance of symptoms

insidious very gradual and unnoticeable progression of disease

inspection careful observation of a patient to detect signs of pathology

interstitial space space between cells containing extracellular fluid

ischemia [iss-KEE-mee-ah] loss of blood flow to a tissue

jaundice [JAWN-dis] yellow discoloration of the sclera, skin, and mucous membranes; also called **icterus**

lability [lah-BILL-ih-tee] instability, unsteadiness, particularly used to refer to mood

lethargy [LETH-ar-jee] a profound sleep or extreme fatigue accompanying or following disease state; differentiated from coma in that the person can be aroused

leukocytes [LEW-koh-siyts] white blood cell (phagocytes, eosinophils, etc)

libido [lih-BEE-doh] normal hormonal and emotional sex drive

lipolysis [liy-POLE-eye-sis] metabolic breakdown of stored fat in response to energy demand (eg, during exercise)

lymphadenitis [LIM-fad-ih-NIH-tiss] swelling of the lymph nodes

lymphadenopathy [lim-fad-ih-NOP-ah-thee] enlargement of the lymph nodes; a sign of possible infection

malaise [mah-LAYZ] general discomfort; "not feeling well"

malignant [mah-LIG-nant] severe and harmful; resistant to treatment; highly invasive and pervasive

medical history the status of the person, past and present, related to the current illness

melena [mel-EE-nah] black stools with the consistency of tar

menarche [meh-NAR-kee] first menses

meninges [meh-NIN-jeez] protective layers of connective tissue surrounding the central nervous system

menses [MEN-seez] sloughing of endometrial lining, consisting of mucous and blood, from uterus through the vagina

metabolism interrelated biochemical functions and processes of the organ-systems

metaplasia [met-ah-PLAY-zee-ah] replacing of one cell type by another

metastasis [mih-TASS-tah-sis] migration of malignant cells to organs and systems other than thoses of origin

myalgia [my-AL-jee-ah] muscular aching

myocardial infarction ischemic damage to the myocardium; a "heart attack"

myocardium muscle tissue which comprises the heart, as distinct from striated (skeletal) and smooth (organ) muscle

myoglobulinuria [MY-oh-GLOHB-oo-lin-OO-ree-ah] myoglobin in the urine, a result of excessive exercise and muscle breakdown

myotomal [my-oh-TOH-mal] refers to groups of muscles controlled by a single nerve root

necrosis [nih-KROH-sis] metabolic death in a group of cells

neoplasm [nee-oh-PLAH-zum] tumor; abnormal cell proliferation

nociceptor [no-see-SEP-tur] a receptor that responds to potentially harmful (painful) stimuli

nocturia [nock-TOO-ree-ah] unusual urgency to urinate, waking the victim from sleep

occult [oh-KULT] hidden, undetected, or undiagnosed

oligomenorrhea [AHL-ee-goh-men-oh-REE-ah] three to six menstrual cycles per year, with cycles in excess of 35 days

oliguria [AHL-ee-GOO-ree-ah] very infrequent urination

orthopnea [or-thop-NEE-ah] dyspnea (shortness of breath) exacerbated when the trunk is upright (as in sitting or standing)

overdose ingestion of toxic amounts of a chemical compound, usually used to indicate poisoning as a result of drug use or abuse

ovulation [oh-voo-LAY-shun] release of an ovum from the ovary; part of the menstrual cycle

pain a sensory and emotionally unpleasant symptom, usually associated with tissue damage

pallor [PAL-or] general paleness of skin caused by vasoconstriction of fever or vascular collapse

palpation manual touch or manipulation conducted during the physical examination

palpitation [pal-pih-TAY-shun] uncomfortable sensation of forceful, rapid, or fluttering heartbeats

paresthesia [pair-es-THEE-zee-ah] abnormal cutaneous sensation, including numbness, tingling, burning, etc

pathogenesis the cause of a particular disease or morbid process

pathology medical science concerned with all aspects of disease; the structural and functional changes that result from disease

pathophysiology the physiology of disease

pectus carinatum [kar-NAY-tum] abnormal convexity of the sternum and anterior ribs; also called "pigeon-chest"

pectus excavatum [ex-kah-VAH-tum] abnormal concavity of the sternum and anterior ribs; also called "funnel-chest"

percussion striking to cause vibration in the internal structures of the body

pericardium a double-walled sac of connective tissue which surrounds the heart and its great vessels; contains the pericardial fluid; attaches endocardium to thorax

peritoneum [PAIR-ee-toh-NEE-um] connective tissue lining the abdomen and abdominal organs

peritonitis [pair-EE-toh-NIH-tis] inflammation of the peritoneum, usually a result of infection (primary) or trauma (secondary)

phagocyte [FAHG-oh-siyt] white blood cells that destroy and ingest foreign microorganisms and cell debris

phagocytosis [FAHG-oh-siy-TOH-sis] process of ingesting foreign microorganisms and cell debris

piles hemorrhoids; varicose veins in the rectum or on the anus

pleura [PLOOr-ah] the sacs of connective tissue lining the thorax and the surface of the lungs; contain fluid to reduce the friction between the inspiring lung and the chest wall

pleurisy [PLOOR-ee-see] pain resulting from inflammation of the pleura; sharp and localized, occurring over the affected region

pleuritic pain pain similar to that caused by pleurisy; pain over the affected pleural region of that worsens during respiration

pneumoconiosis [NEW-moh-coh-nee-OH-sis] lung disease resulting from chronic inhalation of insoluble or semisoluble particles causing fibrous scarring within the lung

pneumothorax air or gas in the pleural space (between visceral and parietal pleura of the lung) causing widespread collapse of the aveoli

polydipsia [pahl-ee-DIP-see-ah] excessive thirst, usually a result of dehydration or loss of blood volume

polyphagia [pahl-ee-FAY-jee-ah] excessive intake of food

polyuria [pahl-ee-OO-ree-ah] excessive frequency or volume of urine

postprandial [post-PRAN-dee-ahl] relating to the period following a meal

prandial [PRAN-dee-ahl] relating to the period during a meal
preparticipation examination physical screening, survey medical history, and review of systems conducted before allowing participation in athletics
prodromal [pro-DROH-mal] relating to a symptom preceding onset of an illness
prognosis predicted outcome of injury, illness, or disease
prostatitis [prahs-tah-TIY-tis] inflammation of the prostate gland
proteinuria [pro-tay-ee-NOO-ree-ah] presence of protein in the urine
pruitis [proo-RIY-tis] severe itching
ptosis [TOH-sis] sagging of the upper eyelids as a result of muscle or nerve dysfunction
purulent [PYEW-roo-lent] the presence of a thick fluid (also known as pus) containing leukocytes, dead cells, and other tissue debris

rales [rahlz] also called crackles; abnormal auscultation of a series of distinct pops during inspiration
rebound tenderness pain elicited upon sudden release of a manually depressed abdomen
relapse recurrence of active disease that was previously in remission
remission absence of detectable or active disease in a person who previously demonstrated the disease; often used to refer to recovery from cancer
renin [REE-nin] hormone secreted by the kidneys; renin increases vasoconstriction and thus raises blood pressure
respiration exchange of oxygen and carbon dioxide between the circulatory system and the atmosphere; occurs in the aveoli of the lung
review of systems screening examination of each major organ system; usually conducted by survey or during the medical history
rhonchi [RON-ky] abnormal auscultation of continuous rumbling during inspiration and expiration
rigidity "splinting"; protective muscular spasm, particularly of the abdominal wall

sanguineous [san-GWIN-ee-us] describes bloody discharge or drainage of body fluid
seizure sudden electrochemical discharge in the brain causing interruption or alteration of normal cerebral activity
septicemia [sep-tih-SEE-mih-ah] presence of an infectious organism in the blood
septum a wall of tissue that divides an organ, such as the heart, into chambers or sections
serosanguineous [SEE-roh-san-GWIN-ee-us] describes a combination of watery and bloody discharge or drainage of body fluid
serous [SEER-us] describes watery discharge or drainage of body fluids
shock sudden and severe impairment of the life-sustaining functions of the body; signs include tachycardia, hypotension, diaphoresis, and altered level of consciousness
sign any indication of pathology observed by the clinician
smooth muscle muscle tissue of various internal organ systems, such as the gastrointestinal system
spasm involuntary continuous contraction of skeletal or smooth muscle
spirometer [spir-AHM-a-tur] instrument used to measure ventilatory volumes
splenomegaly [SPLEH-noh-MEG-ah-lee] pathological enlargement of the spleen

sputum [SPYOO-tum] fluid expelled from the mouth during spitting, coughing, or sneezing

stool feces

stria [STRY-ah] longitudinal cutaneous discolorations caused by a constant stretch on the skin, such as occurs during pregnancy

striated muscle muscle tissue which moves the bony skeleton

stridor [STRY-dur] raspy sound upon inspiration, usually indicative of a partially obstructed airway; usually detectable without auscultation

stroke volume amount of blood ejected into the aorta during a single ventricular contraction

symptom any departure from normal function, appearance, or sensation experienced and reported by the patient

syncope [SIN-koh-pee] complete loss of consciousness and postural tone, caused by a sudden reduction in blood supply to the brain

systole [SIS-toh-lee] active contraction phase of the cardiac cycle

tachycardia [tack-ee-KAR-dee-ah] rapid heart rate, usually in excess of 100 beats per minute

tachypnea [tack-ip-NEE-ah] rapid respiration rate; may be in excess of 20 breaths per minute

thrombosis formation of a blood clot in a blood vessel

thrombus a clot of blood attached to the wall of a blood vessel

triage [TREE-ahj] initial examination of a patient to determine the severity of his or her condition

tumor neoplasm; abnormal cell proliferation

tympanites [TIM-pah-NEE-teez] abnormal air or gas within the abdomen

urinalysis [yu-rih-NAL-ee-sis] laboratory analysis of the chemical composition of urine

urolithiasis [YU-roh-lih-THI-ay-sis] kidney stone

urticaria [UR-tree-KAR-ee-uh] hives; lesions of the skin characterized by red, raised regions, usually widespread in reaction to anaphylactic or allerigic reaction

varices [VAR-ih-seez] pathologically dilated veins; "varicose veins"

varicoceles [VAR-ih-koh-seel] varicose veins in the scrotum

varicose [VAR-ih-kohss] describes permanently dilated veins

vector an organism, usually an insect or animal, that passes an infectious organism from one host to another without being affected

ventilation physical movement of air into and out of the lungs

verrucae [veh-ROO-kah] warts; tumorous skin lesion caused by papillomavirus

virulence [VEER-yu-lint] the relative severity, progression, noxiousness, or toxicity of a disease

vital signs heart rate, respiration rate, blood pressure, and body temperature

wheals [wheelz] hives; inflammed, raised areas of skin, generally in reaction to an immune response

whispered pectoriloquy [peck-toh-RIL-oh-kwee] abnormal ausculation; whispered sound is clearly heard

withdrawal physical and psychological condition produced by the cessation of chronic use of a physically addicting substance

Normal Lab Values

Normal Lab Values*

Blood Chemistry	Normal (Reference) Range
pH	7.35 to 7.45
Bicarbonate	22 to 26 mEq/L
Red blood cells	3.6 to 5.4 million/μL
White blood cells	5000 to 10,000/μL
Platelets	150,000 to 350,000/μL
Hemoglobin	Males: 14 to 18 g/dL Females: 12 to 16 g/dL
Hematocrit	Males: 40% to 50% Females: 37% to 47%
Sodium	135 to 142 mEq/L
Potassium	3.8 to 5.0 mEq/L
Calcium	4.0 to 5.0 mEq/L
Magnesium	3 mEq/L
Chloride	95 to 102 mEq/L
Total protein	6.0 to 8.6 g/dL
Albumin	3.2 to 4.5 g/dL
Glucose (fasting)	70 to 110 mg/dL
Total iron	60 to 150 μg/dL
Total lipids	400 to 800 mg/dL
Cholesterol	150 to 250 mg/dL
Triglycerides	75 to 160 mg/dL
High-density lipoproteins	>40 mg/dL
Low-density lipoproteins	<180 mg/dL
Bilirubin (direct)	0.1 to 0.4 mg/dL
Creatinine	0.6 to 1.2 mg/dL
Uric acid	Males: 2.4 to 7.4 mg/dL Females: 1.4 to 5.8 mg/dL

**Most laboratory reports highlight low and high values and provide normal ranges.*

Normal Lab Values*

Urinalysis	**Normal (Reference) Range**
pH	4.5 to 8.0
Hemoglobin or cells	0
Sodium	75 to 200 mg/24 hours
Potassium	25 to 100 mEq/L
Protein	0 to 150 mg/24 hours
Glucose	0
Bilirubin	0
Creatinine	1.0 to 2.0 g/24 hours
Uric acid	0.6 to 1.0 g/24 hours
Urea	25 to 35 g/24 hours
Ammonia	20 to 70 mEq/L
Acetone	0

**Most laboratory reports highlight low and high values and provide normal ranges.*

Index